DEVELOPMENTS IN ENVIRONMENTAL CONTROL AND PUBLIC HEALTH—2

THE DEVELOPMENTS SERIES

Developments in many fields of science and technology occur at such a pace that frequently there is a long delay before information about them becomes available and usually it is inconveniently scattered among several journals.

Developments Series books overcome these disadvantages by bringing together within one cover papers dealing with the latest trends and developments in a specific field of study and publishing them within *six months* of their being written.

Many subjects are covered by the series, including food science and technology, polymer science, civil and public health engineering, pressure vessels, composite materials, concrete, building science, petroleum technology, geology, etc.

Information on other titles in the series will gladly be sent on application to the publishers.

DEVELOPMENTS IN ENVIRONMENTAL CONTROL AND PUBLIC HEALTH—2

Edited by

ANDREW PORTEOUS

B.Sc., M.Eng., D.Eng., C.Eng., F.I.Mech.E., M.I.Chem.E., M.I.S.W.M.

Reader in Engineering Mechanics, Faculty of Technology,
The Open University, Walton Hall, Milton Keynes, UK

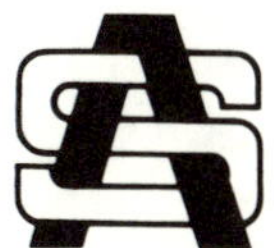

APPLIED SCIENCE PUBLISHERS LTD

LONDON

APPLIED SCIENCE PUBLISHERS LTD
RIPPLE ROAD, BARKING, ESSEX, ENGLAND

British Library Cataloguing in Publication Data

Developments in environmental control and public
health.—(Developments series).
2
1. Environmental health
I. Porteous, Andrew   II. Series
614.7   RA565

ISBN 0-85334-941-X

WITH 24 TABLES AND 63 ILLUSTRATIONS

© APPLIED SCIENCE PUBLISHERS LTD 1981

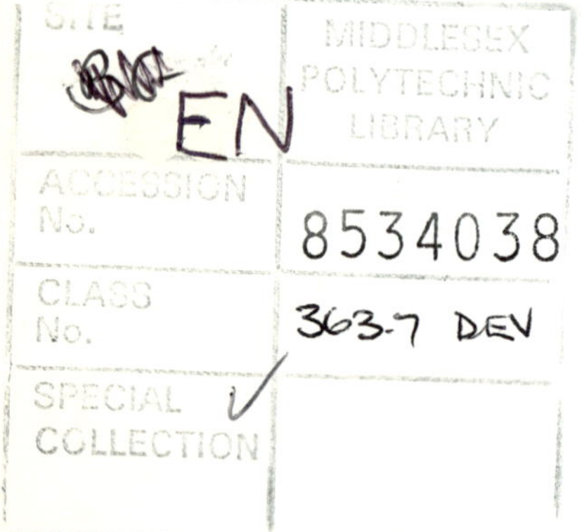

Printed in Great Britain by Galliard (Printers) Ltd, Great Yarmouth

PREFACE

This text is the second in the present series, and deals with specific areas of environmental concern which complement the general ones covered in the earlier volume. The major emphasis is on the maintenance and control of the physical environment and the safeguarding of public health thereby.

The individual contributions, nine in all, are written by experts in the respective areas. The text has an applied bias and gives a thorough grounding in the selected topics to those who wish or need to know about either an individual subject or the components which together form the inter-related environment which engineers, public health officers and scientists need to manage and husband for future generations. References to the literature and reading guides are also provided. An outline of each contribution follows.

Messrs A. Parker and G. M. Williams discuss the selection and operation of landfill sites for municipal and hazardous waste disposal. A key feature of this contribution is the emphasis on hydrogeological assessment and leachate behaviour in the landfill, thus aiding the improved landfilling of wastes.

Mr L. E. Baker's contribution is on non-landfill methods of hazardous waste disposal which complements the preceding chapter. Recovery, recycling, incineration, ultrafiltration and biological and chemical treatment methods are reviewed and economic guidelines presented.

Professor P. O. A. L. Davies and Mr A. H. Middleton review industrial noise and vibration control. Their contribution embraces legislation, codes of practice, principles of noise and vibration control and personal noise and vibration protection. Building design and examples of low noise and vibration machinery are also included.

Mr J. R. Tagg's contribution is on the measurement and control of sulphur dioxide emissions and contains a wide ranging review of the methods employed for measuring ambient concentrations. Potential methods of control are also examined and an extensive literature survey is included.

Dr J. M. Harrington examines asbestosis and other dust related diseases with particular reference to health effects, plus prevention and control measures for this important environmental area.

Dr R. Briggs extensively reviews the instrumentation and systems for the monitoring and control of water quality. Examples of existing installations are given as well as methods of interpreting the results.

Mr G. F. G. Clough takes a broad look at water supply resources, treatment and distribution. The UK reorganisation of water supply administration and the essentials of good water supply management are also reviewed.

Dr E. G. Bellinger considers environmental monitoring by biological means and gives both examples and data for aquatic monitoring.

Dr J. J. Colls describes the environmental monitoring practices at two divisions of the British Steel Corporation and gives two very comprehensive case studies, backed by on-site data, of sulphur dioxide and particulate emissions for selected plants.

CONTENTS

LIST OF CONTRIBUTORS

L. E. BAKER

Director, Re-Chem International Limited, 80 Shirley Road, Southampton SO1 3EY, UK.

E. G. BELLINGER

Assistant Director, Pollution Research Unit, University of Manchester, Oxford Road, Manchester M13 9PL, UK.

R. BRIGGS

Consultant Research Associate, Water Research Centre, Stevenage Laboratory, Elder Way, Stevenage, Hertfordshire SG1 1TH, UK.

G. F. G. CLOUGH

Consultant Engineer, Allmeadows, Wincle, Macclesfield, Cheshire SK11 0QJ, UK.

J. J. COLLS

Pollution Control Engineer, Scunthorpe Division, British Steel Corporation, PO Box 1, Scunthorpe, S. Humberside DN16 1BP, UK.

P. O. A. L. DAVIES

Professor of Experimental Fluid Dynamics, Institute of Sound and Vibration Research, University of Southampton, Southampton SO9 5NH, UK.

J. M. HARRINGTON

Professor of Occupational Medicine, The Birmingham Hospital Saturday Fund, Department of Medicine, The University of Birmingham, Birmingham B15 2TT, UK.

A. H. MIDDLETON

Technical Manager, Wolfson Unit for Noise and Vibration Control, Institute of Sound and Vibration Research, University of Southampton, Southampton SO9 5NH, UK.

A. PARKER

Section Leader, Landfill Research, Environmental Safety Group, United Kingdom Atomic Energy Authority, Harwell Laboratory, Harwell, Oxfordshire OX11 0RA, UK.

J. R. TAGG

Lecturer in Engineering Mechanics, The Open University, Walton Hall, Milton Keynes MK7 6AA, UK.

G. M. WILLIAMS

Team Leader, Landfill Studies, Institute of Geological Sciences, Environmental Protection Unit, Harwell Laboratory, Harwell, Oxfordshire OX11 0RA, UK.

Chapter 1

LANDFILL SITE SELECTION AND OPERATION FOR MUNICIPAL AND HAZARDOUS WASTE DISPOSAL

A. PARKER, B.Sc., F.R.I.C., M.Inst.S.W.M.

*Section Leader, Landfill Research, Environmental Safety Group,
United Kingdom Atomic Energy Authority, Harwell Laboratory,
Oxfordshire, UK*

and

G. M. WILLIAMS, B.Sc., M.Inst.S.W.M.

*Team Leader, Landfill Studies, Institute of Geological Sciences,
Environmental Protection Unit, Harwell Laboratory, Oxfordshire, UK*

SUMMARY

*Landfill of waste in UK currently accounts for 90 % of the total production of
45 million tonnes/annum and is by far the most economical disposal option.
The Control of Pollution Act (1974) regulates the deposit of waste on land
and has led to an improvement in disposal standards. Research into the
behaviour of hazardous wastes has identified that there is considerable
potential for wastes to be attenuated by interaction in the landfill, and in
migrating away providing the hydrogeology is favourable. Many diverse
factors require consideration in selecting and engineering a landfill
depending on whether wastes are to be contained or allowed to migrate and
disperse naturally in the environment, and due precautions should be taken to
ensure the safety of personnel on site especially if co-disposal of hazardous
wastes is practised. Gas generation and migration, and methods of leachate
treatment, may also require evaluation especially with respect to after use of*

*the site and where landfills are located near housing or in hydrogeologically
sensitive areas.*

1. INTRODUCTION

Controlled waste production in UK amounts to about 20 million tonnes of
domestic and commercial waste and more than 25 million tonnes of
industrial waste per annum. Only 4–5 million tonnes of industrial waste are
hazardous or toxic and landfill disposal accounts for more than 90 % of the
total solid waste arising. Mine and quarry wastes (110 million tonnes/annum)
and pulverised fuel ash from electricity generating stations (12 million
tonnes/annum) are not classed as controlled wastes and are excluded from
these figures.

Disposal of wastes onto land by controlled methods was first advocated
in Britain in the 1930s.[1] Basically, controlled landfilling consists of
depositing waste in layers of limited depth which are then covered with inert
material; providing screens to prevent waste blowing away; generally
carrying out a tidy operation and taking precautions to avoid water
pollution.

Past experience and recent research[2] has recognised landfilling to be an
effective, economic and environmentally acceptable method of reclaiming
mineral excavations or derelict land if carried out correctly. The practice of
building landfills above natural ground level is occasionally carried out
where the land is low lying, and badly drained, e.g. in a tidal estuary, but
predominantly landfills are established in disused mineral workings.

Since the majority of wastes are potentially polluting, poor landfill site
selection or operation can produce hazards due to smells, dust, vermin or
flies, and may impair groundwater or surface water quality and in some
cases pollute potable supplies.

In the past, waste disposal came under the control of the public health
engineer employed by the local authority, to which legislative control was
granted by the Public Health Acts of 1936 and 1961. Additional control was
possible under various planning Acts and, in the case of water pollution, by
the Water Acts of 1945 and 1973, and the Water Resources Act 1963. More
recently, the Deposit of Poisonous Wastes Act 1972 provides control over
hazardous or toxic waste disposal while the Control of Pollution Act 1974
consolidated the previous controls vested amongst numerous Local
Government departments by creating new Waste Disposal Authorities
within the County Councils of England, and the District Councils in Wales
and Scotland.

The Control of Pollution Act places the following responsibilities on a Waste Disposal Authority.

1. To ensure that adequate means exist for the safe and acceptable disposal of all controlled waste produced or transported into their areas.
2. To conduct surveys of the quantity and nature of the waste arising in their areas.
3. To produce and publicise a plan to show how wastes will be disposed of in the future.
4. To license all waste disposal facilities including landfills, incinerators, treatment plants and transfer stations.

Any proposal to deposit waste must initially have the approval of the Planning Authority and secondly be granted a licence by the Waste Disposal Authority whose duty it is to take into consideration comments by District Council, the Collection Authority, the Health and Safety Executive, and the Regional Water Authority.[3] Where controlled wastes are disposed of into geological formations, i.e. either injected under pressure or allowed to drain by gravity into fractures, fissures or intergranular pores via shafts, galleries, wells, boreholes, or pipes the Insititute of Geological Sciences should also be consulted. Licences cover in detail the type and quantity of waste that can be deposited, the method of operation and the preliminary engineering works that may be needed to prepare the site for disposal operations or to minimise the water pollution impact. These include the creation of screening embankments, fences, surface drainage ditches, culverts, leachate collection or treatment facilities, etc.

Although the conditions are sometimes obvious, site licences can include as many as 60–70 separate conditions specifying how the site should be operated. Needless to say, it may take at least three years from the instigation of negotiations for a site to the first deposit of waste, sometimes much longer, especially if there is a conflict of interest between the Waste Disposal Authority and Water Authority. In this case a dispute may be referred to the Secretary of State for the Environment for his decision.

Since site licensing there has been a decrease in the number of landfill sites mainly due to the fact that the new Waste Disposal Authorities find it more economical to operate larger but fewer sites since more capital is needed for the improved basic level of operation.[4]

The following sections deal with the selection of landfill sites, their subsequent design requirements and management methods to minimise any environmental impact.

2. SELECTION OF LANDFILL SITES

2.1. Location

Landfill sites are ideally located near the areas where wastes are produced in order to minimise transportation costs. However, as available landfill space is used and towns and cities expand around them wastes have to be transported further from the production areas and transfer loading stations often with railway links may be used to transport wastes up to 100 miles to the disposal point. Consequently, sites near the areas producing waste previously rejected as landfills due to problems such as access, risk of water pollution, visual intrusion, etc., may be reconsidered as economically viable even though large financial expenditure may be required on preliminary preparation works to upgrade the site and minimise the impact of the disposal operation.

All sites have certain advantages and disadvantages as landfills and the final selection is often based on weighing numerous complicated factors against each other. However, it is important that landfills should be chosen primarily on the basis of their hydrogeological suitability for the waste to be deposited as, although other factors may be changed, the hydrogeology is more or less fixed.

2.2. Hydrogeological Assessment

Once wastes have been deposited in a landfill the principal mechanism for their mobilisation and possible return to the surface environment is through leaching by percolating water and transport away from the site in solution. The ability of the underlying rock to transmit fluids, which is governed by the local geology and hydrogeology, is therefore fundamental in evaluating the pollution potential of the disposal site to ensure that ground or surface water will not be affected. Geologically, sites can be classified on their ability to contain wastes or conversely on their ability to allow leachates to migrate from them. Where the underlying geological formation is permeable, leachate will migrate and thereby interact with the rock minerals or groundwater, so that natural processes may occur to attenuate or reduce the concentration of contaminants in the leachate. On this basis three types of site can be identified but in reality sites rarely fall completely into any one category and often possess combined characteristics.

1. Sites in relatively impermeable strata which afford significant containment of wastes and leachate, e.g. clay or marl pits.

2. Sites where leachate is allowed to migrate away slowly with significant attenuation, e.g. a site above the water table underlain by silts or fine sand and clay.
3. Sites where leachate migrates away relatively rapidly with little potential for attenuation, e.g. quarries in fissured crystalline rocks or limestones.

Classification of sites in this way introduces the concept of whether wastes should be concentrated and contained within a site or whether they should be diluted and dispersed into the environment. There is no simple answer to this question since whether a particular waste is acceptable at a non-containment site depends on its physical and chemical character, the size of the landfill, the local geology and hydrogeology, waste-rock interactions, local use or potential use of groundwater or surface water, the method of landfill operation and so forth.

Each option has advantages and disadvantages which must be evaluated with respect to individual sites and waste. Clay pits, marl pits, or quarries in fine grained compact formations such as slates may constitute containment sites and these are commonly flooded since there is no way for rainfall to escape except either by overflowing on the surface, or, if the low permeability material which forms the base of the site is overlain by more permeable rocks, then water may rise until it can escape through the permeable strata.

Alternatively, the water level may rise in the landfill until the hydrostatic head is capable of transmitting input volumes of water through the low permeability containing medium and a steady state is achieved. Although clays or shales are often regarded as impermeable they do have a finite permeability albeit low which, over long periods or under high hydrostatic pressure can transmit significant volumes of water.

Consequently, wastes in a containment site, even if the site is pumped dry before disposal takes place, eventually become saturated. Unless provisions are installed to reduce infiltration into the site and to collect and otherwise dispose of the leachate in its treated or untreated form, any escape of leachate may result in the pollution of surface water or groundwater. In addition, saturated domestic refuse or other wastes, e.g. calcium sulphate in plaster board, can produce obnoxious smells due to biodegradation in anaerobic conditions and may constitute health hazards. Furthermore, saturated landfills are difficult to reclaim for building development and if they contain hazardous wastes which do not naturally degrade to a stable inert form may sterilise the ground for development or future mineral extraction and, depending on their chemical character, the site may require perpetual surveillance.

In contrast, sites where leachates are allowed to migrate rarely present leachate management problems, but require detailed hydrogeological investigations in the site selection stage to ensure that leachates are attenuated by natural processes and do not produce unacceptable impairment of water resources. Fine grained unsaturated formations such as sands or silts in which water moves slowly through the pore spaces between the sand grains or minerals are examples of formations through which leachates migrate slowly. Because of the intimate and prolonged contact between the rock and the leachate, attenuation interactions e.g. ion exchange or adsorption may result. Where a landfill is sited above a fissured formation such as limestone or fractured igneous rocks (granite, basalt, etc.), leachate migration may be rapid, and the opportunity for interaction of leachate and rock minerals correspondingly poor. Wherever possible the dilute and disperse strategy is to be preferred on the grounds of economy, ease of operation, and absence of long term problems. It is particularly appropriate to biodegradable wastes such as domestic refuse which, although producing a highly mineralised leachate, does not release significant amounts of toxic species which would render water unfit even if present in trace amounts.

Toxic substances which are not attenuated by normal processes within the landfill or groundwater system should be prevented from migrating. Concentration of such wastes in containment sites is therefore appropriate and economically it is sensible to conserve such sites for hazardous or toxic waste rather than allowing |them| to be filled with waste which could be satisfactorily disposed by dilution and dispersion.

In particular, containment sites seem to be eminently suitable for the disposal of toxic liquid wastes following pre-treatment by chemical fixation to form a stable inert product which eventually sets into a solid.[5]

2.3. Attenuation of Leachates

In evaluating landfill sites the mechanisms controlling the migration and attenuation of leachates must be understood. The behaviour of hazardous wastes in landfill sites has been the subject of recent research in the UK[2] where the movement of leachates from 20 toxic waste landfills in differing geological and hydrogeological environments was studied by drilling boreholes within and around the landfills. In addition controlled field irrigation experiments, simulated landfill leaching experiments and laboratory scale tests were undertaken using specific toxic wastes. Research is still continuing in this respect.

Wastes, once deposited are subjected to three environments in which attenuation may occur:

(1)   in the landfill,
(2)   in the unsaturated zone of the aquifer, and
(3)   in the saturated zone of the aquifer.

2.3.1. *Interaction in the Landfill*

If wastes from manufacturing industries are landfilled it is unusual for the site to accept only one type of material. Normally a wide range of wastes is dealt with and in very many instances these wastes are landfilled in sites which also contain domestic refuse. Provided that interactions between certain specific wastes are avoided, e.g. sulphides with acids, then co-disposal is beneficial. Reactions can occur between potentially hazardous materials and domestic waste which can either destroy the former or render them insoluble so that they do not escape from the landfill site. Such reactions have been studied in detail in the Department of the Environment research programme, but some examples are given below.

Cyanide. Various decomposition mechanisms have been identified. Thus conversion to volatile hydrogen cyanide, formation of complex cyanides, hydrolysis to ammonium formate and formation of thiocyanate may take place. Pilot scale experiments showed that when cyanide waste was sandwiched between domestic waste and then irrigated, less than 3 % of the cyanide appeared in the leachate.

Heavy metals and acids. Research has shown that important mechanisms which will help to prevent escape of heavy metals from a domestic landfill, include precipitation as sulphides, hydroxides or carbonates under the near neutral pH conditions which normally prevail. The valency of the deposited metal is important since, for example, hexavalent chromium is more mobile than the trivalent form. However, co-disposal can be beneficial for this element in that the anaerobic reducing conditions within the site will assist in the reduction to the trivalent form. Obviously the addition of excess acid to a site containing heavy metals should be avoided since if the buffering capacity of the waste is exceeded then dissolution of metals will occur with risk of possible escape of these from the site. It has been found that 1 kg of waste can neutralise between 22 g and 33 g of sulphuric acid depending on the age of the waste.

2.3.2. *Unsaturated Zone*

Once leachate is produced it will either build up at the base of the landfill if the underlying strata is of low permeability, or will migrate through the unsaturated zone assuming that the site lies on permeable strata above the water table. The factors governing water or contaminant flow in the unsaturated zone are complex and are subject to much research at present. The term unsaturated means that the voids present between the rock minerals contain both gas and liquid phases, and in such conditions there will be surface tension forces acting. When the voids are completely filled with liquid then the formation is 100 % saturated with maximum moisture content, and the hydraulic conductivity will also be at a maximum. If the formation is allowed to drain under gravity for a long enough period so that downward movement of water essentially stops a certain volume will be retained in the rock by surface tension. The formation in this condition is said to be at field capacity.

Before significant downward movement can take place in an unsaturated formation the field capacity must be exceeded. It has been found that the hydraulic conductivity in unsaturated conditions depends primarily on the moisture content and the effective hydraulic conductivity decreases markedly by many orders of magnitude once a formation becomes unsaturated.

As a result, migration of liquids through the unsaturated zone is very much slower than through the saturated zone of the aquifer, and since it is primarily influenced by gravity, movement is predominantly vertical so that lateral movement may be neglected.

A mathematical expression for unidirectional flow in a homogeneous unsaturated granular formation under isothermal conditions is:

$$V = k\lambda \left(\frac{\mathrm{d}\theta_z}{\mathrm{d}z} + 1 \right)$$

where $V = $ flow per unit area in unit time,

$\mathrm{d}\theta_z/\mathrm{d}z = $ change in matric potential (or soil suction) with depth,

$k = $ saturated hydraulic conductivity, and

$\lambda = $ function relating hydraulic conductivity with degree of saturation.

Therefore, estimation of water movement requires a knowledge of the matric potential, the moisture content and the characteristic curve relating conductivity to moisture content. Evaluation of these parameters in the field is extremely difficult and time consuming and the establishment of a landfill site may appreciably alter the conditions in the underlying unsaturated zone as measured before the commencement of landfilling. A major disturbance caused by the landfill is the change in the temperature gradient in the underlying strata due to the heat generated in the landfill as a result of biodegradation. Since temperatures of up to 70 °C are often found in landfills, the movement of volatile organics, water vapour or gas may be significant especially in the early stages of landfilling.[6]

Because of these difficulties it is often better to estimate migration in the unsaturated zone by direct measurements, e.g. by profiling the vertical distribution of a chemical tracer for which the input characteristics are known, e.g. tritium, nitrate or introducing radioactive tracers.[7,8] However, if fissure flow takes place in the unsaturated zone leachates may reach the water table rapidly and in advance of times inferred from chemical profiling. Fissured formations are generally unfavourable for leachate attenuation if rapid migration can occur but chalk or Bunter sandstone, which although fissured have a high intergranular porosity may not necessarily be unfavourable if the moisture content or irrigation rate is low enough to prevent significant fissure flow occurring.

Because of the generally slow rate of migration in unsaturated formations there is significant opportunity for leachate/rock interactions to occur which lead to leachate attenuation.

The potential for rock/leachate interaction obviously depends on the mineralogy. Formations containing clay minerals which often have adsorptive or ion exchange properties are likely to attenuate cations far more than a sandstone composed principally of quartz. Other mineralogical compositions such as a high carbonate content may buffer an acid leachate and maintain a neutral pH so that heavy metals are precipitated.

This is illustrated in research into the migration of a synthetic leachate containing heavy metals (Ni, Zn, Pb, Cu, Cr, Cd) each at 100 mg litre^{-1} in an acid solution (pH 5) of short chain carboxylic acids (acetic, propionic and butyric) in a lysimeter of Lower Greensand at Uffington near Harwell, Oxfordshire[9] (see Fig. 1). The Lower Greensand contains silica (60 %) clay, mainly calcium montmorillonite (up to 30 %), calcite and aragonite (8 %) and free hydrated iron oxides (goethite).

The variation in composition of interstitial water in the unsaturated formation was monitored over several years at different depths in the lysimeter by the use of suction probes.

Results (Fig. 2) suggest that the organic content of the leachate is attenuated principally by biodegradation and conversion to carbon dioxide and methane since there is a cyclic variation in organic carbon, lowest concentrations being observed in the summer months when the temperature is more favourable to microbiological activity.

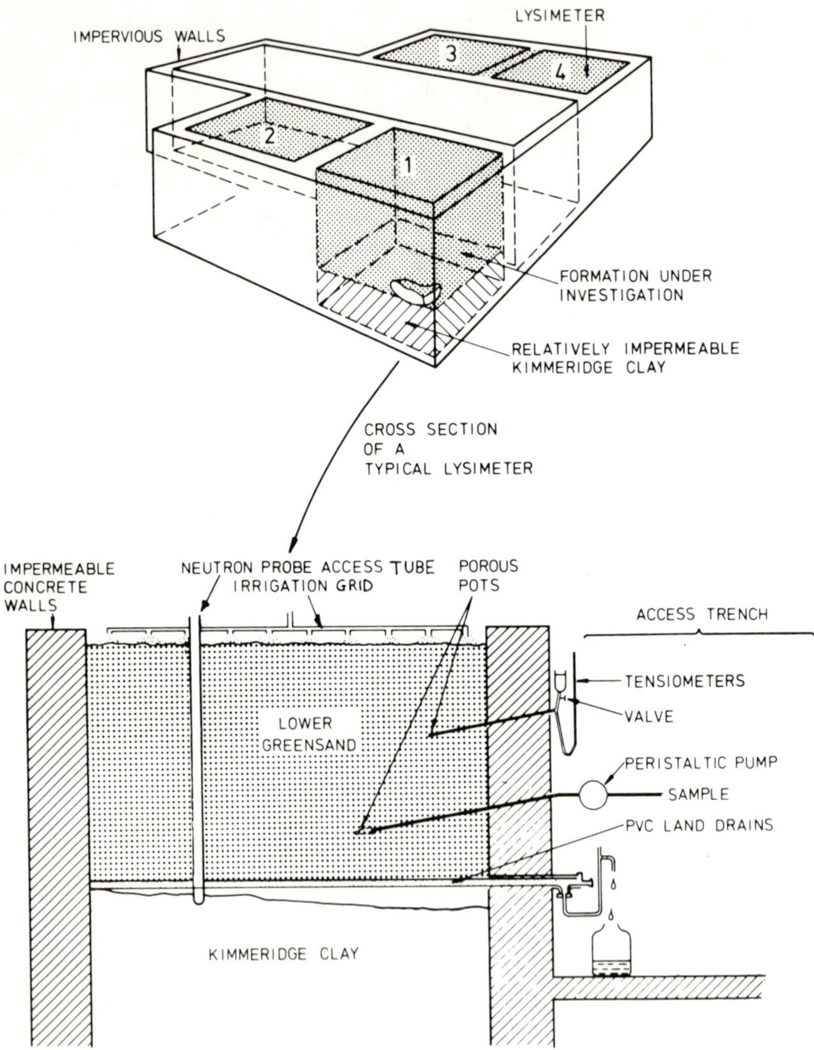

FIG. 1.   Uffington lysimeters—construction details. After reference 13.

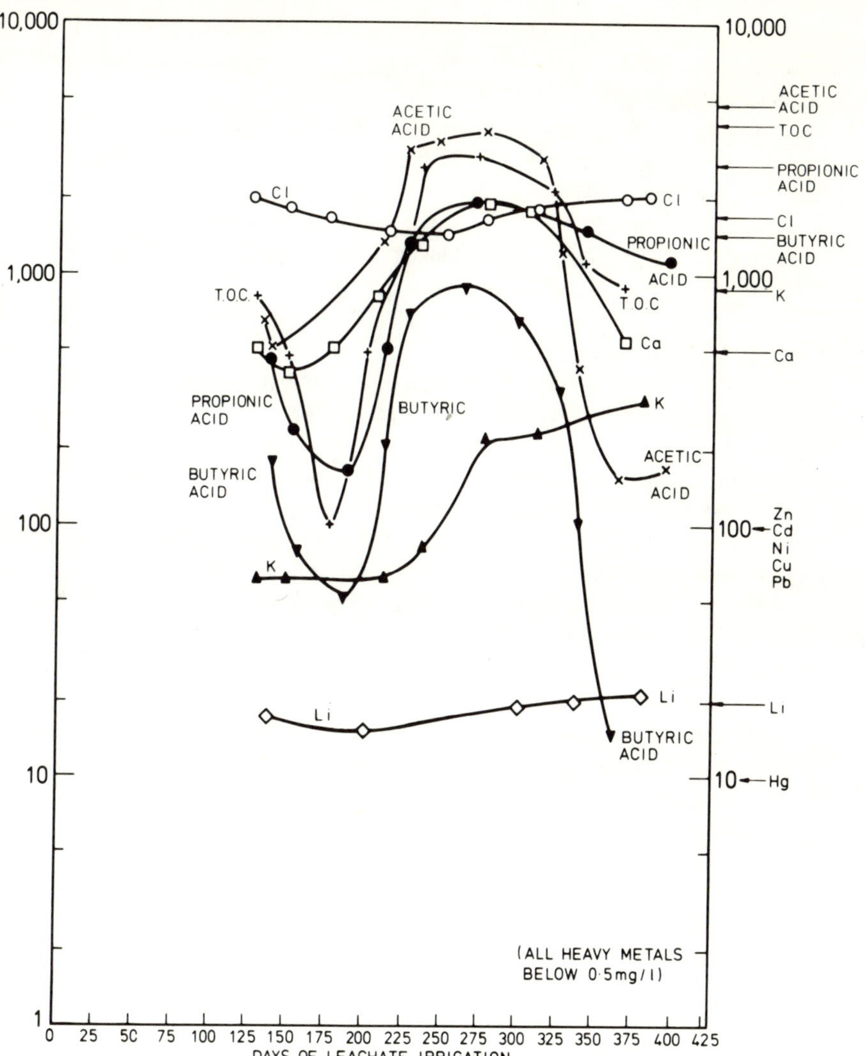

FIG. 2. Concentration of chemical species (mg litre^{-1}) in lysimeter 4 probe 8 (400 mm below surface). After reference 13.

Heavy metals have been significantly attenuated and retarded in their rate of migration through the lysimeter. Mechanisms for attenuation are complex but heavy metals appear to be attenuated in the clay, iron oxide, organic and sulphide phases within the formation, and once attenuated are not easily re-mobilised.[10]

The diffusion of oxygen into the unsaturated zone is also important in aiding attenuation especially by creating aerobic conditions for biodegradation of organics. A fissured system may be superior in this respect than an inter granular medium especially since water table variations in fissured formations may be large and cause piston displacement of the soil atmosphere.

2.3.3. *Saturated Zone*

On reaching the water table in the aquifer, leachates will flow with the groundwater in the direction of the hydraulic gradient and in doing so will be diluted as a result of the pollution front spreading due to hydrodynamic dispersion and chemical diffusion. The last mechanism will occur whether or not there is groundwater movement but generally hydrodynamic dispersion due to mechanical mixing of the leachate as a result of the tortuous flow paths through the aquifer predominates.[11] Dispersion within the saturated zone depends on a number of factors especially on whether the contaminant is miscible with the groundwater. For example, oils which are immiscible may form a separate phase and move on the surface of the groundwater. Other contaminants of significantly greater density than the groundwater may sink to the bottom of the aquifer and the true hydraulic gradient within the aquifer will not necessarily be that determined by the level of water in a borehole.

Flow through the aquifer may occur either as a result of movement through fissures or by movement through microscopic pores between the grains or rock minerals. Fissure flow can be very rapid, of the order of tens of metres per day, while intergranular flow is commonly much slower at rates of much less than $1\ \mathrm{m\ day^{-1}}$. Complicated flow patterns may occur in dual porosity aquifers, i.e. where there is intergranular flow and fissure flow, for instance Bunter sandstone or chalk. In these cases diffusion of contaminants between the fissure and pore water will occur, depending on concentration gradients, and this will have the effect of delaying the advance of a pollution front but of extending the period of the contamination at any one point.

Chemical and biological reactions similar to those occurring in the unsaturated zone may take place in the saturated zone, but because of faster flow rates, complete chemical equilibrium may not be attained between the aquifer and the leachate.

A common observation is the reduction in dissolved oxygen in groundwater beneath and down gradient of a landfill from that in groundwater up a hydraulic gradient. Where insufficient oxygen is able to diffuse into the unsaturated zone beneath a landfill to aerobically degrade the organic or ammoniacal constituents of the leachate, oxygen within the groundwater may be utilised and these constituents are often found to be reduced to background concentrations immediately on entering the saturated zone.

Changes in physico-chemical conditions in the saturated zone, e.g. pH–Eh changes may also cause precipitation of heavy metals as hydroxides and lead to attenuation.

Because of the complexity of chemical and biochemical processes and the difficulty of predicting leachate attenuation, it is easier to calculate the dilution of leachate in groundwater or in a borehole or spring discharge, based on a worst case where such attenuation is disregarded. In this way any chemical or biochemical attenuation provides a safety factor in the calculation.[12]

2.4. Site Investigations and Monitoring

In line with legislation controlling landfill operations, greater emphasis is also placed on investigations into the geology and hydrogeology of potential sites prior to disposal operations. This is especially pertinent to the selection of larger landfill sites in areas where there is an increasing need to conserve groundwater and surface water resources.

Unfortunately, many constraints besides those involving water pollution influence the waste disposal operator in selecting a site and it is rare for a site to be chosen primarily on the basis of its hydrogeological suitability. Very often because of land availability, sites may be purchased with very scant information about the hydrogeology and detailed investigations may only be possible or practicable after the site has been purchased. Considerable time is then required to drill boreholes, analyse water and rock samples, or to collect data on seasonal variations in stream flows, groundwater levels and chemistry sufficient to adequately define the hydrogeology. If the risk of water pollution is unacceptable, engineering works may be necessary to improve the site or, alternatively, the method of landfill operation or nature of the waste to be deposited, may need to be modified.

The exact hydrogeological information required for landfill site evaluation will obviously be site specific, and the degree to which the investigation is carried out will depend on how hydrogeologically sensitive a site may be. In this respect many water authorities in England have developed aquifer protection policies which attempt to divide their catchments into zones of differing sensitivities to groundwater pollution.[13] For example, the zone immediately surrounding a major groundwater abstraction for public water supply from an unconfined aquifer may be regarded as highly sensitive to any activity which may give rise to polluting leachates and any landfill site proposed in this area would require extensive investigation to ensure that unacceptable pollution of the supply would not ensue. Conversely, a relatively minor hydrogeological investigation may be appropriate to a landfill sited in an area remote from surface water courses and devoid of groundwater resources, or where existing groundwater was of poor quality.

A first stage in any landfill site assessment is the collection of all published information on the area and the acquisition of an accurate topographic map not only of the site but of the surrounding area. Initially a scale of 1:10 000 may be adequate but as more detailed hydrogeological information is gathered a smaller scale, e.g. 1:500 may be necessary. Aerial photography is often used to produce detailed topographic maps of a site and if a number of sites are surveyed in one sortie then the technique is faster and more economical than conventional ground based surveys.

Geological information is usually available from maps on the 1:50 000 scale or equivalent, published by the Institute of Geological Sciences and, normally, maps of 1:10 000 are also available for consultation.

A number of hydrogeological maps have also been produced which although valuable do not provide sufficient detail to obviate the need for local hydrogeological surveys. A *National Inventory of Wells and Boreholes* under the auspices of the Institute of Geological Sciences is also a source of geological information and, together with the Regional Water Authority, provides information on the location of groundwater abstractions. Even so, a study of the local geology is essential and this will usually entail drilling boreholes.

For containment sites investigations may be relatively simple since they are usually aimed at establishing the permeability of the containment medium, e.g. clay, and its presence in sufficient thickness beneath and around the landfill. Where leachates are expected to migrate away then the investigation may be more extensive, usually requiring a number of boreholes from which hydrogeological information can be obtained.

Boreholes provide information on the depth to the water table, which can be used to infer the hydraulic gradient in any underlying aquifers, as well as providing samples of groundwater and rock for chemical and mineralogical analysis. Physical properties such as effective porosity, permeability and moisture content may also be determined in the laboratory from rock samples, and the extraction and analysis of pore water from the unsaturated zone of the aquifer may provide valuable information on the rate of migration of solutes to the water table.

The drilling method used must not cause contamination of the geochemical samples and for this reason air flush rotary or dry percussion drilling are to be preferred to water or mud flush methods.[14]

Where hazardous or toxic wastes are to be landfilled it is important to investigate their interaction with the underlying geological formations. As already mentioned research lysimeters have been employed for this purpose but, on a smaller scale for unconsolidated sediments, repacked laboratory columns, and 'monolith' lysimeters (which consist of large cores of sediment retrieved in a glass fibre tube 0·8 m diameter and 1 m long, driven hydraulically into the ground) can be irrigated with leachate of the expected composition. Sampling interstitial fluids by means of suction probes at various depths in the column or lysimeter provides information on the rate of migration and attenuation of particular leachate constituents.[15]

Pumping tests or injection tests on boreholes can yield *in situ* information on the permeability of the aquifer and its capacity to store water. These are essential parameters in assessing the dilution and rate of movement of pollutants in the saturated zone. Measurement of dispersion in the saturated zone requires sophisticated field techniques and may necessitate the use of radioactive tracers. Few determinations of dispersion coefficients have been undertaken in the UK[16] and consequently conservative estimates have to be made in assessing dilution in the saturated zone.

Additional information on flows in adjacent streams may be obtained from gauging records held by water authorities or may require measurement by installing a temporary flume or weir, or by flow measurements using an impeller device. Rainfall data is usually available from the Meteorological Office as are figures for potential evaporation which together provide an estimate of the volume of leachate likely to be produced.

Investigatory boreholes to define the geology and groundwater conditions may be used to monitor the natural variations in the hydrogeological regime prior to landfilling and provide essential background data to which subsequent changes can be related. Additional factors to be monitored will depend on the characteristics of the site but invariably will include measurement of surface water flows, groundwater levels in boreholes and the collection of groundwater or surface water samples for chemical analysis. It is essential that a routine is established for water sampling or measurement since a water system is continuously changing and because density contrasts between contaminants and groundwater may lead to stratification within a borehole column. The act of drilling a borehole may also upset the natural flow in the aquifer and induce vertical flow in the borehole which obviously confuses interpretation of chemical sampling. To overcome these problems, several boreholes may be required, perforated at different depths in the aquifer, or small diameter piezometer tubes installed at different isolated positions in a larger diameter borehole.[17] Several chemical parameters need measurement at the time of sampling, e.g. pH, Eh and alkalinity; other parameters should be determined within a few days, e.g. organics and calcium, while after acidification samples containing some constituents, e.g. heavy metals, can be preserved for several months before analysis.[18]

If adequate sampling procedures are not maintained, correlation of analyses is not valid and any conclusions drawn may be subject to gross error. However, once the basic water chemistry has been determined, routine sampling may be less frequent or involve determination of fewer chemical species or may be limited to *in situ* measurement of electrical conductivity or dissolved oxygen of the groundwater, by lowering a probe into the borehole.

3.   DESIGN OF LANDFILL SITES TO REDUCE THEIR ENVIRONMENTAL IMPACT

3.1. Past Experience

Environmental pollution from landfill sites can be separated into two groups:

(1)   pollution of ground and surface waters by leachate, and
(2)   general pollution above the surface which will include smell, noise, dust, gas emissions, vermin and increased traffic on access roads.

Pollution of surface waters can be minimised by good management techniques mainly involving leachate control and treatment. However, if pollution of an aquifer occurs then restoration of groundwater quality may involve considerable effort and money and may not, in fact, be possible. In the UK aquifer pollution due to landfill has been very limited but serious incidents have occurred in the United States. As an example Clark[19] has described groundwater contamination from the Army Creek landfill in an abandoned sand and gravel pit in Delaware. Refuse thickness over the 19 ha site ranged from 2 m to 12 m. Deposition ceased in 1968 but by 1971 water in a well some 300 m from the site became contaminated and it became apparent that a significant pollution plume had developed. The main attenuation mechanism appeared to be dilution. Various options to lessen the environmental impact were considered including transport of the waste to another landfill, incineration of the waste, increasing the rate of decomposition by recirculating leachate over the landfill, and pumping air into the site to produce aerobic conditions. However, these and some other possible remedies were rejected either on cost grounds or technical uncertainties. The recommended permanent control measures are as follows:

(1) minimisation of leachate production by decreasing rainfall infiltration and groundwater flow, and
(2) recovery of leachate by drilling and pumping wells close to and within the landfill.

The initial costs are estimated to be approximately 4·4 million dollars with annual operating and maintenance costs amounting to about one million dollars. Examples of leachate plumes are described by Kimmel and Braids[20] in two sites in New York State where these extended 3200 m and 1500 m down the hydraulic gradient.

It should be emphasised that aquifer clean-up, if it is possible, is likely to prove to be an expensive operation. Such problems can be prevented from occurring by proper site selection in which hydrogeological factors are carefully considered before development takes place. For example, in an alluvial site excavated in sand/gravel and with nearby water abstraction points the only two options available may be either the installation of an impermeable liner or the abandonment of the site for landfill purposes altogether. It should be pointed out that the number of cases where significant aquifer pollution has occurred is very small compared with the many thousands of landfill sites which have been in operation in the UK and other countries. However, the importance of good site selection will be more crucial in the future if the phasing out of small sites continues, accompanied by concentration of refuse disposal at sites accepting at least 1000 t day^{-1}. Obviously if problems occur at very large sites they could make a very serious environmental impact.

In addition to pollution of groundwater, environmental problems may occur due to lax site management but because of more stringent licensing requirements this is less likely to happen nowadays in the UK. An example of landfill causing problems in South Yorkshire has been described by Khan.[21] The site had an area of 2·6 ha, was situated in a series of sandstone quarries, and had been used for the deposition of acid tars, oil contaminated fullers earth and other industrial wastes. The total quantity involved was though to be about 10 000 t. The whole site was considered to be dangerous especially for children from nearby houses and complaints had been made about dust and smells. Various disposal options were considered including removal to other landfill sites, incineration, encapsulation but these all presented problems so on-site neutralisation using lime was chosen. The waste was treated in batches with the resulting innocuous material being compacted and covered with subsoil. The total cost of the operation was about £200 000. An example of past inadequate management is given by a site in Scotland receiving acid tars and also oils which formed a lagoon. The oily layer, which was present above an acidic aqueous phase, was set alight on several occasions. Problems with this site have been largely overcome but other countries have experienced trouble with sites in which hazardous chemicals have been deposited. For example, in New York State, a disused canal known as Love Canal was used from 1947–1952 for toxic wastes disposal. In 1976 heavy rains caused the underground channel to overflow allowing chemicals to spread into land occupied by houses and a school. Many people claimed that their health had been adversely affected and property values have dropped. Legal battles over the site and allocation of responsibility continue. It has become apparent that the disposal of hazardous wastes can be a serious problem and generally the disposal of such materials by dumping them in a hole in the ground should be discouraged. Other routes, e.g. co-disposal with domestic waste, incineration, chemical treatment, encapsulation or storage in underground salt mines should be considered.

Smells from landfill sites can cause a nuisance to inhabitants of any nearby houses although there is no firm evidence of any long- or short-term health risk. Smells can originate from the decomposition of solid wastes, from co-deposition of industrial wastes or chemicals or from any leachate produced by the landfill. Research has been carried out to identify odiferous compounds in gases produced during decomposition. Use of gas chromatography/mass spectrometry has led to the isolation and identification of many tens of compounds including alcohols, esters and sulphur-containing compounds which are probably mercaptans. The latter are present at concentrations of less than one part per million. Evidence suggests that the range of compounds varies with age of the refuse and that smell from leachate is different to that from solid refuse. Attempts to overcome smell problems by using oxidising or masking agents have not been entirely successful. The recommended procedure for landfill operations is to cover the refuse surface with a layer of soil about 150 mm thick at the end of each day's work. This layer also helps to prevent trouble with vermin and flies. Spraying with an insecticide during refuse deposition may be necessary in hot weather to control flies. Seagulls and, to a lesser extent, other birds can be a nuisance on sites especially if these are near airport runways. Bird scarers, e.g. small detonators, have not proved adequate although falcons have been a useful deterrent. The use of fine wires spread between poles has been claimed to give good results.

Dust on roads within a landfill site is a common problem during dry months but can be minimised by lightly spraying with water. The use of rubble on porous synthetic |sheeting| such as 'Terram' for site roads rather than compacted soil or clay will tend to reduce the nuisance. Mud carried onto public roads by lorries is unpopular with other users but can be largely eliminated by the provision of wheel washes at the site entrance. Wind-blown paper or plastic can be a problem particularly at exposed sites but can be trapped by the installation of movable mesh fences around the operating area. Labourers are employed at some sites to collect such debris. This problem can also be minimised by baling refuse prior to delivery to site (see Section 4.4.).

3.2. Leachate Control

Once a landfill site has been selected then action may be required to improve conditions to meet hydrogeological criteria which may have been laid down by the Water Authority and the Waste Disposal Authority prior to the issue of a site licence. For a containment site the most important of these is the prevention of leachate escape. This problem can be greatly reduced by minimising water ingress into the site by the provision of suitable bunds to intercept and divert surface run-off. Use of relatively impermeable cover materials and a high rate of refuse deposition may enable sections of the site to be completed before the field capacity of the refuse is exceeded, thus reducing leachate production.

It must be recognised that as it will be impossible to prevent leachate production in most landfills, especially those situated in areas having a high rainfall, it may be necessary to prevent infiltration into underlying strata. This can be accomplished by lining the inside walls and floor of landfill sites with an impermeable material. The materials used or proposed can be divided into two main groups: natural and artificial. Natural liners, e.g. clays, have been widely used for years to retain water in canals, reservoirs and for holding lagoons in various factory operations. One such material, bentonite, has been used as a landfill liner since it swells on contact with liquid thus giving a good seal and also tends to adsorb heavy metal cations from leachate. This factor will give some attenuation if leakages occur in the liner. Another example of the use of natural materials is given by the use of naturally occurring chalk in puddling experiments. In these, the floors of disused chalk quarries have been pulverised and then compacted, thus reducing the permeability to such an extent that they may be considered for use as landfill sites having good containment characteristics.[22]

In recent years there has been great interest in the use of synthetic materials, e.g. polyethylene, polyvinyl chloride, butyl rubber and ethylene propylene diene monomer (EPDM) for lining purposes. These have the advantage that they are of uniform thickness and composition and are also available in large rolls which can be joined together on site to form large sheets. They suffer from disadvantages particularly in that the site has to be carefully prepared before installation to prevent puncturing on uneven ground. Prior to refuse deposition they are normally protected from penetration by sharp objects by a layer of soft material, e.g. sand or pulverised fuel ash. The integrity of the liner is important since leachate leakage from a limited area of the site may cause a more significant environmental hazard than if no liner were used and leachate were allowed to migrate naturally.

The long-term resistance of synthetic liners to landfill leachate is very important since the material should remain unaffected throughout the period during which significant decomposition of refuse is occurring. This may extend up to 20–30 years. This information is not yet available since the use of synthetics for landfill liners is a fairly recent innovation. However, work by Haxo[23] indicates that the behaviour of polyethylene and PVC is encouraging. Attempts are also being made to judge the behaviour of potential liners under strain when subjected to accelerated tests under elevated temperature and pressure. It should be emphasised that liner behaviour is normally assessed in terms of resistance to leachate from domestic refuse. If liners are to be considered for use on industrial disposal sites then their good resistance to organic solvents and other chemicals will be important.

Other liners based on asphalt or concrete have also been used. Mixed asphalt–cement sealants are not always completely impermeable and may require surface sealing. Portland cement and fine-grained soil mixtures can result in hard, low strength concrete having a permeability of $< 10^{-6}$ cm s^{-1}. Some degradation can be expected under acid conditions. Soil–asphalt mixtures can be prepared *in situ* with their permeability depending on the asphalt content. Such liners are resistant to cracking and more flexible than asphalt–concrete or soil–cement. They are acid resistant but their behaviour in the presence of oils is suspect. Asphalt can also be sprayed onto the landfill walls giving a flexible membrane.

Two questions must be answered before a landfill site is to be lined. First, is the considerable financial outlay involved justified or should the prospective site be abandoned and an alternative one sought? Costs of lining can be up to about £5 m^{-2} (1980 prices) and additional capital costs for installing an under-liner monitoring system for leaks may be necessary. These costs may render the use of the site uneconomic. The second question must be—do the operators want a containment site? While a containment site will probably satisfy the Local Water Authority, the problems which can be encountered with leachate build-up during its operation should be recognised.

The number of domestic landfill sites in the UK which have been lined is small, especially when compared with some European countries, e.g. West Germany. While liners may be necessary in some sites, the need for them should be clearly thought out and they should only be installed where absolutely necessary since they will increase the cost of landfill waste disposal.

4. LANDFILL SITE MANAGEMENT

4.1. Health and Safety

In the UK, the health and safety of landfill site staff and others who officially use the site, e.g. waste collection vehicle drivers, is affected by the Health and Safety at Work Act (1974). The chief areas in which the Act can operate are given below.

1. Washing and toilet facilities. Adequate facilities should be provided; these are normally situated in the site offices. Obviously this is important since on large landfills many workers will eat food on site.

2. Protective clothing. Items could include waterproof clothing and protective footwear. Wellington boots with flexible steel soles can eliminate foot injuries due to sharp objects, e.g. nails projecting from pieces of timber. Ear protectors are to be recommended for

      drivers of heavy machinery, e.g. compactors. On many modern machines air conditioned cabs ensure good working conditions.

3. Site roads should be of a high standard without sharp curves and steep drops at the sides. Signs clearly showing routes to be taken are desirable.

4. Smoking should be prohibited to prevent fires due to methane accumulations or ignition of refuse. Deposition of hot materials, e.g. cinders, should not be allowed.

5. Special care should be taken when dealing with hazardous chemicals. Protective clothing should include rubber gloves and also goggles to protect eyes. Operators should be aware of the potential dangers of inhaling certain chemical vapours. Care should be taken to avoid the mixing of some chemical wastes especially if wastes are being discharged into trenches. For example, a fatal accident occurred when acid was discharged on to sulphide waste when toxic hydrogen sulphide was evolved.

6. Accidents can occur when workers are in close proximity to heavy machinery, e.g. compactors, bulldozers and lorries. Cases have been reported of operators being crushed while attempting to release jammed release mechanisms, e.g. on skip lorries. Other accidents have occurred when workers have been trapped by reversing lorries. Provision of 'hard-hats' is desirable during some unloading operations.

7. Liquids are often discharged into trenches or shallow lagoons. Posts with warning bunting or ropes should surround such excavations.

8. In order to obtain a site licence, the management should normally provide a security fence to keep children and totters from entering the site. However, this is not always successful since cases have occurred when sections of the fence have been cut away and stolen! Also children have been known to enter sites and drive around in machinery causing considerable damage.

Very little work has been carried out on a study of the general health of workers employed on landfill sites. Some worries have been expressed as to the long-term effects of organic impurities present in the gases evolved during the decomposition of the putrescible fraction of domestic waste. In addition, the possible presence of pathogens in dust commonly encountered on landfill sites requires investigation especially if sewage sludge is co-deposited. As a further precaution anti-tetanus injections for operators are desirable.

4.2. Operational Strategy

If a landfill site is to operate in an acceptable manner considerable thought should be given to management strategy before starting the project. We suggest that this can be done by posing a series of questions. Examples are given below.

1. What daily input of waste is expected?

   In practice, forecasts are often exceeded.

2. How will the waste be transported to the site?

   Rail or road or possibly a combination of both.

3. Will private contractors' vehicles be allowed on the site?

   These may be less suitable than vehicles designed for site.

4. Will waste arrive in containers?

   Travelling cranes will be required for unloading and slave vehicles needed to take containers to working face.

5. What machines will be required to handle waste input?

   For example, rubber tyred loading shovels for low inputs and steel wheeled compactors for high inputs.

6. What type of weighbridge, wheel washes, mess rooms, offices will be needed?

7. How many permanent staff will be required to operate the site?

8. What charge should be made for waste disposal?

   This should cover items such as site purchase or rent, wages, equipment and depreciation.

9. Are the access roads to the site and in the site suitable?

10. Is sufficient top cover available?

    If it has to be brought to the site, how much will it cost?

11. Should water ingress, e.g. from springs, be diverted? Is there excessive surface water drainage into the site? If so, can this be diverted?

12. How should the waste be deposited in the site?

    For example, should only one area be initially worked and this be brought up to final level as soon as possible?

13. Are complaints from local residents likely on such matters as excessive traffic movements, odours, noise? | Can a public relations exercise be carried out emphasising the temporary nature of the operation and beneficial land reclamation?

14. Does methane evolution and diffusion through the sides of the site pose a threat to nearby houses?

15. Is it safe to practise co-disposal of industrial wastes which may be hazardous? If so, what is the maximum loading of hazardous material to domestic waste?

Such a list is not exhaustive but additional questions will depend on local conditions and possible environmental impact.

4.3. Methods of Waste Deposition and Landfill Machinery

Before the introduction of controlled landfill techniques waste was simply deposited in holes in the ground, e.g. disused quarries, with little or no regard for any effect on the environment. Waste was tipped into such sites usually from lorries, little attempt was made to compact the material and it was fairly common practice to deliberately set fire to the waste to extend the life of the site. Such dumping often gave rise to local protests and much effort has been required to improve the image of disposal by landfill. The concept of 'sanitary landfill' as it is known in the United States has been developed. In this, waste is deposited in layers up to 2 m thick which are covered at the end of each day's operation with a layer of inert cover material some 150–300 mm thick. The type of cover is not critical and may be sub-soil, broken builders' rubble or bricks, colliery shale, etc., in fact any material that is cheap and readily available. Most site operators welcome such cover and make no charge for its deposit. The cover fulfils several functions viz. smell prevention, discouragement of vermin and birds and the prevention of refuse becoming wind-borne.

The machinery required for successful landfill operations is becoming more costly and sophisticated especially as sites are becoming larger. This machinery can be divided into two groups. The first will only be required during the initial site preparation while the second group will operate throughout the life of the site. The first group could include drag-line excavators, bucket excavators or graders to contour the site, create access roads and to dig ditches to divert surface water and possibly install leachate collection ditches and holding/treatment lagoons. After a site has been prepared then the type of machinery to be used subsequently will depend on the daily input of waste. In a small site dealing with under $100\,t\,day^{-1}$, a rubber tyred loading shovel will be adequate (Fig. 3). It should be able to

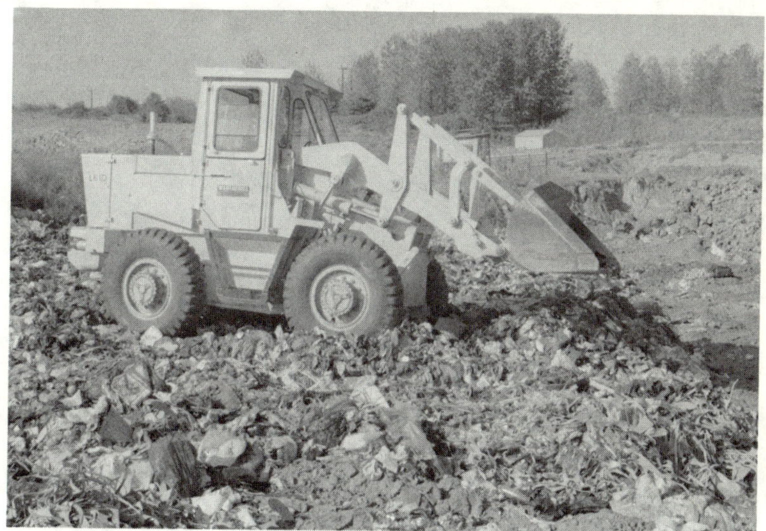

FIG. 3.   Rubber tyred loading shovel.

spread the waste efficiently, having reasonable traction, and has the great advantage that it can collect cover material easily. The fitting of heavy duty reinforced tyres is advisable to reduce punctures. An alternative is to use a small tracked vehicle with a bucket but this will be slower than a rubber tyred machine (Fig. 4). As the daily input rate increases then the type and number of machines will change. On sites having intermediate capacity (100–500 t) then large track vehicles fitted with a blade are popular. Obviously these are not suitable for bringing in cover material so that an additional machine will be required. For larger sites (800–1000 t and over) heavy steel wheel compactors are widely used. These are fitted with a blade, their wheels have strong plates or teeth projecting from the surface so that refuse is chopped and compacted as the machine traverses the waste (Fig. 5). It is claimed that these machines can give high bulk density to the waste and

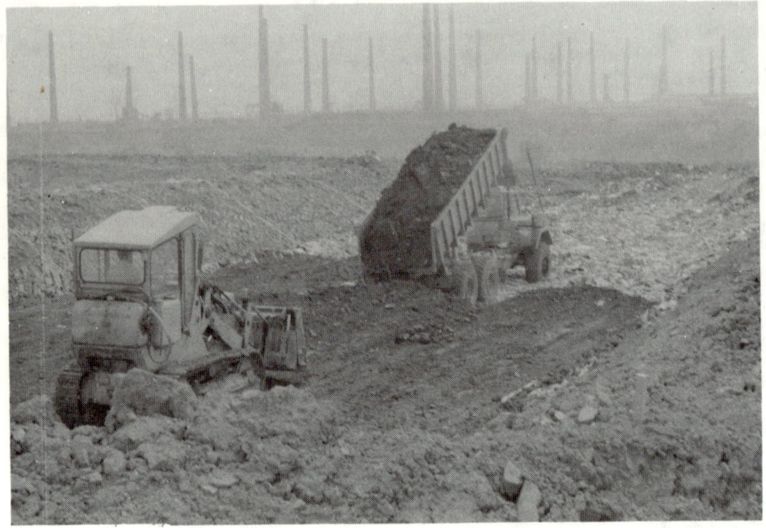

FIG. 4.　Small tracked machine.

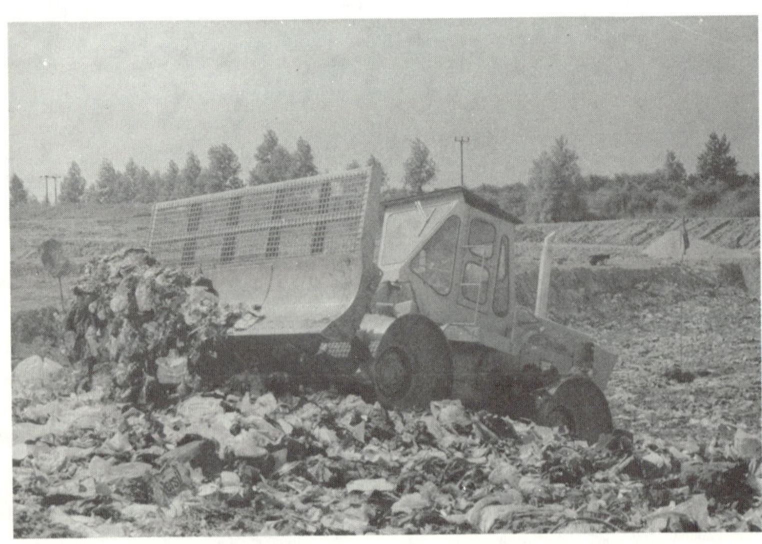

FIG. 5.　Steel wheeled compactor.

that they are less prone to mechanical trouble than a tracked vehicle. Even so, especially for large sites, several machines will be required and adequate spare capacity must be available in case of machine breakdown. On large sites it is becoming common for the waste to be delivered to the site in steel containers containing 13–15 t of waste either by road or rail. These are normally off-loaded using a travelling crane and transferred to a 'slave vehicle' which takes them to the operational sector of the site. These powerful vehicles have deeply ribbed tyres to obtain maximum grip on site roads and can raise and tilt the containers thus discharging their contents. The advantage of this transfer system is that the road delivery vehicles do not suffer extra wear and tear and also remain cleaner.

When waste is delivered to the tipping face it may be placed at the top from where it is pushed over the edge. Compaction, which is desirable to get the maximum amount of waste into the minimum void space, is largely obtained by running over with landfill machinery or by the delivery lorries. It has been found that these methods give a refuse density of 0.5–$0.6\,t\,m^{-3}$. Higher densities can be achieved if the compactor runs over the face of the waste but in many sites with high input rates there is insufficient time to carry this out efficiently. An alternative method is to place the refuse at the foot of the face and to push the material in thin layers up the face. This technique gives densities of about $1\,t\,m^{-3}$.[24] The advantage of achieving high initial density is that the amount of subsequent settlement is minimal although it must be remembered that high densities may inhibit the rate of decomposition since water inflow into the refuse may be reduced. Initial high density is important in shallow sites since in deep sites the weight of the refuse will cause natural compaction to occur eventually. The main advantage of steel wheeled compactors is that they are able to place quantities of refuse rapidly and that they crush bulky items, e.g. refrigerators or furniture, effectively.

4.4. Pulverising and Baling Prior to Landfill

During recent years it has been suggested that pulverising or baling of waste is advantageous before disposal, and various plants have been built in the UK. Pulverisation can be carried out using dry refuse in a hammer mill of which there are various types available. Bulky items and ferrous metals are normally removed prior to treatment. Advantages claimed are that landfilled pulverised waste only requires the minimum of cover, is unattractive to birds and vermin, is easy to transport and decomposes rapidly. However, pulverisation increases waste disposal costs by a factor of two to three and there is some evidence that fires on sites filled with the material are more prevalent. Wet pulverisation plants are an alternative—examples are the Dano or Shear rotating drums. In these, refuse is introduced into the top of a gently sloping drum which rotates at 3–4 r.p.m. Water or wastewater from sewage plants is added at a controlled rate. The residence time in the drum is 4–5 h. Approximately 60–70 % of the waste is pulverised while the remaining coarse fraction is separately landfilled. As with dry pulverisation treatment, costs are much higher than with conventional landfill and many existing plants are being phased out.

Baling prior to landfilling has been claimed to have significant environmental advantages. Two main groups of plant have been marketed. These can be divided into the type which gives medium density bales which are tied with wire to prevent disintegration. The more popular type gives 'high density' bales each 1 m^3 in volume and weighing about 1 t, which do not require wiring. The bales are usually transported to the landfill by lorry and placed in position using a fork-lift truck. In practice about 20 % of the bales break during transport or placement. The main advantage claimed is that leachate produced is less polluted than that obtained from normal landfill since any water entering the site should percolate through the cracks between bales and hence should not leach out such large quantities of material from the waste. Although more experience in large scale operation is required to substantiate this claim, baling drastically reduces problems with wind-blown litter. Costs of baling are similar to those of pulverisation which may again limit the acceptance of the technique.

4.5. Co-disposal of Hazardous Wastes

Examples of beneficial reactions which can occur between domestic and hazardous wastes have been given in Section 2.3.1. This idea of co-disposal is attractive both on the grounds of simplicity and economics since no additional capital costs are required as would be the case if the hazardous wastes were to be incinerated. In practice the co-disposal of liquids presents little problem since the waste is discharged into trenches and shallow lagoons excavated in the domestic waste. The amount and composition of the waste liquid which can be deposited per day is closely defined in the site licence which should ensure that the absorptive capacity of the solid waste is not exceeded. Organic solvents can be landfilled in small quantities but recovery or incineration are to be preferred.

Sludges are often co-disposed in landfill sites either in trenches dug on domestic waste or by being spread in thin layers prior to their incorporation. A manual dealing with all aspects of disposal of municipal sludges on landfill has recently been issued by the US Environmental Protection Agency.[25]

Where there are no safety problems hazardous solids can be spread over the working face of a landfill and then covered with a layer of domestic waste. This has the advantage over trench deposition in that attenuation mechanisms are more likely to work effectively than if the hazardous wastes were deposited in discrete pockets. An exception to the technique of spreading prior to disposal is the landfilling of asbestos. This material is received on site in sealed plastic bags which are buried in trenches and immediately covered with other waste.

Thus co-disposal of many hazardous wastes is a safe and economical disposal route provided that several very important criteria are observed.

1. The site should be hydrogeologically suitable. Obviously site selection is of great importance in the disposal of domestic waste and if the introduction of hazardous wastes is to be allowed then this is of even greater significance.
2. The site should not be overloaded, i.e. the ratio of hazardous/ domestic waste must be carefully controlled. In many respects the determination of what is the maximum rate allowable is one of the most difficult aspects of co-disposal. Government departments are in the process of issuing guidelines to site operators covering this topic.
3. It should be recognised that not all hazardous wastes are suitable for landfill co-disposal. For example, PCBs and some pesticides are probably best incinerated rather than landfilled and chemical destruction of cyanides is preferable to direct landfill.

It should be pointed out that many European countries have yet to be persuaded that co-disposal is an environmentally acceptable waste disposal route since many have invested in expensive treatment plants. However experience in the UK indicates that co-disposal is not only cheap but also efficient.

4.6. Gas Control and Recovery

The anaerobic decomposition of organic material in waste has been studied by various workers. It has been established that organic materials decompose at different rates with, for example, vegetable matter degrading more rapidly than cellulosic materials, e.g. paper and wood. In fact on excavation of landfills newspapers can often be exhumed even after burial for 10 or 20 years especially if the site has a low moisture content. Research by Farquhar and Rovers[26] indicates that decomposition involving gas formation occurs in four stages. The composition of the gases shows wide variations with time (Fig. 6).

In the first stage any oxygen present is rapidly used up and the principal gases found are hydrogen (up to 15%), nitrogen and carbon dioxide. As decomposition continues nitrogen concentrations gradually decrease

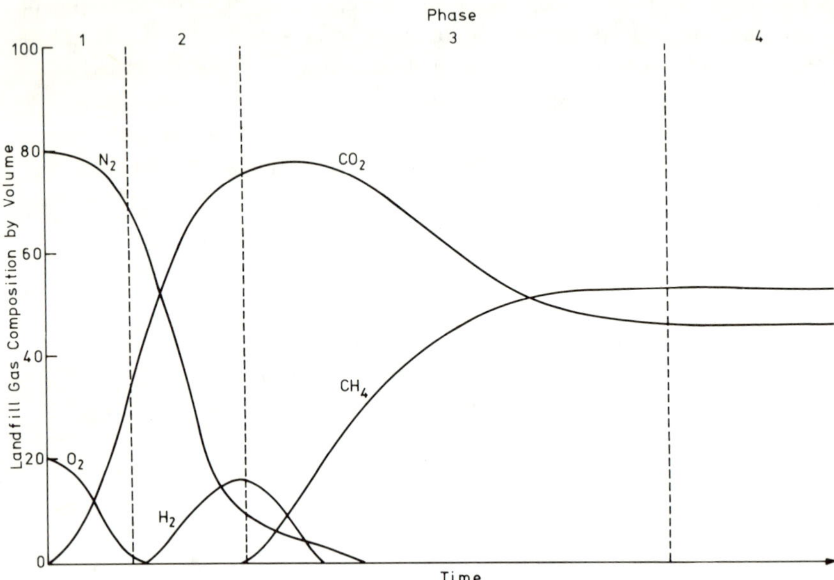

Fig. 6. Sanitary landfill gas production pattern. After reference 26.

accompanied by an increase in carbon dioxide; hydrogen drops to negligible levels. As methanogenic bacteria increase in number methane is generated and carbon dioxide is less prevalent. During the most active stage which can last for a 2–10 year period depending on moisture content methane is the predominant gas at about 60–65%, while carbon dioxide accounts largely for the remainder with traces of other hydrocarbons, nitrogen and a wide variety of organic compounds being present. As the activity of the landfill subsides gas evolution rates drop but traces of methane have been detected in sites even after 80 years.

Methane is the main hazard due to its inflammable nature and the formation of explosive mixtures with air in concentrations of 5–15% methane. In most sites this gas will diffuse harmlessly through the cover material but high concentrations may be found in cracks between the fill and surrounding ground. Problems have been encountered when buildings have been erected on completed landfill sites when methane has diffused into basements and other areas usually through service ducts, soakaways or drains. Explosions and fires have occurred[27] but now that the potential hazard is more widely recognised venting systems can be incorporated at the design stage, largely overcoming the problems. Buildings adjacent to the site may also be at risk since methane can diffuse laterally in certain circumstances up to a distance of several hundred metres. This is most likely to occur when landfills are in worked-out sand or gravel pits where loosely compacted material can allow gaseous diffusion. The problem can be overcome by the installation of an interceptor trench filled with rubble or coarse aggregate around the perimeter of the site. However, this remedy is not likely to be satisfactory for deep sites in which gaseous diffusion can only be prevented by the installation of pumped gas wells either in the refuse close to the site boundaries or in the area immediately adjacent.

Nowadays as landfill sites become larger there is considerable interest, especially in the United States, in the possibility of extracting the methane for use as a fuel. Gas wells are drilled in a grid pattern in the refuse and are pumped at suctions of a few inches of water. The distance separating the wells for effective collection varies from site to site depending on density and moisture content of the refuse but a distance of about 100–150 m appears to be satisfactory. Tests are carried out to determine the maximum gas extraction rate without sucking significant quantities of air through the surface of the landfill and hence lowering the calorific value of the gas. Values of 22–$45\,\text{ml}\,\text{kg}^{-1}\,\text{day}^{-1}$ have been quoted by Constable $et\ al.$[28] for some sites in the United States. The extracted gas can be purified, e.g. by passage through molecular sieves to remove carbon dioxide and some other impurities after which the gas can be injected into pipelines containing natural gas. A simpler and more economically viable approach is to condense out water vapour and use the impure gas as a fuel directly since its calorific value is similar to town gas. Other suggestions for its use are on-site electricity generation or in the production of methanol. It should be emphasised that this is a new but growing area of technology and not surprisingly some difficulties have been experienced particularly with corrosion to pipework and pumps. Methane recovery should be considered if the landfill is at least 10 m deep and the amount of refuse present is at least one million tonnes.

4.7. Leachate Treatment

Once waste in a landfill has become saturated, i.e. its field capacity has been exceeded then leachate will be produced. This liquid can cause an environmental hazard since although near neutral it is characterised by its high organic loading due mainly to carboxylic acids which present problems during treatment. Leachate from freshly deposited refuse will have a high BOD/TOC ratio but this will drop as the concentration of the more readily degradable organics decreases with time. Various options are available for leachate treatment but as already mentioned, good site management should significantly decrease any leachate generation.

The simplest treatment method is either to pipe or tanker the leachate to a local sewage works. However, landfills are often in sites not served by main drains so the former may not be possible and tankering, if volumes are large, may be prohibitively expensive. Treatment at sewage works also requires adequate handling capacity and this may not be available.

Some work has been done on leachate treatment by spraying over waste or pasture land. For instance, in Cornwall it has been demonstrated that 5000 gallons of liquid per day per acre can be sprayed and lost by evapotranspiration. Intermittent pumping is desirable. Another scheme involved pumping leachate through perforated horizontal pipes placed along a tree-planted hillside and allowing liquid to flow slowly downhill along the surface. The leachate had no adverse effect on vegetation. Such schemes are suitable when land is available and population is sparse, since smell problems can arise. An alternative approach is to spray leachate over the surface of the landfill itself. Evaporation will occur which will be aided by the elevated temperature within the landfill. Some liquid will penetrate the waste and will eventually reappear as leachate at the base of the fill. Experimental work has shown that the concentration of pollutants in this leachate is considerably higher than in the original sprayed leachate so that overall a much reduced volume of more highly polluted liquid is obtained. However, this can reduce any tankering costs and there is the additional advantage that the increased moisture content of the waste will increase the rate of decomposition thus ensuring that the duration of leachate generation will be much reduced.

Purification of landfill leachate under aerobic conditions is being investigated both in the laboratory and under field conditions. One approach is to collect leachate in a holding lagoon and then either spray the leachate back into the lagoon, or blow air and/or oxygen through the liquid or treat with hydrogen peroxide or ozone. It appears that retention times of some tens of days are necessary and that the addition of nutrients such as nitrogen or potassium may be beneficial. Trickling filters have also been tried but with varying success since leachate flows and impurity contents are variable. In addition, problems have been encountered due to blocking with precipitated ferric hydroxide.

Anaerobic treatment of landfill leachate is attractive in that methane gas would be produced which might be formed in sufficient quantity, if the leachate were grossly polluted, to enable the gas to be burnt and used to increase reaction temperatures which in turn should increase plant efficiency. However, this technique has only been tested in the laboratory and in pilot plants and would require a fairly constant source of leachate having a high BOD for its successful operation.

Leachate production, composition and treatment have been reviewed[29] with reference to various physical and chemical treatment methods. Treatment with oxidants such as hydrogen peroxide and ozone has already been mentioned; in addition to diminishing the concentration of organics, hydrogen sulphide which is normally found in leachate will be oxidised to innocuous sulphate. Use of precipitants or coagulants such as lime or alum have little effect on highly polluted leachates in reducing organic loadings but removal of colour, suspended solids and metals can be satisfactory. Activated carbon shows promise for 'polishing' leachate after preliminary biological treatment but tends to become blocked if used on untreated leachate. Other methods such as ion-exchange or reverse osmosis have been considered. Reverse osmosis requires preliminary treatment of the leachate or else clogging of the membrane will occur. The main advantage of physico-chemical methods appears to lie in their flexibility and fast reaction rates compared with biological treatment.

4.8. Landfill in Countries Other Than the UK

Disposal of wastes in uncontrolled sites is widely practised throughout the world, using the minimum of equipment and at negligible expense. However, in developed countries such as the United States and those in Western Europe this basic approach has been superseded by the sanitary landfill designed to reduce the environmental impact and danger to health, and in a number of countries the concept of the sanitary landfill is only now being introduced. For example, Ribeiro da Luz[30] has recently described the introduction of four such sites in Sao Paulo, Brazil, and many rapidly developing cities, e.g. Lagos in Nigeria, and those in Saudi Arabia are receiving aid from British and European contractors to improve their methods of waste collection and disposal.[31]

In countries where sanitary landfill is well established, there are some differences at present in their attitude to co-disposal of potentially hazardous wastes. In some parts of the United States there is legislation to allow disposal of a wide range of hazardous wastes only in containment sites. This contrasts strongly with the philosophy in the United Kingdom where the co-disposal of hazardous and domestic waste is not necessarily discouraged and the use of containment sites is not obligatory. The merits of a carefully thought out co-disposal policy are at present being discussed in many Western European countries, while current research[32] will probably resolve some unanswered questions. Landfill is not the favoured disposal route in all European countries. Denmark, for example, favours incineration of domestic wastes coupled with district heating schemes since there is both a shortage of suitable landfill sites and of indigenous fuel supplies. Finally, mention should be made of the use of waste in land reclamation schemes, and this approach has been developed extensively in Tokyo Bay, Japan where many millions of square metres have been reclaimed in recent years.[33] Many other countries have had similar schemes although not necessarily on such a large scale.

5. CONCLUSIONS

Landfilling of wastes has been widely practised by man for thousands of years so that middens from the past have proved a fruitful hunting ground for archaeologists. At present, in the UK, landfill is the preferred method for waste disposal since it is very significantly cheaper than other disposal options, e.g. incineration. It has been estimated that the cost of landfilling using a local site is about £3–4 t^{-1} compared with at least £15 t^{-1} for incineration. However, considerable changes are taking place in waste disposal technology especially in the transport of waste. Now that many landfill sites on the outskirts of towns and cities have been filled, waste disposal authorities are considering or have already implemented schemes in which waste is transported, often by rail, to sites up to 100 miles distant. This increases costs significantly but still remains below those of incineration.

Discussion is taking place in the waste disposal industry as to the merits of pre-treating waste before landfilling. The most popular options at present are baling or pulverisation. The exponents of these claim significant environmental advantages but at present costs approximately double those of landfilling untreated refuse.

Consideration is now being given to various waste separation schemes in which components are separated and then used as raw materials in their own right. Demonstration plants have been built in the UK at Doncaster and Bowker so that within a few years it should be possible to determine whether they are economically viable. Fluctuations in the market price of the separated components will obviously affect such recovery schemes. Landfill has advantages in its own right. For example, it can be used to reclaim otherwise derelict land and on the larger sites recovery of methane from decomposing organic material may prove worth while.

When the large numbers of landfill sites are considered, the fact that the vast majority have had little or no adverse effect on the environment is significant. However, it must be remembered that in the past most sites have been relatively small so that effects of leachate generation or even of refuse burning have been very limited. This is now changing with emphasis being placed on the use of fewer but larger sites which, because of their size, could have a more marked adverse environmental impact. Thus site selection with special emphasis being placed on hydrogeological suitability, sound landfill design and good operating practice including a long-term filling plan, are paramount in ensuring that landfilling remains environmentally acceptable.

REFERENCES

1. BEVAN, R. E. *Controlled Tipping*, Institute of Public Cleansing, W. & J. Mackay, Chatham, 1967.
2. Department of the Environment. *Final report on the behaviour of hazardous waste in landfill sites*, HMSO, London, 1978.
3. Department of the Environment. *The licensing of waste disposal sites*, Waste management paper No. 4, HMSO, London, 1976.
4. WILLIAMS, G. M. Implications of changes in landfill practice, *J. Inst. Water Engnrs. Scientists*, 1980, **34**(2), 153–60.
5. CHAPPELL, C. L. Disposal technology for hazardous wastes, *Surveyor*, 1973, **142**(4247), 42–3.
6. CARY, J. W. Water flux in moist soils: thermal versus suction gradients, *Soil Science*, 1965, **100**(3), 168–75.
7. SMITH, D. B., WEARN, P. L., RICHARDS, H. J. and ROWE, P. C. Water movement in the unsaturated zone of high and low permeability strata by measuring natural tritium, *Proc. Symp. Isotope Hydrology*, International Atomic Energy Agency, 1970, 73–7.
8. YOUNG, C. P., HALL, E. S. and OAKES, D. B. *Nitrate in groundwater—studies in the chalk near Winchester, Hampshire*, Technical Report No. 31, 1976.
9. REES, J. F., PARKER, A., ROSS, C. A. M., KING, J. W. and CAMPBELL, D. J. V. *Uffington lysimeters, operation and results (part 4)*, Department of the Environment, WLR Report No. 60, HMSO, London, 1979.
10. ROSS, C. A. M. *Extractive characterisation of heavy metal distribution in contaminated Lower Greensand*, Department of the Environment, WLR Report No. 61, HMSO, London, 1978.

11. FRIED, J. J. Groundwater pollution, in *Developments in Water Science*, Vol. 4, Elsevier Scientific Publishing Co., Amsterdam, 1975.
12. OAKES, D. B. *Dilution of landfill leachates in groundwater* Department of the Environment, WLR Report No. 53, HMSO, London, 1976.
13. ANON. *Aquifer protection policy*, Severn Trent Water Authority, Birmingham, 1978.
14. HARRISON, I. B. Construction of investigatory boreholes in landfill sites, *Surveyor*, 1976, **147**(4383), 22–4.
15. STUART, A. *Monolith lysimeters in the landfill research programme* Department of the Environment, WLR Report No. 48, HMSO, London, 1976.
16. OAKES, D. B. and EDWORTHY, D. J. Field measurements of dispersion coefficients in the United Kingdom, in *Proc. Conf. Groundwater Quality—Measurement, Prediction and Protection*, Water Research Centre, Reading, 1977, 274–97.
17. NAYLOR, J. A., ROWLAND, C. D., YOUNG, C. P. and BARBER, C. *The investigation of landfill sites*, Technical Note TR91, Water Research Centre, Medmenham, UK, 1978.
18. WOOD, W. W. Guidelines for collection and field analysis of groundwater samples for selected unstable constituents, in *Techniques of Water Resources Investigations in the United States Geological Survey*, United States Dept. of the Interior, Washington, DC, 1976.
19. CLARK, D. C. Remedial action activities for Army Creek landfill, in *Proc. 5th Ann. Research Symp. on Municipal Solid Waste: Land Disposal*, Orlando, Florida, EPA-600/9-79-023a, 1979, 343–57.
20. KIMMEL, G. E. and BRAIDS, O. C. Preliminary findings of a leachate study on two landfills in Suffolk County, New York, *J. Res. US Geol. Survey*, 1975, **3**, 273–80.
21. KHAN, A. Q. in *Proc. of Eastbourne Conf. on Reclamation of Contaminated Land*, Oct. 1979, (to be published).
22. SMITH, A. C. S. Chalk puddling in Kent—a review, *Solid Wastes*, 1979, **69**, 338–55.
23. HAXO, H. E. Liner materials exposed to MSW landfill leachate, in *Proc. 5th Ann. Research Symp. on Municipal Solid Waste: Land Disposal*, Orlando, Florida, EPA-600/9-79-023a, 1979, 241–67.
24. BRATLEY, K. J. A description of comparative performance tests of mobile plant on a major landfill site, *Solid Wastes*, 1977, **67**, 57–80.
25. USEPA. *Process design manual: municipal sludge landfills*, EPA-625/1-78-010, 1978, various pagings.
26. FARQUHAR, G. J. and ROVERS, F. A. Gas production during refuse decomposition, *Wat. Air Soil Pollut.*, 1973, **2**, 483–95.
27. BROMLEY, J. and PARKER, A. Methane from landfill sites, *Internat. Environ. Safety*, Aug. 1979, 9–11.
28. CONSTABLE, T. W., FARQUHAR, G. J. and CLEMENT, B. N. Gas migration and modeling, in *Proc. 5th Ann. Research Symp. on Municipal Solid Waste: Land Disposal*, Orlando, Florida, EPA-600/9-79-023a, 1979, 396–412.
29. ROBINSON, H. D. and MARIS, P. J. *Leachate from domestic waste—generation, composition and treatment. A review*, Water Research Centre, Medmenham, UK, Report TR108, 1979, 38 pp.

30. RIBEIRO DA LUZ, F. X. Development in the methods of treatment of urban wastes. *Paper presented at the ISWA Conf.*, London, Jun. 1980.
31. HEWITT, M. R. British waste disposal expertise at work abroad, *NAWDC News*, Apr. 1979.
32. NATO Committee on the Challenges of Modern Society. *Disposal of hazardous wastes. Landfill*, PB-276 811, NATO/CCMS-64, Brussels, Belgium, May 1977.
33. SHIGEO MORITA. Reclamation of land from the sea by tipping. *Paper presented at the ISWA Conf.*, London, Jun. 1980.

Chapter 2

NON-LANDFILL METHODS OF HAZARDOUS WASTE DISPOSAL

L. E. BAKER, B.Sc., C.Chem., M.R.I.C.
Director, Re-Chem International Ltd, Southampton, UK

SUMMARY

The terms 'non-landfill' and 'hazardous waste' are clarified and a general background to the hazardous waste processing industry offered. It is shown that the great majority of such wastes are still disposed of by landfill methods. Setting aside recovery and reclamation possibilities which are felt to be too extensive for inclusion in this chapter, the main 'non-landfill' alternatives are seen as being incineration, solidification and chemical treatment. Each is covered in some detail, dealing with the process philosophies and technologies, their strengths and weaknesses, and the commercial implications of employing them. Consideration is also given to a few other processes, such as catalysis and pyrolysis, which are not currently widely used for hazardous waste processing, but which are either extensively used in other waste disposal areas, or offer some prospect of being developed within the hazardous waste sphere.

1. SCOPE FOR THIS CHAPTER

The term 'non-landfill' requires some clarification and is taken to mean processes in which wastes are subjected to some form of treatment, even though the treated material or residues therefrom may nevertheless be deposited on a landfill site. In other words, this chapter excludes those methods involving the discharge of untreated hazardous waste to landfill, to sea or river, to mine shafts, or to deep wells.

39

The definition and classification of hazardous wastes stem from a number of sources which are not entirely consistent. The first UK legislation to cover the disposal of this sort of waste was the Deposit of Poisonous Waste Act 1972 (DOPWA)[1] which offered the following definition.

> 'Subject to...where the waste is of a kind which is poisonous, noxious or polluting and its presence on the land is liable to give rise to an environmental hazard.'

This Act covered all wastes except those listed in an exclusion schedule published in regulations made under the DOPWA.[2]

The Control of Pollution Act 1974 (COPA)[3] introduced site licensing procedures for all disposal sites, irrespective of whether wastes were processed or landfilled. An extensive classification of hazardous wastes was published in supporting literature[4] as a guide to licensing authorities involved in drawing up and defining the scope of each facility. This classification contained nearly 20 main groups, and about 150 sub-groups of waste.

Subsequently, and even as this chapter is being written, plans are being evolved for a 'special waste' class under the provisions of S17 of COPA. The broad intention is to subject certain wastes of a particularly difficult or dangerous nature to additional controls, but both the nature of these controls and the definition of 'special' remain to be finalised.

There are also classifications of hazardous waste devised in connection with transport codes and regulations. The recent regulations concerning tanker labelling[5] and the Health and Safety Commission Consultative Document on further provisions for safety in transport[6] contain schedules in which wastes are broadly classified according to hazard (in a transport context), and which then require the vehicle or container to be labelled accordingly. Disregarding the rather specialist transportation classification, the criteria employed in grouping hazardous wastes generally seem geared more to considerations of suitability for landfill, than in relation to the other options such as process methods. Therefore, this chapter will address the subject by reviewing the process methods available, rather than considering different types of waste individually, and discussing the alternative methods which could be used.

It would be interesting to compare the British approach to that adopted by other countries, and analyse the relative strengths and weaknesses of the alternatives. A number of countries have now produced legislation incorporating their interpretation of what constitutes hazardous waste and in some cases there have also been suggestions as to classification.

The USA Resource Conservation and Recovery Act of 1976[7] offers the following definition of 'hazardous waste' in Section 1004(5).

> 'A solid waste, or combination of solid wastes, which because of its quantity, concentration, or physical, chemical or infectious characteristics may—
>
> (a) cause or significantly contribute to an increase in mortality or an increase in serious irreversible, or incapacitating reversible, illness: or
>
> (b) pose a substantial present or potential hazard to human health or the environment when improperly treated, stored, transported, or disposed or otherwise managed.'

The United States Environmental Protection Agency (USEPA) has published its proposed rules covering various aspects of the Act,[8] and these make most interesting reading for anyone wishing to understand the thinking behind the American approach.

2. THE UK HAZARDOUS WASTE MARKET

If we make the assumption that wastes deemed to be hazardous are also those which require notification under the procedures specified in DOPWA, then there are some broadly based estimates available indicating annual tonnages. These are:

England	3 500 000 tonnes
Scotland	100 000 tonnes
Wales	150 000 tonnes
Total	3 750 000 tonnes

These figures omit wastes which may be subjected to controls under other legislation, such as sea disposal[9] and radioactive materials.[10]

Greater detail is available for the English sector of the market, where the 3.5 Mt year^{-1} can be seen as part of an overall 25 Mt year^{-1} of industrial waste. Industrial waste excludes the 'rubbish' production of industry, but does include a large proportion of slags and furnace wastes, and certain specific chemical waste streams which are exempted or excluded from the notification procedure.

There is no generally available breakdown of the notifiable waste market into more detailed classifications, although some Waste Disposal Authorities produce such data in respect of their own area. Some of the Waste Management Papers[11] dealing with more specific types of waste offer some suggestions as to market size and origins.

There can be little doubt that the great majority of notifiable waste is disposed of by landfill methods, whether at in-house or contractor/authority owned sites. Information suggests that $2.3\,\mathrm{Mt\,year^{-1}}$ is handled by contractors, of which almost $2.0\,\mathrm{Mt}$ is landfilled, $0.1\,\mathrm{Mt}$ incinerated, and $0.25\,\mathrm{Mt}$ chemically treated and/or solidified. The balance of the market is disposed of at in-house facilities, with most being landfilled. Incineration, at $0.2\,\mathrm{Mt\,year^{-1}}$, accounts for a significantly larger quantity than within the private contracting sector, but it should be noted that there are very many more in-house incinerators than contractor operated ones, and that many of the former are comparatively small sized, dedicated units (i.e. an integrated part of the process stream, dealing with the wastes from that process).

In addition to the above figures, some $0.5\,\mathrm{Mt\,year^{-1}}$ of liquid wastes are sea disposed under licencing and permit procedures which do not involve notification under DOPWA. This chapter is not concerned with, and offers no statistics on the disposal of radioactive wastes.

The quantities of waste set out above clearly do not reflect the vast volumes of effluents which may be processed at in-house chemical or biological treatment facilities located at, for example, metal finishing works or food processing factories. Neither do the figures include the volumes passing through oil–water separators or interceptors. Such statistics simply are not available, and the market figures which have been offered, refer to the quantities of waste which may be thought of as requiring final disposal.

3. THE GENERAL BACKGROUND OF THE WASTE DISPOSAL INDUSTRY

3.1. The Structure of the Industry

Within Great Britain, hazardous waste processing facilities, such as incinerators and solidification plants, have been provided and continue to be operated almost exclusively by the private sector. Waste disposal activities in general, including landfill, are under the control of the Waste Disposal Authorities (WDAs), these being departments of the County Councils in England and the District Councils in Scotland and Wales. The WDAs are responsible for the licensing arrangements referred to in Section

1. Central Government is not directly involved in waste disposal control but evolves policy in conjunction with financing research work and waste studies and also acts as a central source of information and advice.

The private sector facilities which exist have generally been conceived, in the case of contract operations, on a regional service basis, and to some extent reflect the geographical areas in which the companies concerned are well established. There is a view held in some quarters that the existing network of facilities is incomplete and that there are large areas of the country which do not have easy access to a plant. In some respects that may be true and is a consequence of the development strategy whereby, in the absence of any central plan, companies have moved to provide plants on an individual basis, when they have seen what appeared to be an attractive commercial opportunity, and have been able to obtain a suitable site.

Plugging these gaps, such as they are, presents a number of problems. A plant must be at least a certain size to have potential viability and there must, therefore, be sufficient waste produced in that area to provide an adequate degree of plant utilisation. Recognising that process charges will invariably be greater than for the principal alternative of landfill, one also needs the will of industry and the resolve of the enforcing authorities to ensure that such facilities, if provided, are adequately used. If they are not, a loss making operation would result and, whether this is in the private or the public sector, could only lead to even higher charges or to the need for subsidies from some external source. The former would inevitably lead to the spiral of diminishing returns and the latter, never previously considered appropriate for Britain, would undoubtedly lead to problems if applied in isolated cases.

Some countries have tackled the problem in a different way—by directly or indirectly stimulating the provision of facilities for processing wastes but ensuring that those facilities were utilised by directing the wastes to them. A range of approaches, including interest free loans, government led consortia, subsidies and tax incentives and equalisation of charges and transport costs, have been employed. Such an approach is not necessarily the best in every respect, but is likely to ensure a better strategic disposition of facilities and a better matching of supply and demand.

3.2. The Waste Industry Through the 1970s

Almost all the process and treatment facilities available within the private contracting sector now (1980), came into being during the 1970s, and in particular, in the early–middle part of the decade. This was a period of great change, during which attitudes had to alter in many ways. Interest in, and ultimately regulation of, disposal of all types of waste forced many companies to sharpen up their practices, invest in modern equipment and techniques, engage technically competent staff and generally prepare for the upsurge in accountability and the scrutiny which was to come from the general public, environmentalists and the newly created regulatory authorities.

An early consequence of the shift toward processing approaches was the need for more detailed analytical data on waste compositions. This was only usually required in the most general terms for landfill activities but where processes were to be carried out concentrations, contaminants and so forth became important considerations.

Analysis of waste is now regarded as an important part of all major contractors' procedures for doing business, whether they engage in the process areas, landfill, or both. New business would not normally be accepted until advance samples had been checked to establish that they were within the scope of the process facility or landfill site. Thereafter, for regular or repeated loads, samples are taken upon receipt to establish a number of factors.

1. Confirm chemical and physical characteristics in relation to process needs, safety precautions required, etc.
2. Establish concentration in readiness for invoicing customers on a strength related basis.
3. Record certain information about consignments to comply with record keeping requirements of both good practice and the regulatory authorities.

Additional analytical requirements for operations involving processing include the regular or continuous monitoring of the processes themselves, and a variety of checks on outgoing residues, including ash, stack emissions and liquid effluent discharges to public sewer or water course.

In general, the industry has had to make great efforts to modernise its image and live down its sometimes less than satisfactory past. This has been achieved by the introduction of a much higher level of professional and technical expertise, focusing on the whole range of management functions within this important, but often forgotten, industry.

4. RECOVERY AND RECYCLING

Recovery, recycling, or whatever term is used, represents an important, although sometimes rather idealistic, option for hazardous waste disposal.

Clearly it avoids, in total or in part, the need for final disposal of the original waste and, furthermore, will contribute to the conservation of natural resources. However, in practice, individual recovery operations will usually only proceed when they are economically viable in their own right, that is to say, when the recovered product can be supplied at a lower price than the equivalent virgin material.

Of course, important factors in the economic balance are the cost of the new material and the cost of disposal of the waste. With sudden, disproportionate increases in raw material costs, such as in the case of crude oil, recovery of oil-based products would be expected to become more attractive. The trend would be helped by tighter controls on disposal, when cheap options such as landfill might disappear to be replaced by relatively expensive incineration services. This has actually happened, to the extent that volumes of solvent and oil wastes requiring disposal have dramatically declined in recent years and many of the remaining sources are regarded by their producers as having some sale value.

The logical conclusion of progressively tightening restrictions on disposal would be that recovery would take place by virtue of being the only 'disposal' method left. There are signs that this could happen in Holland, where restrictions on landfill of mixed metal hydroxide sludges are resulting in extensive development programmes into ion exchange and solvent extraction methods of separating and recovering the metals—not primarily for the sake of recovery, but because it is so difficult to dispose of the sludges by other routes.

5.   INCINERATION

Incineration is a very well established technique for destroying a broad range of liquid, sludge and solid wastes and is likely to remain in wide use for many years to come. The commercial basis for incineration ranges from in-house units handling exclusively the waste producers' own materials, to multi-purpose contract op ations drawing their custom from many sources. Within Britain, this latter approach falls entirely within the private sector and may also be regarded as including sea incineration facilities, which are not based in Britain, but which have collected waste from British clients. In general, the municipal incinerators do not accept hazardous or chemical wastes, although there are limited instances where this may happen on a small scale.

The total installation required for handling any particular selection of wastes (i.e. not just the combustion section of the plant) needs to take account of a number of factors, notably:

(1)   the physical form of the waste (i.e. liquid, sludge, solid),
(2)   the calorific value,
(3)   its chemical composition (halogens, or acid gas producing elements, etc.), and
(4)   the quantity and nature of any ash which may remain.

These factors dictate not only the basic incinerator type, but also the gas cleaning plant that will be required together with storage facilities, pre-treatment needs, etc.

5.1. Types of Incinerator

5.1.1. *The Rotary Incinerator*

In recent years this has firmly established itself as the usual choice for general purpose chemical waste incinerators. Able to embrace a wide range of capacities, they are extremely flexible, are robust, reliable, and can demonstrate a number of distinctly advantageous features. Although rather expensive, it is no accident that most of the larger waste incinerators built in recent years, or being planned now, both in Europe and North America adopt this approach.

The rotary unit can be scaled to embrace a wide range of demands. The size of the rotary barrel itself is usually such that the overall length is some three to four times the diameter which, in the case of some of the larger units, might be as much as $4\,m$. The capacity of the larger units, including liquid or waste gas burners in the subsequent non-rotating parts of the incinerator, can be in the region of $4\,t\,h^{-1}$, with a heat release as much as $100\,GJ$ ($95 \times 10^6\,Btu\,h^{-1}$). Rotating at typically 10 revolutions h^{-1}, (although most units can operate at a range of speeds) and inclined slightly towards its back end, solid wastes introduced into the front of the rotating barrel will slowly move down the inside, to be discharged after a residence time of an hour or more. This rotating motion thus causes ash, slag or other solid residues to be removed but has the added advantage of constantly renewing the surface of solid wastes and preventing them developing a baked, insulating surface layer which would slow down or prevent total destruction. (See Figs. 1 and 2.)

5.1.2. *The Multi-Hearth Incinerator*

These comprise a series of individual hearths, each designed or intended for a particular type of waste, determined on physical or chemical

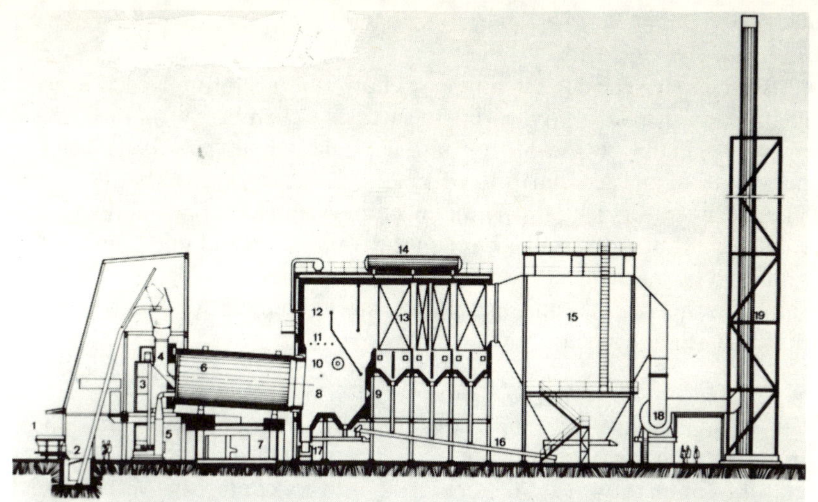

FIG. 1. General arrangement of rotary incinerator, showing waste feed systems, energy recovery plant and electrostatic dust precipitators. Key: 1, feed point; 2, bucket elevator; 3, drum elevator; 4, feed chute; 5, combustion air; 6, rotating drum; 7, control room; 8, secondary air; 9, solvent burner; 10, waste oil burner; 11, secondary air; 12, tertiary air; 13, waste heat boiler; 14, boiler drum; 15, electrostatic filters; 16, ash removal; 17, cinder removal; 18, induced draft fan; 19, chimney. Reproduced by courtesy of Von Roll Ltd, Zurich.

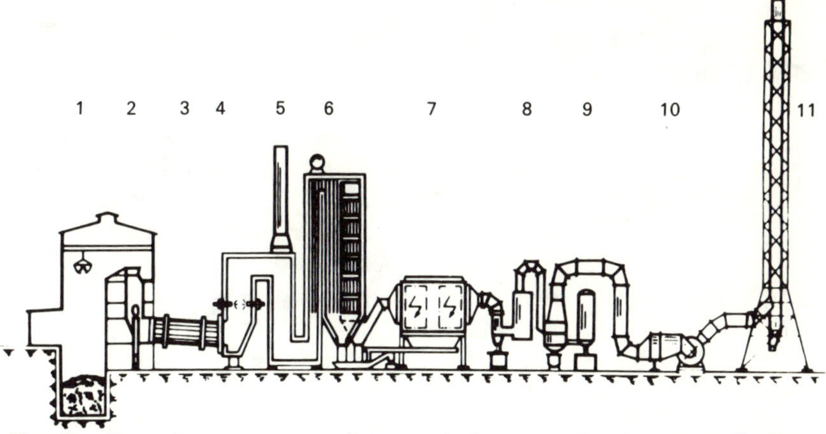

FIG. 2. General arrangement of rotary incinerator, showing waste feeding arrangements, energy recovery plant, electrostatic precipitators, wet gas scrubbing and waste gas reheating. Key: 1, solid waste bunkers; 2, kiln charging system; 3, rotary kiln; 4, liquid waste burners; 5, afterburner chamber with emergency stack; 6, heat recovery boiler; 7, electrostatic filters; 8, flue-gas scrubber (3-stage); 9, scrubber water oxidation; 10, suction blower with heat exchanger; 11, stack. Reproduced by courtesy of Steinmuller GmbH, Gummersbach and Bayer AG, Leverkusen.

considerations. The combustion gases flow in series through each hearth, giving some degree of pre-heating to successive chambers. Combustion air would normally be introduced into each hearth to guard against the possibility of oxygen starvation from overloads earlier in the sequence. These incinerators lack the neat and simple solution for ash removal and solids agitation which is displayed in the rotary unit, and must achieve the same end by mechanical means. Frankly, it is difficult to do as well as the rotary in this respect, and these areas are undoubted weaknesses of the multi-hearth approach.

5.1.3. *The Fluidised Bed Incinerator*

This technique displays many advantages in the continuous agitation of materials in the bed, the intimate contact between the hot bed and the waste and the comparative ease of recovering heat by contact between the bed medium and heat exchange tubes or other plant. However, this approach does not suit the general purpose application, as the fluidised bed material must be carefully protected from residues which might cause it to slag or solidify. The technique can be seen, therefore, as having application with particular, regular feed stocks (e.g. tyre or plastics pyrolysis, but see Section 8.2.) and has been applied to sewage sludges and similar consistent sludge feed stocks.

5.1.4. *Molten Salt Combustion*

This technique is believed to have been developed only to the point of pilot or demonstration scale plant.[12] Having some similarity to the fluidised bed approach, and sharing some of its limitations, the essentials of the process consist of a melt of sodium carbonate at around 1200 K, into which the wastes are introduced. The intimate contact with the hot molten salt assists efficient and effective destruction of the organic species, and the alkalinity of the molten salt will internally neutralise any acidic products of combustion. As with the fluidised bed, care must be taken to prevent anything being introduced which could upset the molten or fluid nature of the melt, and provision must be made to replenish the alkalinity as it is neutralised, and remove any accumulated inert ash.

A multiplicity of possible designs exist for incinerators handling only liquid wastes. In the simplest sense, all that is required is a burner firing into a chamber, although obviously more sophisticated arrangements exist with cyclone burner arrangements, submerged combustion and so forth.

5.1.5. *Sea Incineration*

Although the principle of ship mounted incinerators does not involve any single or particular type of incinerator, this sort of operation has developed characteristics of its own, and merits some consideration in this section. Confined mainly to liquids and sludges, a number of commercially operated vessels have engaged in this activity, taking on board stocks of disposable waste at selected port installations, and then carrying out the incineration itself whilst at sea.

The purpose of this approach is clearly to avoid some of the restrictions and controls which would be imposed on land-based operations, particularly in respect of the scrubbing or cleaning of the gaseous products of combustion. The complete avoidance of this requirement means, in the case of highly chlorinated wastes, that a considerable saving in operating costs can be made in relation to a land based facility. It is in this particular area that sea incineration has made its mark, where it has achieved a wide degree of acceptance and recognition, and where testing and evaluation programmes have been carried out.[13,14]

5.2. Gas Cleaning

Many operators of incinerator plants would take the view that having incinerated or combusted the waste, the most difficult stage is still to come —namely the cleaning or conditioning of the products of combustion prior to emission into the atmosphere.

The first consideration must be the effectiveness of the combustion processes themselves, but thereafter the issue boils down to the removal of particulate, removal of acidic gaseous combustion products, and the various factors which might control the appearance (as opposed to the quality) of the emission.

The effectiveness of combustion, or more precisely, the efficiency of destruction of any particular organic species, will be a function of temperature and residence time, assuming of course that there is otherwise adequate oxygen present for the combustion chemistry stoichiometry. In broad terms, this would require the conversion of carbon and hydrogen to carbon dioxide and water vapour, respectively, and halogens, sulphur, nitrogen, etc. to acidic gases.

The subject is not generally well understood, at least in an exact or quantitative way. The usual practice has been to adopt the 'overkill' philosophy whereby conditions are maintained within the incinerator at well in excess of those proven to have been adequate for the most difficult and persistent species. Thus, a few such chemicals have been subjected to quite comprehensive testing on both laboratory and plant scales in programmes which have extensively varied the waste feed rate and concentration, residence time and operating temperatures. Sophisticated analytical techniques have been employed to measure and analyse the products of combustion, and to establish the destruction efficiencies.

Many incinerator operators have carried out such work for their own information, but the United States Environmental Protection Agency has published the results of its extensive researches into the optimum incineration conditions for materials such as kepone and polychlorinated biphenyls (PCBs).[15,16,17]

Turning to the cleaning or conditioning of the gaseous products of combustion, we are mainly concerned with particulate and acidic gases. The particulate itself will derive from solid or dissolved portions of the feed stock and could include materials ranging from inert ash and water soluble salt crystals, to heavy metal containing particles. The acidic gaseous by-products would most frequently be expected to include hydrochloric acid and sulphur dioxide, although other possibilities can arise with certain wastes.

In general terms, chemical waste incineration is a registerable process under the Alkali Act, and the control of emissions therefore falls under the Alkali and Clean Air Inspectorate. The policy of the Inspectorate is not to operate within a framework of fixed air quality standards, but to apply the concept of 'best practicable means' (b.p.m.) to every registered works. This permits them to take into account a great many factors, including the emergence or development of new technology, in establishing their emission control requirements in each case. There are, nevertheless, a few fixed, or presumptive limits, made in relation to waste incinerators. Quoted in the somewhat quaint, but soon to be metricated,[18] units of grains per cubic foot, the present total particulate level is set at $0.05\,\mathrm{grain\,ft^{-3}}$ $(114\,\mathrm{mg\,m^{-3}})$, and hydrochloric acid at 0.1 to $0.2\,\mathrm{grain\,ft^{-3}}$ (224 to $448\,\mathrm{mg\,m^{-3}}$).

Although there are a great many schemes and processes reputed to be available for gas cleaning and treatment, in practice the number actually in use on commercially or technically successful incinerators is much fewer. As the combustion gases leave the incinerator chamber, they will probably retain a temperature of at least 1300 K, and will need to be cooled before any of the conventional cleaning processes can be applied.

One of the most common approaches is found on a number of the larger units on mainland Europe, and is illustrated in Figs. 1 and 2. It comprises the sequence of heat exchange boiler plant, and electrostatic precipitator. The boiler plant may produce steam or hot water for process needs, electricity generation, or even district heating schemes, and, as such, contributes significantly to the economic basis of the operation. However, it also reduces the gas temperatures into the region of 500 to 600 K, at which level the electrostatic precipitators can function, and remove a large proportion of the airborn particulate load. Such a system clearly makes no provision for removing acid gases, and such emissions can only be controlled by regulating the rate at which they are formed. This in turn requires careful control of the incinerator feed stock, and will usually involve a blending facility in which the problematical materials can be diluted to acceptable levels. Subject to this limitation, the emission will probably be low in particulate matter, and remain hot and dry, features which will combine to ensure that it is scarcely visible to the naked eye.

More recently, there has been some attention directed toward incorporating wet scrubbing acid gas removal stages, prompted no doubt in part by the tightening environmental standards, but also by incinerator operators' needs to handle higher proportions of problem wastes than can be accommodated by mere dilution. The plant to do this poses no great technical problems in itself, indeed a number of arrangements have been shown to reduce acid gases to extremely low levels, but there are consequent disadvantages. The final emission will be cooler, and will contain proportionately much more water vapour as a result of evaporation in the scrubber. It is, therefore, likely to condense to form a visually obtrusive steam plume, which may itself be stabilised by the low residual levels of particulate and acid gases, and result in excessive plume persistence. Some plants now seek to re-heat the cool plume gases, utilising recovered energy from the up-stream boiler plant. This will certainly alleviate the problem, particularly when there is not a high atmospheric humidity, but it is not economically feasible unless cheap, recovered energy is available (Fig. 2).

The overall strategy has been somewhat different in Britain, where none of the hazardous waste incinerators incorporate boiler plant to utilise the incinerator heat output. There are various reasons for this, centering particularly on the considerable additional capital cost of building in such facilities, related to the rather poor terms which usually exist for the utilisation of the recovered energy. District heating schemes are not common in Britain, and the financial attractions of generating electricity are not as favourable as in some other countries. Process steam can often be produced more economically from a separate package boiler system.

The absence of boiler plants has led to water quenching being adopted as the principal gas cooling method. Such saturated, or near saturated gas streams will not respond to electrostatic precipitation and wet treatment methods including particulate agglomeration in a venturi, must be relied upon to remove particulate and acid gases. In fact, this is perfectly able to produce relatively clean emissions, but the quantity of water evaporated will ensure that the same dense steam plume is produced, with the same risk of stabilisation and extreme persistence. In the British plants, plume re-heat simply cannot be considered given the non-availability of cheap recovered heat. The other options which have been or are being looked at invariably centre on trying to eliminate persistence by removing the stabilising influence. There is some prospect that process systems incorporating bag filters could achieve this, but they will inevitably be operating near their limits.

5.3. Other Operational Considerations

Success in the incineration business is dependent on a number of considerations other than the direct operation of the incinerator and gas cleaning plant. In particular, materials handling in the context of operations accepting solid or semi-solid wastes can prove crucial.

Materials handling, including its introduction into the furnace chamber, can be tackled from two directions. The first is well demonstrated at a number of the larger rotary units, where elaborate elevators, double doors, air locks, rams, pistons and so forth are installed to feed solid wastes directly into the incinerator. Materials handled in this way can include canisters and containers of sizes up to 200 litre (although some operators claim that the 200 litre drum should not be more than $\frac{2}{3}$ full), and loose waste conveyed by dumper truck and fed by overhead grab or bucket elevator/conveyer.

In the main, this system avoids any need to open drums of solid or semi-solid wastes and handle the contents prior to introducing them to the incinerator, and thereby offers advantages in minimising the risk of ground level smells, and reducing the frequency of operators having to wear additional protective clothing. Conversely, the practice of introducing large increments of combustible waste into a hot chamber has the disadvantage of creating thermal shock, if not oxygen starvation, and for this reason the '$\frac{2}{3}$ drum' limit referred to previously has sometimes been required. The alternative approach relies on trying to process solid or semi-solid wastes in such a way as to produce a more consistent feed stock, capable of being introduced into the incinerator more or less continuously. Systems incorporating crushers, shredders, pulverisers and macerators have been applied to the problem with only limited success, although development work continues because the advantages of the relatively stable temperatures which would be obtained are felt to be valuable goals.

A high repair and maintenance burden has become a fact of life with all waste incineration operations. Refractory wear and tear is heavy and expensive, and stems from the temperature fluctuations previously referred to, the physical consequences of introducing large and heavy waste receptacles, and deterioration of the refractory as a result of constituents in the wastes. Pumps, filters and pipe runs are prone to blockage, and pump impellers, instrumentation and handling plant subjected to usually heavy wear stemming from the wide range of physical and chemical characteristics of the wastes processed.

Operational monitoring is essential if control and process security are to be maintained. In this context, it is particularly the incineration process itself and the gas cleaning functions which must be monitored, and provision made for fail-safe arrangements and alarms. The incinerator itself requires temperature monitoring, at a number of locations if possible, but certainly at the exit from the primary waste incineration area, and prior to the after-burner chamber. The temperature so recorded can activate as necessary the after-burners to ensure that the highest temperatures are applied to the waste gases. Draught measurement and oxygen levels can also be recorded at critical positions, and could be used to bring about changes in air distribution in the incinerator.

The gas cleaning plant, although initially accepting gases of 1300 K or more, would not normally be designed to withstand such temperatures throughout. Where gas cooling is being effected by water quenching, a water supply failure to the quench unit would subject the subsequent low-temperature sections to uncooled gases, and cause enormous damage. Temperature detectors must, therefore, activate systems to divert such hot gases elsewhere, often out of a 'dump stack'. The measurement of pressure drops across various parts of the plant will also give an indication of operating efficiency, as would flow meters on gas wash liquor systems, pH monitoring, etc.

The ultimate criterion is the quality of the stack emission, and it is a somewhat unsatisfactory fact that on-line, continuous monitoring equipment is not sufficiently well developed to be of real value in measuring what and how much is in an emission.

5.4. Economic Considerations

Incineration is never going to be a cheap option. Some of the most sophisticated units, when taken in combination with the tank storage, administration and support facilities obviously needed as part of a total installation, would undoubtedly require investment in the order of

£5–10 million (1980 prices). Operational costs are also high, with the high repair and maintenance levels needed, the effort directed toward analytical functions, the rising cost and diminishing availability of the fuel type wastes necessary to support combustion of the more difficult materials, and the general attention which must be lavished on controls, both on the process side, and on the administrative and record keeping side to comply with the requirements of the controlling authorities.

Charges for incineration vary across an enormous range, and are dependent on a great many factors. Chemical composition considerations are among the most important, and although the formulae applied will differ from operator to operator, generally speaking, account will be taken of the load being imposed on the gas cleaning facilities, the quantity of inert ash which may have to be removed and disposed of, the calorific value of the waste, and such special factors as obnoxious smells, or particularly high toxicities, both of which may require tailor made plant, or individual handling arrangements. Physical conditions will also be important, notably in relation to the physical form of the waste, where bulk consignments are likely to involve much less effort and administration than the same quantity of material in small drums or packages. The need for pre-processing, such as on a centrifuge or through filtration equipment will also place a premium on the rate.

Some incineration operations cater only for liquid wastes, and some of these further limit their intake to bulk loads. It might be expected that such operation would, by virtue of the essentially cheaper basic incinerator unit and the much reduced need for support personnel and plant and ancillary processes, offer very competitive rates for liquid wastes as compared to the more expensive multi-purpose operations. This is not necessarily so. The liquid waste market has shown signs of decreasing, and the operator who can handle only that kind of waste is clearly in a somewhat weaker position than the general purpose units which can make their revenue from the genuinely difficult and intractable sludges and solids.

It is difficult to give any useful guidelines on actual prices in the space of a few sentences. With a good knowledge of the UK contractor market, and a number of examples of contract and in-house prices in European countries and North America, it can generally be stated that prices vary from a small payment for good quality high CV liquids which are nevertheless wastes, to charges of as much as $£500\,t^{-1}$ (1980 prices) for the most difficult, persistent, highly chlorinated solids. Essentially non-chlorinated solids in 200 litre drums or large packages are unlikely to be much less than $£100\,t^{-1}$ (1980 prices), and materials which present few incineration problems, but where there is a high handling penalty such as with aerosol canisters or small containers and tins, are likely to be at least £200 t^{-1}.

As mentioned in Section 5.1.5., sea incineration can be regarded as something of a special case. It is able to avoid altogether the high costs associated with gas cleaning, and is generally likely to be concerned only with bulk loads. However, these advantages must be offset against the high overheads of maintaining a sea going vessel, and the cost of accumulating and storing wastes at ports awaiting the vessel calling. The balance is usually only in favour of the ship-borne operation when substantially chlorinated wastes are involved.

6. SOLIDIFICATION AND RELATED SYSTEMS

This approach to waste treatment has developed markedly in the last decade, having previously been largely confined to processes dealing with radioactive or nuclear waste. A recently published book on the subject[19] either deals in detail or merely lists over 40 companies offering such a service, and the author is aware of a number of others not mentioned in that publication.

6.1. The Rationale of Such Systems

When applied to the processing of toxic wastes, the object of these systems is to significantly reduce the degree to which toxic constituents of the waste can escape into the environment. In the context of the conventional landfill type operation, such a risk is principally represented by the possibility of toxic constituents being washed or leached from the deposited waste by rain water, flooding or a rising water table.

To be a valid alternative and improvement on conventional landfill, successful solidification systems will display one or more of the following characteristics.

1. Substantially reduce the permeability of the waste such that water will be unable to penetrate into the waste mass, and leach toxic constituents from it.
2. Aggregate the waste into a large, undivided or monolithic mass, significantly reducing the ratio of the surface area to the mass, and thereby presenting a much smaller proportion to direct contact with water and to the possibility of surface leaching effects.

3.   Incorporate toxic elements into the solid matrix by chemical bonding, rather than mere physical entrapment, and thereby render it more difficult to remove those elements by physical processes such as leaching.

6.2. Terminology and Approaches

A number of terms are commonly used in connection with this type of disposal, notably solidification, stabilisation, fixation, encapsulation, polymerisation and cementation. It is a mute point whether there is any significant or real distinction between some of these terms, which can generally be seen as deriving either from the desired objective of the process, or the way of carrying it out. Encapsulation alone perhaps justifies distinction, as it really refers to the wrapping up or enclosing in an inert case, the otherwise unchanged waste. The other terms imply mixing or some other process which affects the raw waste itself.

Technical approaches. The many individual processes available can be reduced to a limited number of basic approaches. A soundly based classification has been suggested by the USEPA in their publications[20] which discuss the relative merits of each class in some detail. Consideration is given to raw materials supply and relative cost, the range of wastes which can be so treated, the volume of solidified product in relation to that of the original waste, capital plant needs, etc. The seven basic classes in the USEPA publication are as follows.[20]

1.   Cement-based techniques.
2.   Lime-based (pozzolanic) techniques.
3.   Thermoplastic techniques (including bitumen and polyethylene).
4.   Organic polymer techniques.
5.   Encapsulation techniques.
6.   Self cementing techniques.
7.   Glassification.

6.3. Criteria for Assessing or Comparing Systems

The three objectives sought from these systems, as listed in Section 6.1., suggest three criteria which may offer some measure of performance (both absolute and comparative). These criteria would be:

(1)   the leaching characteristics of the solidified product,
(2)   the permeability of the solidified mass, and
(3)   the compressive strength of the solidified mass.

Measurement of these three factors, if it is to have real value should be done by carefully conceived standard methods which not only can be interpreted in an absolute sense, but provide for valid comparison between results and systems. Many process owners and operators publish brochures and literature detailing test results in one or more of these areas, but often do not mention the test method used. Further investigation across a range of process claims will probably reveal a variety of test methods being employed, thus making a true comparison between the systems impossible.

The USEPA is intending to standardise the testing procedures (at least within their own sphere of control),[21] and then to lay down guidelines as to the interpretation and significance of the results obtained. Thus, attainment of a particular test result using a standard method would determine whether or not the system could be used in certain conditions.

Leaching characteristics provide some measure of the ability of the solidified material to retain toxic constituents of the original waste, when subjected to wetting, soaking and saturation, possibly in conjunction with fracture and crumbling. Many of the tests employed involve the solidified sample being ground into a fine powder (particle size unspecified) and subjected to column leaching or to agitation in a fixed volume of liquid. Some tests attempt to leach through a solid core of material, or to use larger fragments or chips of solid in agitation or column tests.

Undoubtedly, the tests involving use of a powdered sample offer a more rigorous challenge to the process, and have sometimes been referred to as accelerated weathering tests, giving a very high specific surface area, and representing, it is claimed, a 'worst case'. Distilled water is often used for these tests, but other synthetic leachates have been tried, these being seen by their proponents as more accurately representing the likely realities of a landfill site.

Some strikingly impressive results are claimed for some processes, whereby mixtures containing considerable quantities for various toxic constituents yield only fractions of $1\ \mathrm{mg\ litre^{-1}}$ in leachate collected under test conditions. Naturally enough, many operating companies will publicise only those results which show their process in a good light, so it is perhaps to the independent test programmes that one should look for substantiation of these claims. The largest such programme is probably that being conducted by the USEPA, and involves an extensive range of tests on a number of commercially available systems. To date, the detailed results of the work concerning leaching are not yet published, but preliminary views have been expressed[22] to the effect that some processes can demonstrate a significant improvement in leaching as compared to the unprocessed sludge, whereas others are of limited or negligible worth.

Testing, including X-ray crystallography, has been carried out by the Dutch Research Organisation—Stichting Verwijdering Afvalstoffen (SVA) and the results have been published.[23] The general conclusion was to question the value of the systems tested in chemically reducing the relative leaching between solidified and unsolidified (i.e. raw) sludge waste, and suggests that the value of these processes may rest with physical considerations such as the reduction of permeability.

The German authorities have also engaged in a test programme but have yet to publish the results. However, a preliminary statement has been made suggesting that the results cast some doubt on the value of the processes in reducing leaching.[24]

Permeability is an important consideration with these processes, since if liquid cannot first penetrate into the solidified mass then it cannot leach or affect the toxic components dispersed throughout that mass. In such cases, leaching effects would be confined to the surface of the solid, which in the case of a large monolithic mass would be low in relation to the total mass. The permeability coefficients of the products of a number of commercially operated systems have been tested by the USEPA, and the results published as part of a general study of physical and engineering properties of wastes.[25] Given that the coefficient of permeability is expressed in centimetres per second, the tests displayed a range of values from 1×10^{-4} to $1 \times 10^{-11}\,\mathrm{cm\,s^{-1}}$, although most results were in the range of 1×10^{-5} to $1 \times 10^{-7}\,\mathrm{cm\,s^{-1}}$. Concretes typically yield results around 1×10^{-7}, and sand perhaps around 1×10^{-2} to $1 \times 10^{-3}\,\mathrm{cm\,s^{-1}}$.

The USEPA research work and report referred to above devoted itself to a number of areas connected with the physical properties and performance of solidified sludges. These included the study of compressive strength, as well as the effect of repeated 'freeze/thaw' and 'wet/dry' cycles, on solidified specimens. These properties are considered to be of value in gauging how solidified wastes will perform after they have been deposited in whatever location is chosen. Certain commercial operators claim uses for the solidified products as hard core, tip lining and even a coarse building material, so the ability to stand up to certain types of wear and tear is important. Equally if not more important is the relationship between strength and relative surface area, and the consequent effect on permeability. A material of high strength is less likely to crumble or break up under load, or in adverse weather conditions, and thereby expose a much higher surface area to the effects of surface leaching.

The USEPA tests showed compressive strengths in the range 7–50 $\times 10^4\,\mathrm{kg\,m^{-2}}$ (100–700 psi) for the solidified samples obtained from the same range of commercial processes as were tested for permeability. Concrete would show a result of $30\text{--}35 \times 10^5\,\mathrm{kg\,m^{-2}}$ (4000–5000 psi).

6.4. Economic Considerations

Section 6.2. pointed out the range of processes falling within the general term 'solidification'. Some of these processes are geared to low throughput, highly hazardous materials, such as radioactive wastes; others have established themselves in the high volume market such as with inorganic effluent sludges.

Within Britain it is largely in the latter area where these processes have made their mark. Processes employing both fixed and portable plant have become very well established in certain geographical areas, handling large volumes of predominately inorganic liquid and sludge wastes, at very competitive prices. The competitive edge is gained, at least in part, from the use of waste silicaceous materials, such as pulverised fuel ash (PFA), sewage sludge incineration residues, and pulverised or ground furnace slags. Charges for these processes are believed to start in the region of £10–£15 $\mathrm{t^{-1}}$.

At the other extreme, there are processes for which the charges can be in the range of £100–£200 $\mathrm{t^{-1}}$, or even greater. These may arise from the use of expensive chemical ingredients, expensive and sophisticated equipment, or both. This range of process normally finds application with particularly hazardous or toxic chemicals, and may be regarded not only as offering an advantage in ultimate disposal, but also in making intermediate handling and transportation much safer.

In the end, solidification processes cost money, and are only going to be carried out if they seem to display some sort of benefit. That benefit may take the form of reducing the handling and transportation difficulties of certain wastes, of making available more geographically convenient landfill sites than would otherwise be open to unsolidified wastes, or satisfying the desires of certain companies to use disposal techniques which appear to offer the highest security, even though they may be marginally or considerably more expensive than other options.

7.   CHEMICAL TREATMENT

Chemical treatment is a general or collective term which can be applied to many processes and techniques. Within the context of this chapter, it may be defined as any process which alters the characteristics, composition or properties of a waste, in such a way as to assist with or make more acceptable its ultimate disposal. More specifically, it will usually seek to employ one or more of the following approaches.

1. To chemically break down or destroy the undesired species.
2. To convert these species to less harmful or insoluble forms.
3. To separate them from the bulk of the waste, and thereby produce a relatively small volume of more concentrated waste for special treatment.

Within conventional waste disposal circles, the term 'Chemical Treatment' had developed a rather narrow and specialist use and is taken to mean the processing of essentially inorganic wastes by neutralisation, the precipitation of heavy metals, the elimination of cyanides, etc. However, a consideration of the subject should recognise the existence of other more sophisticated processes, such as ultrafiltration, ion exchange, electrolytic deposition and reverse osmosis. Such techniques belong rather more to the realms of wastewater and effluent treatment, than to hazardous waste disposal, but there is some degree of overlap, and a brief reference to them should be included.

7.1. Chemical Process Methods

Chemical methods have been employed for many years at effluent treatment plants such as would typically be found in the plating industry. Effluent streams comprising rinse liquors, with the occasional more concentrated waste from a plating tank, and containing species such as cyanide, chromium, zinc, cadmium and nickel are processed on a large batch or continuous basis.

The chemistry really is quite simple, cyanide being oxidised to harmless products, and toxic metals converted to insoluble forms, often requiring no more than pH adjustment to produce the hydroxide. A little more sophistication is required where hydroxide is not immediately formed, such as with hexavalent chromium, where reduction to the trivalent state is first necessary. In the same way, where a toxic metal does not have a stable hydroxide, or where that hydroxide is soluble in the aqueous phase (e.g. copper or nickel hydroxides in ammonia containing effluents), some other reaction must be employed. Finally however, the process sequence depends on separating these insoluble toxic species from the bulk of the system, by gravity or filtration systems and allowing the bulk treated effluent to be discharged to an outlet such as the public sewer. The separated sludge or filter cake, containing the insoluble toxic metal compounds, may be disposed of to landfill, subjected to the solidification approaches described in Section 6., or occasionally recovered where the concentrations of metals are suitable.

Although the chemistry is simple, it is also effective, and whereas the principles have been established at in-house plants, often on continuous processing of high volume, dilute effluents they can equally well be applied to batch treatment or to treatment of concentrated wastes on any scale.

It is often the producers of concentrated wastes who experience the most severe disposal problems, particularly where such a production is infrequent or intermittent, or where the nature of the waste is subject to variation. The provision of in-house facilities is unlikely to be economically viable for such occasional or variable demands, and the services of an external service plant will be necessary if tipping of untreated waste is to be avoided.

A number of central plants have been established within Britain in the last decade, ranging from modern, custom-built facilities, some of which also incorporate solidification as a final stage, to lagoons or ponds at landfill sites. However, all will use the same basic chemical reactions, albeit probably on a batch basis to safely accommodate the diversity of concentrations and compositions of wastes received at such installations.

7.2. Ultrafiltration

This is a membrane process, involving filtration at the molecular level. Membranes are typically polycarbonate or substituted olefin based, and are capable of being produced to offer some variety in the size of molecule rejected by the membrane. The rejection level may also be influenced by the temperature, and by conditions, such as pH, which may cause variations in molecular shape, rigidity or degree of association. Membranes used in ultrafiltration are reasonably inert and stable, but must not be abused. Waste streams to be processed in this way must be reasonably guaranteed not to display large variations in composition, or to contain the types of materials which would certainly damage the membrane. This sort of restriction is always limiting in waste disposal applications, where composition guarantees are invariably more difficult to give.

Established applications include the processing of emulsified cutting oils from the engineering industry and the recovery of paint from water soluble bases. In the case of the former application, a contracting central service plant has now been established with a capacity of $c.\ 4\cdot5 \times 10^{7}$ litres annum^{-1} of emulsion, producing typically $2{-}3 \times 10^{6}$ litres of recovered oil.

7.3. Ion Exchange

The principles of ion exchange need little explanation here, save to state that in the process of passing effluent through a resin bed, the object would be to exchange certain ionic contaminants in the effluent for harmless ionic species on the resin. The contaminants would become fixed to the resin, and the original effluent left clean, possibly clean enough for the water to be re-used. The resin itself would eventually need to be regenerated, liberating the contaminants into a very much smaller volume of liquid than they would originally have been collected from.

This concentration of the original contaminants into a much smaller, more manageable volume, is the single most important aspect of ion exchange techniques. The concentrated liquors produced may often be suitable for recovery processes under conditions which would not have applied with the dilute effluent. Even if recovery is not feasible, such as with concentrates of mixed metals, transportation of the liquor to a disposal point will be a much less costly proposition than would have been the case for the entire volume of dilute effluent. A logical extension of this philosophy has been the realisation that instead of the resin user regenerating his resins, and being faced with the problem of recovering or disposing of the concentrated liquor, exchangeable cartridges of resins could be supplied, with regeneration, and processing of the concentrated liquors taking place at a central plant. There is currently some interest in promoting this approach.

7.4. Electrolytic Deposition

Electrolytic deposition, when discussed in the context of hazardous wastes, would most probably be thought of as a tool for the recovery of valuable metals such as nickel, copper, silver, etc. In fact, such recovery routes require fairly pure waste feed stocks, as the presence of other metals, not to mention other dissolved or soluble species, can seriously disrupt deposition.

Recent years have seen the development of a number of cells able to deposit metals from solutions of low concentration. This has made possible the use of electro-deposition as an effluent polishing technique, but one which will convert the contaminants into a fairly pure and, therefore, valuable metal deposit.

7.5. Reverse Osmosis

This is also a membrane technique, essentially capable of separating dissolved solids from water in aqueous systems. It divides the waste stream into two: pure water which has passed through the membrane, and a progressively more concentrated solution which has not.

Reverse osmosis is probably most widely known to the layman for its desalination applications. It is undoubtedly capable of processing metal finishing, and other inorganic aqueous effluents but the problems of waste consistency and predictability touched on in Section 7.2. are even more important with reverse osmosis, where the membrane is more sensitive, and susceptible to damage.

8.   MISCELLANEOUS METHODS

The methods and technologies described in this final section, are not in general or widespread use for the disposal of the types of toxic and hazardous waste which have hitherto been the subject of this chapter. In some cases, the technologies are in widespread use in other fields and impinge only slightly on waste disposal activities; in others the technology has scarcely been developed to an operational or commercial scale, but does demonstrate some prospect of being applicable to hazardous wastes. In all cases, the chapter would be incomplete without some reference to their scope and potential.

8.1. Catalysis

The use of catalysts in a wide variety of chemical reactions will be familiar territory for all those with experience in oil refining, petrochemicals and chemical synthesis. Applications involving the types of hazardous waste covered by this chapter are few in number, probably the most obvious example being the disposal of waste cyanide salts and solutions. In this case, hydrogen cyanide gas is deliberately produced by acidification of the waste, and the gas catalytically oxidised.

Catalytic oxidation provides most of the examples of the environmental control potential of catalysis. Most concern air purification, and will relate to effluent or waste gas streams containing contaminants which pose problems of toxicity or odour nuisance. These may arise typically from glue making, fat rendering, various animal waste processing activities, wire enamelling, tanning and plastics extrusion. Such gas streams can be perfectly satisfactorily processed using direct flame or fume incinerators, such methods requiring the whole of the gas volume to be raised to the temperature at which the offending species will be destroyed. For various practical and safety reasons, the level of contaminant in the gas stream will normally be maintained well below the lower explosive limit (l.e.l.), and often will be below 1000 ppm. Having so small an inherent calorific value, the heat required to raise the gas to the required temperature will have to be supplied from an external source. This could represent a major cost in treating large volumes of contaminated air.

Catalytic combustion may well achieve the same end, but at substantially lower temperatures, the catalyst simply reducing the temperature at which the oxidation reaction takes place. With temperature differences usually of at least several hundred degrees K,[26] major fuel savings will be possible. It should be appreciated that this technique has conventionally only been applied to gas or vapour streams which themselves are produced as an intrinsic or unavoidable part of another process. As such, it is more a tool for emission abatement than for waste disposal in its more widely used sense. Theoretically, it would of course be possible to deliberately evaporate or volatilise organic wastes, and catalytically oxidise the resulting vapour stream. However, it can very quickly be shown that this is totally uneconomic, compared with conventional incineration.

Catalytic oxidation can also be applied to the processing of strong wastewaters, in which the chemical oxygen demand (COD) is higher than would normally permit discharge to a sewer or river.[27]

8.2. Pyrolysis

Pyrolysis has often been viewed as one of the more promising 'energy from waste' technologies, although up to the present time it has only been tried with refuse, scrap rubber including used tyres, and plastic waste. Even so, some prematurely conceived projects, incorporating perhaps over ambitious scaling-up from pilot plants, or a general lack of attention to engineering details, have encountered technical problems and caused something of a setback to pyrolysis development and acceptance.

Pyrolysis, involving the thermal treatment of organic matter in an oxygen free or deficient atmosphere, produces a combustible gas, a hydrocarbon liquid phase, an aqueous phase and a solid char, in proportions which can be varied to some extent by the choice of pyrolytic conditions. A number of techniques have been employed, including a fluidised bed approach, and both rotary and static kilns or grates incorporating direct and indirect heating. There are considerable doubts as to the economic viability of pyrolysing refuse, but feed stocks with better yield potentials, such as used tyres and plastic scrap, appear to offer better immediate prospects of successful commercial exploitation.

As far as the author is aware, there have been no serious efforts directed towards pyrolysing solid or semi-solid organic hazardous wastes, although these materials must, theoretically at least, be capable of pyrolysis. As is so often the case with processing, development of technologies will often be inhibited by a lack of confidence that sufficient wastes of the required type will remain available for long enough to justify that development.

8.3. Waste Derived Fuels (WDF)

Waste derived fuel and refuse derived fuel (RDF) are terms often used interchangeably, usually to refer to a fuel-type product obtained from refuse of domestic or commercial origins. In this context, the processes involved will include sorting to remove metal and glass, followed by some type of conversion by shredding, pulverising, drying, briquetting or pelletising (or any combination of these) to produce a solid fuel. Such processes could theoretically be developed to incorporate selected hazardous wastes, which could significantly improve the calorific value. However, great care would have to be exercised to exclude those wastes which would cause toxic emissions, either before or after firing, or which would present any other sort of safety or environmental problems.

In its widest sense, the term 'waste derived fuel' embraces numerous processes and techniques for extracting energy from waste. Many, such as the fermentation of cereal crop residues to produce methanol, or the collecting of methane from anaerobically degrading refuse in landfill sites, have little bearing on the hazardous waste market under review in this chapter. However hazardous waste type materials are utilised in the production of certain secondary liquid fuels. An increasing number of companies incorporate selected clean waste solvents and oils into their site fuel supplies for steam generation purposes, etc., and a number of contractors now arrange to collect and process such wastes, with a view to producing saleable secondary fuels rather than recovered solvents or oils for re-use as such.

8.4. Biological Treatment

The fundamental principle of a biological treatment process lies in an interaction between bacteria and the species requiring treatment, such that the bacteria consume the waste and in so doing sustain or increase their own numbers. It therefore follows that the only wastes suitable for this form of treatment are those which are not themselves toxic to the bacteria, and which can act as an effective nutrient supply.

In this respect, limits must be applied to certain contaminants and characteristics of a potential feed stock, such as the concentrations of heavy metals, free oil and grease, and chlorinated hydrocarbons. Limitations must also be applied to the degree of variability of the feed stock. The bacteria are capable of mutation to accommodate a certain amount of change, and can even be developed to cope with unusually high levels of some specific species. However, such changes must be gradual, and be within a certain range of values, otherwise retardation or death of the entire system may occur.

All this really suggests that the typical hazardous wastes under consideration here, are not well suited to processing via biological means. This is generally a fair conclusion, at least in relation to the form and concentration in which these wastes would usually arise. Some effluents containing proportions of hazardous waste are biologically processed, but these usually are essentially aqueous materials in which there are dissolved suitable amounts of appropriate soluble or miscible organic species. Theoretically of course, many organic wastes could be pre-treated to remove the problematic contaminants, and produce an effluent capable of being biologically degraded. However, it will probably be apparent that the costs associated with so elaborate a procedure would be uncompetitive with the principal alternatives of incineration or solidification.

REFERENCES

1. Deposit of Poisonous Waste Act, Ch. 21, HMSO, London, 1972.
2. Statutory Instrument No. 1017, *The deposit of poisonous waste* (*notification of removal or deposit*) *regulations*, HMSO, London, 1972.
3. Control of Pollution Act, Ch. 40, HMSO, London, 1974.
4. Department of the Environment. The licensing of waste disposal sites, *Waste Management Paper* No. 4, HMSO, London, 1976.
5. Statutory Instrument No. 1702, *Hazardous substances* (*labelling of road tankers*) *regulations*, Schedule 1, HMSO, London, 1978.
6. Health and Safety Commission. Consultative Document, *Proposals for dangerous substances* (*conveyance by road*) *regulations*, HMSO, London, 1978.
7. Resource Conservation and Recovery Act (Pub. L. 94-580 (Oct. 21 1976)), USEPA, 1976.
8. US Environmental Protection Agency. Hazardous waste, proposed guidelines and regulations and proposal on identification and listing *US Federal Register*, 18 Dec. 1978, Part IV.
9. Dumping at Sea Act, Ch. 20, HMSO, London, 1974.
10. Radioactive Substances Act, Ch. 37, HMSO, London, 1948.
11. Department of the Environment. *Waste management papers*—a series, HMSO, London.

12. YOSHIM, S. J. and BARCLAY, K. M., *Proc. Natl. Conf. on Hazardous Waste Management, San Francisco*, 1–4 Feb. 1977, 146–56.
13. US Environmental Protection Agency. *Disposal of organochlorine wastes by incineration at sea*, Report No. EPA-430/9-75-014, 1975.
14. US Environmental Protection Agency. *At-sea incineration of herbicide orange onboard the M/T* Vulcanus, Report No. EPA-600/2-78-086, 1978.
15. US Environmental Protection Agency. *Laboratory evaluation of high-temperature destruction of Kepone and related pesticides*, Report No. EPA-600/2-78-299, 1978.
16. US Environmental Protection Agency. *Kepone incineration test program*, Report No. EPA-600/2-78-108, 1978.
17. US Environmental Protection Agency. *Laboratory evaluation of high-temperature destruction of polychlorinated biphenyls and related compounds*, Report No. EPA-600/2-77-228, 1977.
18. Health and Safety Commission. Consultative Document, *Proposals for amendments to the lists of scheduled works and noxious and offensive gases.* HMSO, London, 1979.
19. POJASEK, R. B. *Toxic and Hazardous Waste Disposal*, Ann Arbor Science, Michigan, 1979.
20. US Environmental Protection Agency. *Survey of solidification/stabilisation technology for hazardous industrial wastes*, Report No. EPA-600/2-79-056, 1979.
21. US Environmental Protection Agency. *Compilation and evaluation of leaching test methods*, Report No. EPA-600/2-78-095, 1978.
22. US Environmental Protection Agency. *Proc. 1st Ann. Conf. on Advanced Pollution Control for the Metal Finishing Industry*, Report No. EPA-600/8-78-010, 1978, 130–42.
23. Stichting Verwijdering Afvalstoffen. *Comparative investigation on four immobilisation techniques* SVA 2969E/3247E, Amersfoort, Holland, Mar. 1979.
24. ANON. *Chem. Eng.*, Jul. 1979, **86**(14), 28E–28F.
25. US Environmental Protection Agency. *Physical and engineering properties of hazardous industrial wastes and sludges*, Report No. EPA-600/2-77-139, 1977.
26. HARDISON, L. C. and DOWD, E. J. *Chem. Eng. Prog.*, Aug. 1977, p. 31.
27. ROSS, L. W. and CHOWDHURY, A. K., *Catalytic oxidation of strong waste waters*, American Society of Mechanical Engineers, New York, 1978.

Chapter 3

INDUSTRIAL NOISE AND VIBRATION CONTROL

P. O. A. L. Davies, B.E., Ph.D., C.Eng.Aust., C.Eng., F.I.Mech.E., M.I.O.A.

Professor of Experimental Fluid Dynamics,
Institute of Sound and Vibration Research,
University of Southampton, UK

and

A. H. Middleton, M.Sc.(Eng.), F.I.O.A.

Technical Manager, Wolfson Unit for Noise and Vibration Control,
Institute of Sound and Vibration Research,
University of Southampton, UK

SUMMARY

This chapter discusses noise and vibration control for the industrial environment in terms of (1) specification of the standards to be achieved (2) analysis of the particular problem and (3) the adoption of an appropriate control strategy. Analysis of each problem involves identification of the sources. The chapter goes on to describe the basic mechanisms and characteristics of each of the dozen or more sources most commonly encountered in practice. The latter half of the chapter describes and discusses the range of noise and vibration control procedures that can provide a practical solution. These include modification of the source, control of the propagation path, building design considerations and personal protection.

1. INTRODUCTION

Both sound and vibration can provide a hazard to health in the industrial environment. The extent to which the environment at the workplace can be, or is, controlled to ameliorate situations which are potentially damaging depends on a number of factors, some of which are conflicting. One must, therefore, examine each factor individually to achieve that balance which represents the incentive to take appropriate action to control the noise or vibration in each specific instance.

The order in which one considers these must be somewhat arbitrary and their relative importance must differ with different industrial situations. If one lists them, they include:

    (1)   an assessment of the existing hazard to health,
    (2)   legislative controls and restrictions which may be specific either to the workplace or the environment in general,
    (3)   product marketing incentives including the environmental acceptability of a machine or product for a given task,
    (4)   economic factors and the real costs of control measures, and
    (5)   constraints imposed by the manufacturing process.

Noise and vibration control can, therefore, be described most effectively in terms of a succession of rational steps. The first of them is to assess the problem in terms of all the relevant factors to arrive at a specification of the goals or standards to be aimed for. The second is to analyse the problem to isolate the sources of the noise and vibration. The third step is to adopt an appropriate strategy which involves the consideration of several alternatives. These are

    (1)   reduction of noise or vibration at source by component redesign or change of process or technology,
    (2)   isolation or grouping sources to reduce general exposure or modifying the transmission paths between source and receiver, or
    (3)   protecting the operators with personal hearing protection and by controlling their work cycle to limit noise exposure.

The precise assessment of the extent of hazard presented by a given noise or vibration environment is difficult, since the sensitivity of the individual varies widely. Furthermore the resulting damage from excessive exposure to noise and vibration tends to be insidious and, except in the case of a noise or vibration 'accident', only appreciated after long periods of exposure.

Noise induced hearing loss resulting from normal industrial noise creeps on gradually. Once permanent damage has occurred it is irreversible. The damage occurs in the inner ear in the form of degradation of nerve endings. The sensitivity of individuals to hearing loss varies greatly but, so far, no one has found a way of measuring this by a pre-exposure test. It can only be detected after some degree of hearing loss has occurred. Hence the value of regular audiometry, which enables those suffering from the earlier stages of noise induced hearing loss to be spotted before the damage becomes significant and then to be protected from further damage.

Long periods of exposure to vibration, particularly exposure of the hands to mechanical tool vibration, can produce a condition known as 'vibration white finger' in which the blood circulation to the fingers becomes restricted with consequent numbness and discomfort or pain in cold weather. In a few extreme cases where exposure to high levels of vibration has been persistent the circulation has become so restricted that gangrene has set in.

Exposure of the whole body to vibration produces a variety of unpleasant effects ranging from headaches and nausea through temporary loss of manipulative ability and clear vision to actual physical damage at extreme vibration levels.

2. LEGISLATION AND STANDARDS AS INCENTIVES FOR NOISE AND VIBRATION CONTROL

Legislation regarding noise and vibration has developed to different extents in various countries. Most industrialised countries now attempt to protect employees against exposure to excessive levels by means of laws or advisory codes of practice. At the moment there is little legislation controlling the noise or vibration output of machines or devices. West Germany has taken a lead in this matter and many manufacturers are now finding difficulty in selling their products there because they have not put the required effort into noise control. Product legislation is slowly spreading over a range of potentially noisy products and will, before too long, become a major stimulus to noise control activity. Legal requirements for product labelling with respect to noise emission are also on the horizon, although at present there is little agreement between the various authorities on how the noise of a product is to be described.

Legislation affects the levels of noise and vibration which the community surrounding industrial premises should be expected to tolerate. Specific noise and vibration limits have to be set in each instance because of the large number of variables which must be considered. By specifying noise limits and allowable working hours as part of planning permission for industrial premises, local authorities are able to exercise coarse control over neighbourhood noise. Environmental Health Officers have the power to investigate and require the control of community noise or vibration which is causing a nuisance or a hazard.

2.1. Noise at Work

UK legislation in the form of the Health and Safety at Work Act (1974) can be taken as an example of the regulations prevailing in industrialised countries to control health hazards from noise at work.

Except in the case of woodworking machinery noise and tractor cab noise, which is covered under regulations embraced in the Health and Safety at Work Act (1974), the Act has not so far resulted in the specification of any legal noise limits. It gives the appropriate minister the power to make specific regulations if and when he thinks fit. Otherwise the operation of the Act with respect to noise leans heavily on the advisory document, the 'Code of Practice for the reduction of the exposure of employed persons to noise' (1972).[1] In this document it is advised that no one should be exposed to a continuous noise level exceeding 90 dB(A) during a normal 8 h working day. Shorter durations at higher noise levels are permissible provided that the sound energy received does not exceed the equivalent of 8 h at 90 dB(A). Hence the concept of equivalent continuous noise level or L_{eq}, which is a way of describing a fluctuating noise by comparing the total energy received over a given period with that which would be received over the same period from a steady noise level. Thus an equivalent continuous noise level of 90 dB(A) over an 8 h day rates the same as a steady 90 dB(A) for 8 h. Also a steady noise of 93 dB(A) for 4 h, or 96 dB(A) for 2 h, and so on, represents an equivalent continuous noise level of 90 dB(A). Instruments are available which measure L_{eq} directly, including that due to short duration impulsive and transient sounds.

The Code of Practice recognises that an L_{eq} of 90 dB(A) will not protect everyone from noise induced hearing loss (NIHL). The most sensitive 10% of the population could suffer some degree of NIHL after a working lifetime. The most sensitive 1% or so of the population could suffer a hearing loss sufficient to cause social handicap. In the last few years there has been growing pressure for the adoption of an 85 dB(A) limit but no changes have appeared yet in official documents.

The Code of Practice recommends that received noise levels should be reduced to below 90 dB(A) wherever practical, but recognises that this may be difficult in many cases with existing machinery and processes and allows the use of individual hearing protection as a short term expedient. Most legislation worldwide imposes a 90 dB(A) L_{eq} limit for noise at work. Some legislation imposes lower limits for office workers and other categories of employee. In several countries there is growing pressure for a reduction to 85 dB(A) or thereabouts.

In addition to the limits imposed for continuous noise most legislation or codes of practice specify absolute maximum allowable noise levels for short duration transient sounds. These limits are variously specified but are usually of the order of 140 or 150 dB peak sound level.

2.2. Vibration at Work

The Health and Safety at Work Act applies to vibration as well as to noise, and gives the minister power to set vibration limits although this has not so far been done. Recommended limits for hand/arm vibration are given in reference 2 and for whole body vibration in reference 3.

Hand/arm vibration has been a particular problem in forestry where the use of hand-held chain saws is widespread. Much effort has been expended by chain saw manufacturers in finding ways of minimising handle vibration. Problems have also been encountered in the fettling of castings.

3. PRODUCT NOISE AND VIBRATION LEGISLATION AND STANDARDS

West Germany appears to be taking the lead in setting down detailed standards for the measurement of product noise. The various parts of reference 4 define noise measurement methods for a wide variety of types of machinery. These standards need to be studied very carefully because some of the measurement methods are unique to the German standards. These standards are used in conjunction with the German Work Place Noise limits to define acceptable noise levels for individual machines.[5]

The EEC has for some years been deliberating on the noise from various items of construction equipment, such as tower cranes, welding generator sets and earthmoving equipment, with the objective of arriving at agreed maximum noise levels and methods of measurement.

Many East European countries have published strict noise legislation but whilst they seem to require that imported goods meet the required standard, domestic products do not always appear to do so. Despite an elaborate system of accountability and acceptance by signature of safe working conditions there does not seem to be a notably better noise climate than that existing in the West.

There is no doubt that failure to take suitable steps to control noise will be a barrier to sales in many export markets in the near future, although it may be some years before legislation bites in the UK. Very careful study of the relevant legislation in any export market is essential because of the lack of standardisation of requirements. Even the units of measurement used vary from country to country.

4.   NOISE CONTROL STRATEGY

In any noise control investigation a logical approach is essential. Nearly all machines or devices which generate noise contain more than one cause of noise. It is essential that the predominant sources are identified and controlled first. Extensive efforts applied to the control of secondary sources are unlikely to result in a reduction in the overall noise level of a machine, measured in dB(A). In some situations where the need is for the achievement of subjective improvements in the noise output of a machine, when noise levels are too low to constitute a hazard, attention to secondary sources may be justified. A logical investigation of the problem is, nevertheless, still required.

Any noise control exercise, whether carried out on an existing machine or plant or at the design stage must consist of the following stages.

1.   Identify noise source mechanisms.
2.   Quantify source strength, by measurement or prediction.
3.   Identify noise radiating surfaces or devices.
4.   Identify noise transmission paths between the sources and radiating surfaces and between the radiating surfaces and the listener.
5.   Apply noise control to sources, transmission paths, radiating surfaces or listener, as appropriate.

5.   NOISE SOURCE MECHANISMS AND THEIR CONTROL

Anything that moves is potentially a source of noise. In the case of fluid sources the faster it moves the greater the source strength is likely to be. In the case of mechanical sources the greater the instantaneous acceleration the greater the source strength is likely to be. It is often difficult to separate noise and vibration sources into convenient compartments. Most mechanical noise results from an original source of vibration so noise and vibration control are inextricably related.

Examples of fluid dynamic noise sources are: air jet noise, intermittent or periodic discharge of gas, fan noise, hydraulic pump noise, combustion, flow generated noise within pipe and duct systems, and high speed rotation of irregularly shaped bodies.

Examples of mechanical noise sources are: impacts in bearings and slideways, tooth engagement of gears, electromagnetically induced vibrations in electrical machines, stick–slip motions due to friction, chatter of cutting tools and impacts generated as part of the machine process. When identifying sources of noise it is useful to subdivide them into sources of continuous noise and sources of impulsive noise because the control techniques used may be different.

5.1. Jet and Discharge Noise

Many industrial and manufacturing processes employ compressed air for a wide range of factory operations. Jets of compressed air are used for cooling, for moving light objects or dirt, or for maintenance of an air cushion to separate sheets of material. Compressed air is also used for operating tools, presses, clamps, jacks and hammers. The exhaust from such equipment is often a significant, if intermittent source of noise. Valves and air leaks provide other noise sources. Since compressed air is normally supplied at around five atmospheres, or more, free discharges normally reach or exceed sonic flow speeds.

With low speed jets the noise arises from the mixing and entrainment of air producing severe turbulence. At high or sonic flow speeds, shock cells provide additional sources of intense sound often as discrete tones. Mixing noise generally increases as the 6th to 8th power of the jet velocity (i.e. sound level $\propto$ 60 log velocity). Thus a powerful noise control technique is to use the lowest practical flow velocity to accomplish the desired operation, i.e. a large slow jet is quieter than a small fast one.

The turbulent mixing noise covers a wide frequency range with a broad peak centred on a frequency of

$$f = \frac{sv}{d}$$

where s = the Strouhal number, a characteristic constant, v the jet flow velocity and d its diameter. Supersonic jets produce high level additional descrete frequency components as can be seen in Fig. 1. The noise radiation by jets is directional, being greater towards the sides than along the jet axis. At angles of about $45°$ to the jet axis the value of s is about $0·8$.

Subsonic jets are very efficient amplifiers of upstream flow disturbances. Any disturbance or soundfield upstream of the jet will enhance the noise

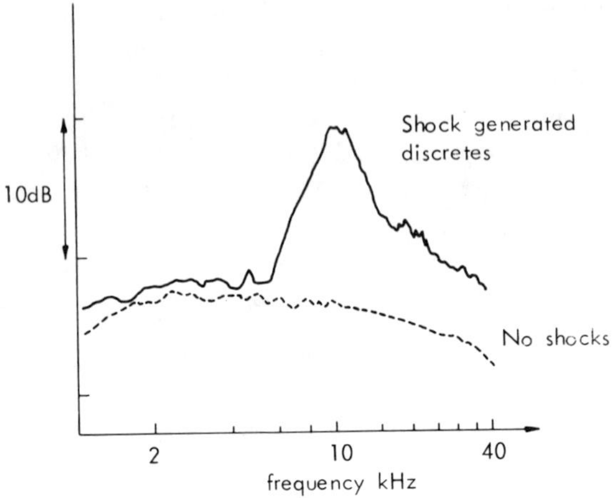

FIG. 1. Typical spectra of supersonic jet noise.

significantly and may change the Strouhal number of the sound. Impingement on sharp edges or cavities can also enhance the sound generation dramatically. The former is a consequence of the generation of edge tones and the latter enhancement by cavity resonance producing discrete tones. In such cases the frequency is governed by the local geometry.

It is often possible to reduce the noise of cooling jets by improving the heat transfer characteristics of the surface to be cooled, or by using a larger diameter, lower velocity jet moving the same mass flow of air. When a jet is used for thrust generation the minimum jet velocity required to do the work in hand should be used. A variety of low noise nozzles for industrial jets are available commercially. Most of these appear to suffer some loss of thrust as a result of the noise control measures applied.

Jet noise phenomena are also the cause of noise in gas flow control valves. These valves used industrially on air, gas or steam systems are often causes of substantial noise (see Fig. 2). Noise radiated directly from the valve is not the only problem. Noise from the associated pipework can often be more serious. At subsonic throat velocities noise will be radiated equally from upstream and down-stream pipework. At sonic throat velocities noise will be radiated mainly from downstream pipework. The noise emitted, although generated by the jet from the throat of the valve, is modified in character by the transmission characteristics of the pipe walls. A variety of low noise valves are available commercially. Alternatively acoustic lagging of the valve and pipework or the installation of inline silencers may be considered.

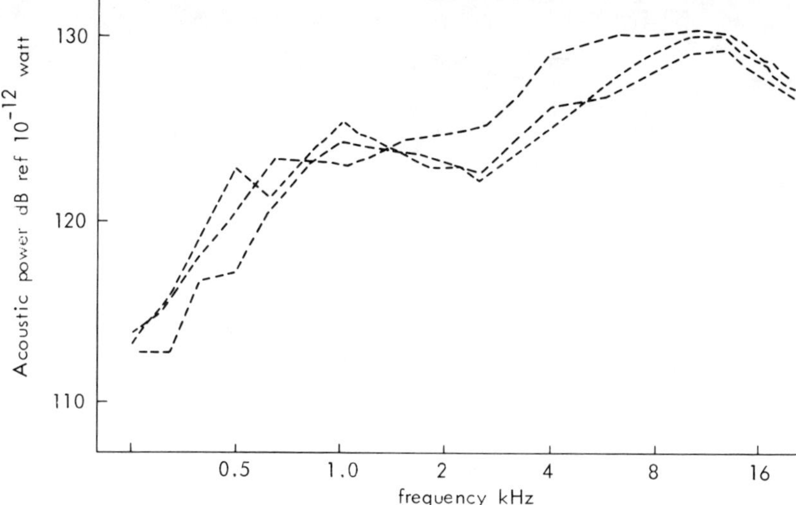

FIG. 2.   Typical $\frac{1}{3}$ octave band spectra of valves of the same size but different geometry operating at the same flow and pressure drop.

5.2. Fan Noise

Fan noise is again a result of turbulence generation, and is very dependent upon fan tip speed. Thus, for low noise, large low speed fans are to be preferred. The aerodynamic lift generated by the fan blades gives rise to noise over a wide frequency range. The frequency spectrum shape tends to depend on the type of fan as shown on Fig. 3. Centrifugal fan noise is usually biased towards the low frequency end of the spectrum, whereas axial flow fan noise usually peaks in the mid frequency range. A second phenomenon of fan noise is the discrete frequency or blade passing frequency noise caused by the interaction of the individual turbulent blade wakes with fixed obstacles or the interaction of the wakes of fixed obstacles in the inlet air flow with the moving blades. To reduce this particularly annoying noise stator to rotor clearances must be maximised. This can lead to a loss of performance so a compromise clearance is often necessary. The problem arises particularly in high performance centrifugal or axial compressors, where the pressure rise which can be generated is critically dependent on rotor to stator clearance.

Motor noise can form a significant part of the noise of commercially available fans. This noise may consist of electromagnetically generated tones which may be radiated directly via airborne paths or via structural paths. Motor cooling fan noise may itself be a problem.

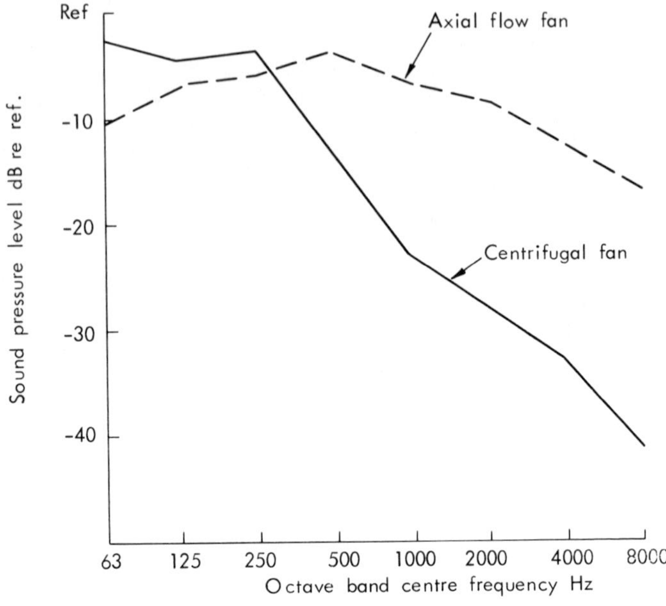

FIG. 3. Typical in-duct spectrum shapes of centrifugal and axial flow fans. (Reference level depends on fan power and size.)

Fan noise control at source involves the use of low speed fans with aerodynamically shaped blades, relatively large blade numbers, and operation of the fan on or near its design point, where its efficiency is greatest and the blades are producing least turbulence. Operation of a fan close to stall will nearly always cause increased broad band noise plus low frequency noise resulting from flow instability.

5.3. Hydraulic Pump Noise

Most hydraulic pumps produce a typical whine, which, incidentally, is usually radiated more from the piping system than from the pump itself because the pump body is much more massive and stiff than the pipes. The noise results from sudden pressure changes imposed on the fluid by the action of the pump. Assuming unimpeded fluid entry to the pump the action of a non-adjustable pump imposes a predetermined pressure rise on the fluid passing through the pumping cycle, whether it be a rotary pump or a piston pump. Only at one outlet pipe pressure condition will the pressure of the slug of fluid emitted from the pump into the outlet pipe be at the outlet pipe pressure. At all other outlet pressures the slug of fluid will be subjected to a sudden pressure change as it leaves the pumping chamber with the result that a pressure wave is set up in the outlet pipe which causes the pipe walls and pump to vibrate and radiate noise. To control the noise steps are taken to reduce the rate of pressure change of the slug of fluid, either by regulating the internal pressure rise of the pump by varying its pumping action or by arranging for a gradual bleed back of outlet pipe pressure into the pumping chamber during the pumping process.

Other sources of noise in hydraulic pumps are cavitation of the fluid at the inlet due to restriction of inlet flow, which causes noise due to the sudden collapse of cavitation bubbles; ingestion of aerated fluid due to poor reservoir design, which changes the compressibility of the fluid; trapping of unwanted volumes of fluid between working parts of the pump, for instance the engaging gear teeth of gear pumps, which gives no useful output but causes unwanted cyclic distortion of the pump structure.

5.4. Combustion Noise

Combustion noise occurs in burner systems, usually in conjunction with turbulence generated noise from the combustion air being drawn into the burning zone through some form of flow regulating device. Combustion noise is usually broad band in character and its level is related to the rate of burning of the fuel droplets in the combustion zone. Periodic noise can also be generated as a result of instability in combustion rate. This can arise from a variety of feedback mechanisms related to flow conditions at the combustion air inlets, periodic fuel flows, resonance in fuel supply pipelines, resonance in combustion or chimney spaces, resonance in air inlet ducting or unsuitable choice or operation of air supply fans. Industrial tunnel burners and package boiler systems often have resonance problems which are difficult to eliminate because it is very difficult to predict which of the many possible resonant systems will be excited in any operating condition.

Combustion noise in internal combustion engines is a special case of combustion noise. Fuel burning takes place very rapidly once every firing stroke. The rate of fuel burning has a profound effect on the engine noise as can be heard by contrasting the knocking noise of rapid combustion in a diesel engine with the slower combustion in a petrol engine. The airborne noise emitted is distorted by the response of the engine structure to the pressure changes in the combustion chamber and the response of the inlet and exhaust systems to the sudden ingestion or emission of slugs of gas. Substantially lower noise levels are claimed for Sterling engines, which whilst having similar reciprocating features to the normal internal combustion engine, use continuous combustion outside the cylinders.

5.5. Flow Generated Noise in Duct and Pipe Systems

This arises in air, gas and liquid flow systems and results from turbulence generated at points where pressure losses occur in the system or aerodynamic drag or lift forces are generated. The noise generated is generally broad band in character and its magnitude is related to the pressure drop incurred. Flow generated noise can travel long distances along air and gas pipes with little attenuation, thus causing a powerful source of pipe wall noise radiation, or pipe exit noise. Where solids in the form of powders or granules, or liquids in droplet form are conveyed substantial attenuation can occur along the pipe.

Flow regulatory vanes or dampers are common causes of noise, both as a result of the air flow over them and of their ability to change the flow conditions of a fan and perhaps make it operate in the stall regime. The presence of the nearly closed damper can then, if the normal degree of bad luck exists, form a resonant length in the pipe system which is excited by the flow instability of the stalled fan.

Where discrete obstructions, such as vanes or bars at right angles to the flow occur, discrete frequency noise at a frequency of approximately $0.2\,v/d$ (v = fluid velocity, d = effective diameter of obstruction) can occur. This can be a particular problem in tube heat exchangers, resulting in unwanted noise and fatigue failures of tubes. For problems to occur it is usually necessary for the vortex generation frequency to coincide with the natural frequency in bending of the tubes or with the frequency of a transverse mode of the airspace contained in the heat exchanger. Flow regulating valves in liquid systems can cause broad band noise due to turbulence generation at points where pressure is dropped. This can be minimised by 'streamlining' the flow passages. Discrete frequency noises can be generated by instability of valve spools caused either by the design of feedback mechanisms or the presence of unwanted friction forces. Low noise is a matter of good basic design and good matching to the rest of the hydraulic system.

5.6. High Speed Rotation of Irregularly Shaped Bodies

High speed rotation of irregularly shaped bodies can produce noise of two types. In the absence of any obstructions close to the rotating body the oscillation of the surface presented to a stationary observer acts as a noise source in its own right.

Rotating bodies act as inefficient air displacement devices because air close to the surface is accelerated by friction forces and thrown off by centrifugal action, thus requiring further air to be entrained to maintain equilibrium. Should the surface irregularities of the rotating body be of periodic shape the displaced air will be discharged in discrete streams which will interact with nearby objects and produce noise in a way similar to the blade passing phenomena with fans.

5.7. Bearings

Significant noise from bearings normally arises from the response of the structure supporting the bearings to impacts within the bearings. Occasionally direct airborne noise will be radiated, for instance from the cage of a rolling element bearing. Whilst the impact process is common to most bearing systems the way in which the impacts arise differs from one bearing type to another.

The quietest types of bearings are usually journal bearings, pressure lubricated with gas or liquid lubricant. The journal runs on a continuous film of lubricant between the journal and bush or shell, which prevents metal to metal contact and evens out any minor irregularities in shape of the bearing parts. In hydrodynamic bearings the 'wedge' of fluid between journal and bush is generated by the rotation of the shaft itself. If the shaft is subjected to oscillatory loads causing it to move rapidly across its clearance in the bush, it is likely that some degree of impact noise will occur as it reaches the limit of travel, because the lubricant wedge takes a finite time to build up and may not be able to become fully developed before metal to metal contact occurs. Hydrostatic lubrication systems should reduce this problem because of the continuous presence of a pumped lubricant film all around the bearing and the greater stiffness of the bearing film. Instability of shaft systems running within journal bearings is often a cause of noise, which itself can be a sign of bearing wear. Even in non-reciprocating machinery shaft and rotors can be subjected to forced motions which cause radial movements within bearings.

Rolling element bearings may appear superficially to offer the best chance of achieving low noise operation. This may be so if high precision bearings are used under well controlled conditions. However, any irregularities in bearing, housing or shaft manufacture which cause departure from true circularity introduce oscillatory forces into the system. Any damage caused to the rolling elements introduces a repetitive impulsive input. There is the possibility of excitation of five different frequencies and their harmonics due to rolling element bearing action. It is most unlikely that all of these would appear in the noise signature of a machine. All machine structures act as frequency selective amplifiers and will accentuate some frequencies at the expense of others. Rolling element bearings are very susceptible to damage caused by careless fitting, dirty lubricants or corrosion, the remedies for which are obvious.

Placement of bearings within a machine structure can affect noise radiation. It is poor practice to put a bearing in the middle of a large panel-like structure which would act as an excellent 'loud-speaker'. Additionally, if bearings are positioned in parts of the structure which are of low stiffness they will fail to provide adequate support for their shafts which could cause excessive noise generation from, for instance, gears.

5.8. Gears

An ideal involute gear pair, perfectly machined, and mounted on infinitely stiff shafts in an infinitely stiff housing should produce little noise because no impacts or sliding between gear teeth should take place, only rolling of one gear face on another, These ideal conditions never occur and to a large extent the noise of gears is determined by the accuracy with which they are made and supported. Typically gear noise is radiated at tooth contact frequency (input shaft speed multiplied by number of teeth on input gears) and its harmonics, indicating the presence of a train of impacts or short duration events as the teeth engage. Gear noise is usually radiated via structure-borne transmission to the casing. In the case of non-enclosed gears it may be radiated from the gears themselves. Insufficient or excess lubrication can also cause excessive noise.

Strategies for the control of gear noise are: new helical gears rather than straight spur gears, provide rigid supports and rigid shafts, relieve gear tooth tips, grind tooth faces with convex shape to control contact position, and avoid having casing natural frequencies at or close to gear tooth mesh frequencies.

5.9. Electrical Machines

Electrically induced vibrations can be divided into two sub-sections.

1. Magneto strictive noise arises in transformers as a result of core lamination vibration. It also arises in motors on start-up. With a 50 Hz supply frequency it is predominantly at 100 Hz.
2. Noise due to rotating electric fields occurs in electric motors. The motive force causing rotation of the rotor of an electric motor is not

constant. It varies with time depending on the design of the rotor and stator windings. This can induce vibration of the motor casing which causes noise, especially if the frequency of generation of the forces coincides with a resonance of the motor structure or casing. A motor designer should ensure that this does not occur.

Direct current motors tend to suffer from brush noise, which is a mechanical impact problem caused by the brushes bouncing off the irregular surface of the commutator.

5.10. Stick–Slip Motions

The main example of motions which may be put into this class is brake and clutch squeal. Many theories have been advanced as to exactly how this squeal is generated, but all seek to explain how the sliding friction between a moving object and a stationary one can change rapidly from a condition of gripping to a condition of slipping. These rapid changes cause the structure to vibrate and radiate noise. In the case of a vehicle disc brake it is primarily disc vibration which generates the noise but the brake calliper supporting structure also vibrates. Lack of rigidity of pads or shoes tends to promote noise. Such squeals and squeaks tend to be very difficult to investigate because they often depend on the establishment of exactly the right conditions for their onset. Merely removing parts and replacing them can easily make the noise disappear, at least temporarily.

5.11. Impacts Generated as Part of Machine Operation

Noise is radiated by a number of mechanisms during impact, amongst them expulsion of air from between the impact faces and vibration of the structure supporting the impacting elements. The latter is usually the predominant source of noise. The magnitude of impact noise is closely related to the duration of the energy transfer between impacting surfaces. This can be enhanced by the subsequent resonant 'ringing' of the structure. Where possible, then, the duration of an impact should be as long as possible to reduce noise and any associated structure should be as heavily damped as possible. All impacts which are not essential for the performance of useful work should be eliminated.

Figure 4 shows the time history of noise radiated by a typical press. The presence of noise caused by the useful event can be seen, and also noise caused by other events in the press cycle which make no direct contribution to the forming of the product.

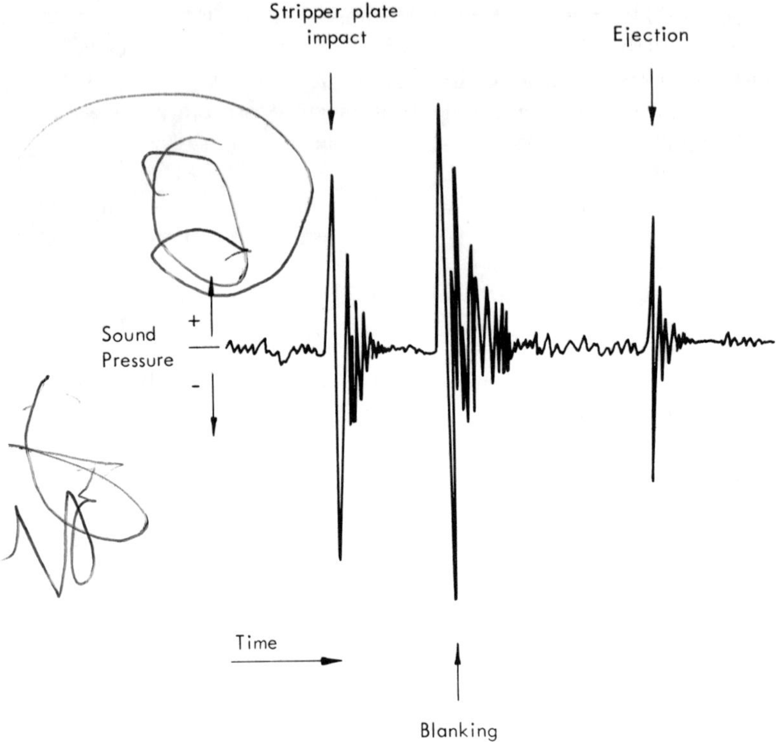

FIG. 4. Simplified oscillogram of noise measured during one stroke of a blanking press, showing three noise events per stroke.

6. NOISE CONTROL BY EXTERNAL TREATMENT

With the present state of the art it is quite often impossible or impractical to control noise at source so external means must be sought.

6.1. Enclosures

To enclose a noisy machine in a box is a superficially simple exercise but abounds with potential problems, such as the need for ventilation, access for personnel and materials and prevention of build-up of combustible or toxic gases.

Fundamental requirements of an enclosure are that its walls must have adequate mass, and sometimes stiffness, to stop sound getting through, that it must be supplied with adequate internal acoustic absorption to prevent the build-up of high levels of reverberant sound inside the enclosure, and that it must be isolated from vibrations produced by the enclosed machine. The transmission loss of heavy impervious materials which would be used for enclosure walls is frequency dependent, being least at the resonant frequencies of the panels of the walls. Figure 5 shows the way transmission loss varies with frequency. Thus enclosures are usually most effective at

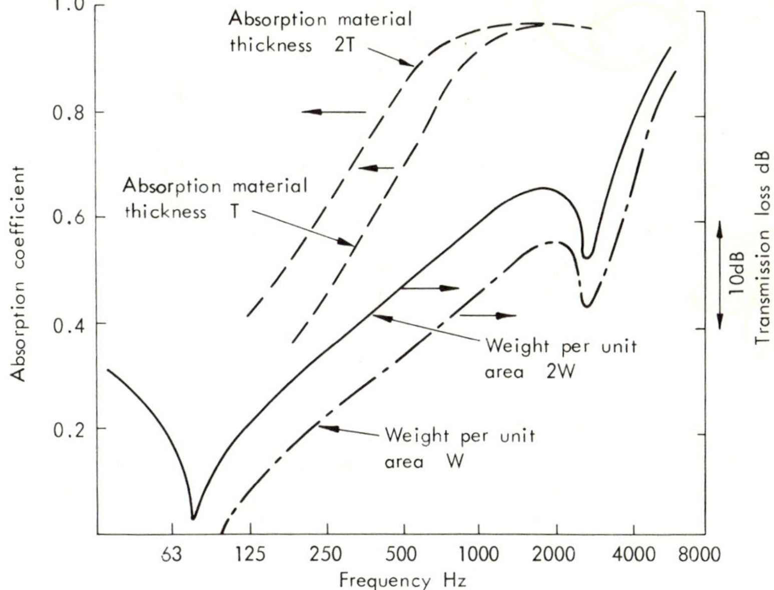

Fig. 5. Typical frequency dependence of absorption coefficients of porous materials and transmission loss of non-porous panel materials.

higher frequencies, and when they have heavy walls. When enclosing sources of very low frequency sound it is sometimes advantageous to concentrate on providing a high wall stiffness, to raise the panel resonance frequencies, rather than high mass.

The absorption characteristics of porous materials, such as mineral or glass wool or open cell plastic foams, are also frequency dependent, as shown in Fig. 5, which again means that the enclosure is likely to be most efficient at higher frequencies. To lower the frequency of effective absorption the thickness of absorption materials must be increased, or they can be fitted over an air space. Absorption materials must be chosen with care to avoid possible problems with combustibility, fibre fall out, emission of toxic fumes when burnt, fluid absorption, cleanability, temperature resistance, cost and mechanical strength.

In most cases it is possible to protect the absorption material with a perforated sheet or metal mesh without significant loss of effectiveness. It is sometimes possible to prevent fluid contamination or improve cleanability by facing the absorbent with a very thin plastic film.

6.2. Silencers

When ventilation is required it is no good just leaving a hole in the side of the enclosure. A small hole will cause a very great degradation in enclosure performance. An adequate silencer must be fitted. This would normally be some sort of duct lined with absorption material and possibly fitted with longitudinal baffles or 'splitters' of absorption material. The performance of such a device depends on the thickness of absorption material, the ratio of airway width to absorption material thickness and the length of the silencer. Several varieties of silencer are shown in Fig. 6. Many types and sizes are available as proprietary items from noise control hardware companies. When air is blown through a silencer some turbulence is

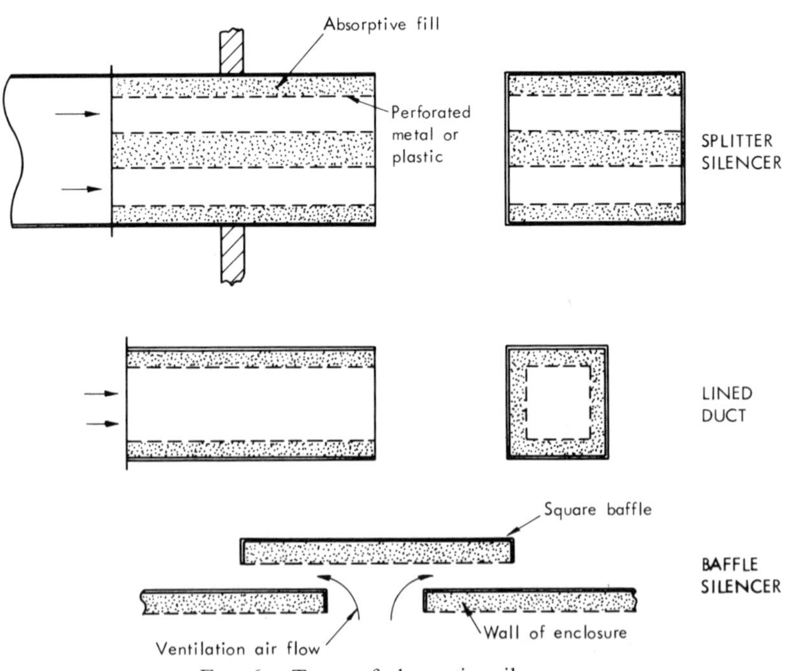

FIG. 6.   Types of absorptive silencer.

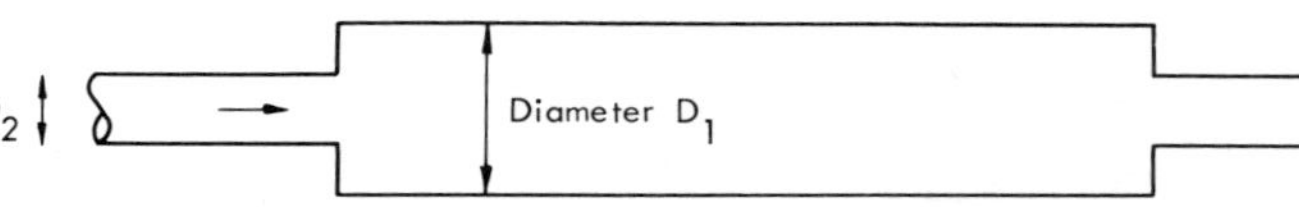

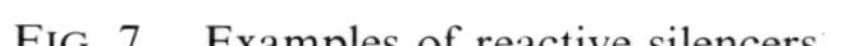

FIG. 7. Examples of reactive silencers.

generated which causes silencer self noise. A silencer should be selected such that the self noise is not significant.

The performance of silencers is frequency dependent, being relatively poor at low frequencies. The choice of silencer is usually dictated by the silencing requirement in the 125 or 250 Hz octave band. This often results in substantial 'overkill' at higher frequencies.

Special low frequency silencers can be made on the reactive principle (Fig. 7), in which expansion chambers of specific sizes are inserted into duct systems. These are frequency selective devices, which amplify some frequencies and reflect others back towards the source. The dimensions must be chosen so that the rejection frequencies coincide with peaks in the frequency spectrum of the noise to be silenced. Single expansion chambers are usually only of use to deal with tonal noise sources with only one predominant frequency component. Suitably designed multiple expansion chambers can provide varying degrees of attenuation over a wide frequency range.

Large expansion chambers lined with absorption material (usually called plenum chambers) can act as efficient silencers over a wide frequency range.

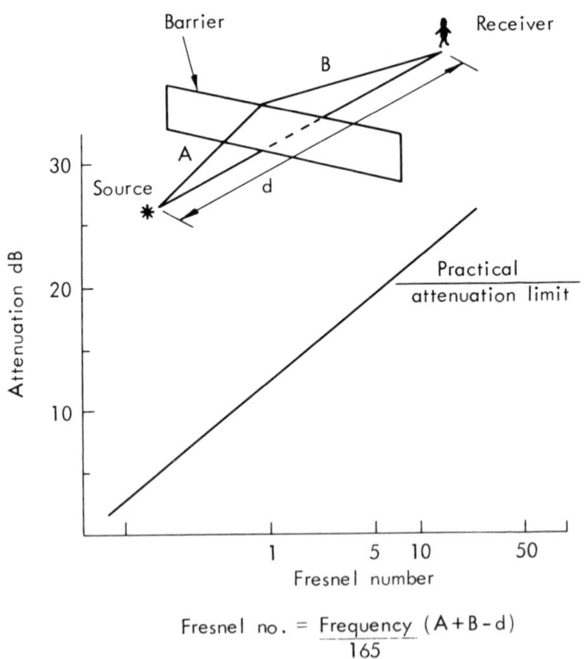

$$\text{Fresnel no.} = \frac{\text{Frequency } (A + B - d)}{165}$$

Fig. 8.   Chart for calculation of barrier attenuation.

6.3. Barriers and Incomplete Enclosures

Except in highly reverberant spaces some form of barrier between a noise source and receiver to interrupt the passage of direct sound can be beneficial. Such barriers are only effective where the direct sound is appreciably louder than sound arriving via reflected paths which would not be intercepted by the barrier. The attenuation of direct sound given by a barrier depends on the difference in path length between sound travelling over the barrier and the shortest path between source and receiver, see Fig. 8. The performance is also frequency dependent, being poor at low frequencies.

The simplest barrier consists of a simple wall, but may be improved in some cases by being wrapped round the source to form sides and a roof, i.e. an open ended box. This will effectively attenuate direct sound on the closed sides but will increase the amount of sound radiated in the direction of the open end. Addition of absorption inside the box will reduce this amplification. An open ended enclosure usually does not need to be specially ventilated but is only useful in a non reflective environment.

7. PERSONAL NOISE PROTECTION

In the absence of any better ways of protecting personnel from noise either the people themselves may be shut into a box or control cabin, which can provide a low noise haven where appropriate, or they can be provided with hearing protectors.

A wide range of ear plugs and ear muffs are available on the market. They vary tremendously in their sound attenuating properties, their durability and their comfort of use. In common with most other noise control devices their attenuation is frequency dependent, relatively poor at low frequencies, better at mid and high frequencies. Typical attenuations of ear muffs and ear plugs are shown in Fig. 9.

The actual attenuation achieved also depends on the quality of fit on the user. This variability of attenuation must be borne in mind when selecting hearing protectors for any application. The standard method of test BS 5108[6] is intended to give a measure of variability of attenuation as well as average attenuation. Hearing protectors should be selected such that the average attenuation minus one standard deviation of attenuation is sufficient to reduce the noise impinging on the wearers ears to a level less than the hearing damage risk criterion.

To avoid risk of infection great care must be taken over cleanliness of hearing protectors.

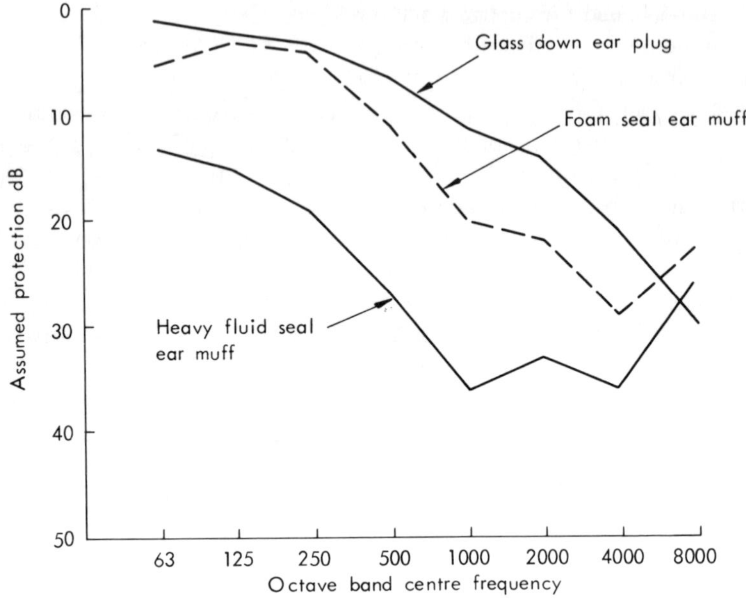

FIG. 9.   Assumed protection given by various types of hearing protection. (Mean attenuation is generally 4 to 6 dB greater than the assumed protection.)

Ear plugs tend to produce relatively low attenuation and may be considered suitable when the noise is up to 5 dB(A) higher than the damage risk criterion. At noise levels above that it is safer to assume that ear muffs will be required.

The most difficult aspect of hearing protection is the enforcement of its use, but no hearing protector can provide efficient protection unless it is used, and used all the time that the noise is present. Because of the discomfort and nuisance value of hearing protection and the need for constant supervision it is most desirable to institute noise reduction measures as soon as possible.

8.   BUILDING DESIGN OR MODIFICATION IN RELATION TO INDUSTRIAL NOISE

The design and layout of an industrial building can have a substantial influence on noise and vibration inside and outside the factory. The noise to which people working in the factory are exposed will depend on the juxtaposition of noisy and quiet machines and processes. Wherever possible noisy machines or processes should be grouped together and isolated from other activities. This minimises the number of people exposed to high or annoying noise and eases the burden of supervision in enforcing the use of hearing protection if it is necessary. Even the presence of a parts storage area with stacked parts containers can form a surprisingly effective barrier between noisy operations and quieter areas.

The amount of acoustic absorption in the factory space controls the way sound is propagated around the space. With little absorption the sound level will tend to be fairly uniform and the noise from noisy machines will be significant everywhere as a result of multiple reflections from wall and ceilings. In a highly absorbent space the sound received by a listener will only be direct sound and will decay at 4 to 6 dB per doubling of distance from the source. This shows us that if the workshop concerned contains a large number of machines each producing a similar level of noise for its operator the addition of acoustic absorption will have relatively little effect (1–3 dB(A)) on the noise exposure of the operators. However, in a space with a few machines and with other people involved in quiet tasks the addition of absorption could have a significant effect on noise received by the quiet operations. It would not have much effect on the noise received by the machine operators. Whether the addition of absorption would be the correct solution in this case depends on the relative costs and convenience compared with, say, enclosure or relocation of the few noisy machines. Addition of absorption often tends to have a greater effect on the subjective acceptability of factory spaces than it does on the measured noise level. The addition of large amounts of absorption in large buildings such as car assembly halls has been claimed to have brought substantial benefits, although at considerable cost.

To prevent noise radiating outside the factory it is necessary to ensure that the transmission loss of the walls and roof is sufficient. This may mean bricking up windows and strictly controlling opening of doors. Roofs and eaves are often weak points. Lightweight corrugated or profiled sheet walls may have insufficient transmission loss unless backed up by an inner skin of plasterboard or similar heavy sheet material. Similar acoustic reinforcement of light roofs may be necessary. Acoustic absorption inside the factory can be of benefit to external noise if it reduces the sound level falling on the inner surface of the wall.

Failure to control peripheral noisy activities outside an otherwise well designed quiet factory can nullify efforts made elsewhere to control noise. Inadequately silenced cooling fans, fork lift trucks, delivery vehicles and noisy waste handling are common causes of complaint. Radiation of ground borne vibration from factories tends to be difficult to predict and difficult to analyse in detail. Propagation can be via surface waves or body waves in the soil, all of which travel at different velocities and can be reflected by subsoil interfaces and surface features. Ground borne vibration problems are likely to be encountered within a few hundred feet of large impact machines such as drop forges, unless suitable precautions are taken.

9. VIBRATION CONTROL

In many cases noise and vibration control are intimately related because noise results from vibration. At the lower end of the frequency scale, particularly below a frequency of 20 Hz, the noise radiated is unlikely to be a problem but vibration felt by people may be. Limits for vibration have already been mentioned. Possible means of reduction of vibration are described in Sections 9.1. to 9.5.

9.1. Balance
It is likely that all rotating machinery will need to be balanced. Dynamic (multi-plane) balancing is often necessary. Reciprocating machinery should also be balanced. This may be achieved to some degree with reciprocating or rotating weights, but complete balance is sometimes difficult to achieve.

9.2. Avoidance of Excitation of Structural Resonances
It is essential that structural resonance frequencies fall outside the range of frequencies generated by rotation or reciprocation of out of balance masses. To prevent annoyance of a surrounding community by ground borne vibration the resonant frequencies of the machine and its foundations on the spring of the soil should also be outside the operating frequency range.

Any processes which involve high levels of impact are likely to produce ground borne vibration problems because the resonant frequency of the machine and its foundations on the soil is bound to be excited to some degree. Vibration isolation of the foundation block may be necessary. Design of such systems is highly specialised.

9.3. Vibration Isolation
Vibration isolation may be desirable in many instances. It consists essentially of the interposition of a resilient link between the source of the

vibration and the receiver. The stiffness of the resilient link has to be chosen carefully such that the resonant frequency of the isolated system acting on the resilient link is below about half the input frequency, in the case of regularly repeating inputs, or as low as possible in the case of impulsive inputs. Particular difficulty arises if the supporting structure for the whole system is resilient or of insufficient mass. Here lies the problem when the isolation of ground borne vibration is attempted. The natural frequencies of equipment on the ground tend to be in the range from 5 to 20 Hz, as do the natural frequencies of buildings (the houses in which complainants live). It is, therefore, necessary to use very low frequency isolation systems to provide effective attenuation and these can cause problems with lack of stability and excessive movement.

The resilient links in vibration isolation systems may consist of rubber mountings, metal springs, air springs, cork or other resilient materials. For systems with natural frequencies below 5 Hz metal springs or air springs will usually be necessary. The lowest practical natural frequency is about 1 Hz. For systems above 5 Hz rubber springs are suitable. For systems above 10 Hz less resilient materials such as cork composition may be suitable as well.

In the selection of resilient materials consideration must be given to temperature and corrosion resistance, fluid contamination resistance, long term creep, load carrying capacity, overload capacity and available ratios of stiffness in mutually perpendicular directions. The design parameters of vibration isolated systems are commonly described by the natural frequency in a vertical direction, but most practical vibration isolated systems have six natural frequencies which need to be considered.

9.4. Damping

The role of damping in noise and vibration control is commonly misunderstood. The application of damping to a system limits the amount of amplification which occurs when that system is vibrated at its resonant frequency and also increases the rate of decay of free vibration after the stimulus is removed. Damping is, therefore, useful in the control of vibration from impulsive sources. It is also useful to limit the motion of a system which is inescapably vibrated at its resonant frequency. Limited damping is useful in vibration isolation systems during starting and stopping of machines, when the excitation frequency inevitably runs through the mounted resonance frequency, but an excess of damping reduces the vibration isolation available during normal running.

Damping can be provided by friction, relative motion of the surfaces of visco-elastic materials or displacement of fluid through orifices or valves. In most cases friction damping is the least desirable option.

9.5. Dynamic Absorbers

A special case of motion limitation, analogous to damping, is the application of dynamic absorbers. These consist of a subsidiary mass spring system attached to a body and vibrating at its resonant frequency. By choosing the subsidiary mass to be 5 to 10% of the main mass and the subsidiary spring to give a sub-system resonant frequency approximately the same as the main system resonance, considerable limitation of motion of the main mass occurs. The subsidiary mass moves in antiphase to the main mass and over a large amplitude such that the inertia forces acting on the small mass balance those on the large mass. This provides very substantial reduction of the motion of the main mass over a narrow band of frequency. Addition of damping to the subsystem increases the frequency range over which it is active but reduces the maximum effect at the tuned frequency. Such systems always exhibit two small peaks in vibration response at frequencies either side of the original main system resonance. The relative magnitudes of these small peaks depend on details of the dynamic absorber design.

10.   PERSONAL PROTECTION AGAINST VIBRATION

Where vibration cannot be controlled at source it may be necessary to control it close to the receiver. Examples of such techniques are the suspension seats used in agricultural tractors and some commercial vehicles, flexible mats for operators who must stand on vibrating platforms, and resilient hand grips or handle systems for hand-held vibrating machines such as chain saws.

In no way can these devices produce magical solutions to problems. Isolation of low frequency vibration can only be achieved with systems which allow large deflections. The tractor seat allows deflections of several centimetres and so can isolate the driver from the large amplitude low frequency motions of the tractor. The seat must be equipped with substantial damping to prevent violent excitation of resonant motions caused by sudden jerks of the tractor. A device such as a floor mat or tool handle cannot provide low frequency isolation because its available deflection is limited to a few millimetres.

11. NOISE AND VIBRATION SPECIFICATIONS

When purchasing machinery or equipment it is not prudent to merely hope that it will not be too noisy or produce too much vibration. In the same way that the machine's required operating performance (e.g. horsepower, speed, etc.) may be detailed in a specification so should its noise output. When examined in detail the requirements for a comprehensive noise or vibration specification are numerous and too detailed to mention here. This arises because of the large number of so called 'standard' methods of measurement there are, the possible influences of other noise or vibration sources and the continuing lack of knowledge of many suppliers in noise and vibration matters.

As an example of the need to think carefully about noise specifications consider the case of the purchase of machine tools for a workshop in which the noise level must not exceed 90 dB(A). It would be no good merely to purchase machines whose noise output did not exceed 90 dB(A), because the operator of one machine would receive noise from his own machine and from all the others in the workshop, depending on how far away they were and on the acoustical conditions in the workshop. It is difficult to measure noise with an accuracy of better than ± 1 dB(A), so to be sure of not exceeding 90 dB(A) in our completed workshop the individual machine specification must allow for this. Machine tool manufacturers build machines but do not often supply the tools to be used on them and may not know that components are to be machined. Noise radiated from the component during machining may be greater than the noise of the machine itself, but the machine manufacturer could hardly be blamed for that. As a result of these and many other considerations it is necessary to specify that for an average workshop the noise of any one machine running alone shall not exceed 83 dB(A) if the noise in the workshop is not to exceed 90 dB(A). Noise measurements are usually made at 1 m from the machine. It is most important that the measurement distance is specified but 1 m may not be relevant in all cases.

12. EXAMPLES OF LOW NOISE AND LOW VIBRATION MACHINES AVAILABLE

The list below is a selection of equipment which is now normal or may be purchased 'off the shelf', with a brief note as to how noise has been reduced. The list does not include everything available and it is to be hoped that it soon becomes out of date as a result of the advances in noise control engineering.

> Fans—better aerodynamic design of impellors, lower tip speeds, silencers.
>
> Electric motors—quieter cooling fans, fan silencers, improved structural design techniques to reduce electromagnetic noise radiation, improved lamination steel.
>
> Air compressors—packaged units with enclosures and silencers, antivibration mounting.
>
> Road drills—exhaust silencers and drill jackets, damped tools.
>
> Generator sets—enclosure, engine silencers, fan noise reduction, antivibration mounting.
>
> Teletypes, typewriters, etc.—enclosures, control of impact noise, fan and motor noise.
>
> Gas control valves—redesign of internal parts to raise the frequency of noise generation to one in which the pipe walls give greater attenuation: redesign of internal parts to produce pressure loss by viscous friction rather than turbulent expansion through a nozzle.
>
> Commercial Road Vehicles (internal cab noise)—vibration isolation of cabs and engines, improved induction and exhaust silencers, application of damping materials and absorption materials inside.
>
> Chain saws—vibration control by handle design and resilient hand grips.

REFERENCES

1. Code of practice for the reduction of exposure of employed persons to noise, HMSO, London, 1972.
2. (a) DD43 *Guide to the evaluation of exposure of the human hand arm system to vibration*, British Standards Institution, London, 1975. (b) DIS 5349 *Principle for the measurement and evaluation of human exposure to vibration transmitted to the hand* VDC 534.1: 614.872.5, International Organisation for Standardisation, 1979.
3. ISO 2631-1974 *Guide for the evaluation of human exposure to whole body vibration* UDC 534.1: 612.014.4, International Organisation for Standardisation, 1974.
4. DIN 45635 *Gerauschmessumg an Maschinen*, Beuth Vertrieb GmbH, Berlin, 1978.
5. Section 15 Workshops Ordinance, Federal Republic of Germany, 20 Mar. 1975.
6. BS 5108 *Method for the measurement of real ear attenuation at threshold of hearing protectors*, British Standards Institution, London, 1974.

Chapter 4

MEASUREMENT AND CONTROL OF SULPHUR DIOXIDE EMISSIONS

J. R. TAGG, B.Sc.(London), C.Eng., M.I.E.E.

*Lecturer in Engineering Mechanics, The Open University,
Milton Keynes, UK*

SUMMARY

The emission of sulphur dioxide from burning fossil fuels continues to rise, and European countries are now more ready to recognise the significance of the resulting environmental damage. A knowledge of ambient concentrations is obviously necessary for effective control of emissions at source, and here descriptions are given of the methods for surveying average daily ground level concentrations, for reference and for measurement over shorter periods. Methods for removing sulphur dioxide from flue gases are still being actively developed. Here outline descriptions have been given of a representative selection of methods that may ultimately prove to be the basis of practical success.

1. INTRODUCTION

Of all the gaseous pollutants which affect air quality, compounds based on sulphur are the most widespread and generally considered to be the most important. Of these, sulphur dioxide (SO_2) is produced by most fossil fuels when they are burnt for generating electric power, for heating or for road transport. Lesser amounts are released during the refining of petroleum, the smelting of sulphur-contaminated metal ores, especially copper, lead and zinc, the manufacture of industrial products, e.g. paper, sulphuric acid, etc., and the incineration of refuse.

97

Many different estimates have been made of the total amount of sulphuric acid discharged into the atmosphere, but they all seem to fall within the range of 100–150 million tonnes per year from man-made sources. Most of these emissions arise from industrial areas; some six million tonnes per year are discharged into the air over the United Kingdom, whilst the corresponding total for the United States is more than 33 million tonnes. Yet vast as these emissions are, it has been estimated that natural emissions of sulphur dioxide from volcanoes, the decomposition of organic material and sea spray, may amount in total to more than double the quantity discharged from man-made sources.

Sulphur dioxide, a colourless gas, can be detected in air by taste at a concentration between 1 and 3 milligrams per cubic metre ($mg\,m^{-3}$). At higher concentrations most people find it has a pungent irritating smell. Sulphur dioxide is extremely soluble; at normal temperatures, water will dissolve over 10% of its own weight of sulphur dioxide. When discharged from combustion sources, sulphur dioxide is usually accompanied by a small proportion of sulphur trioxide (SO_3). Once discharged into the atmosphere, oxidation of SO_2 to SO_3 continues. As water droplets or vapour are invariably present this leads to the formation of sulphuric acid. The processes involved include photochemical reactions in the presence of hydrocarbons, catalytic oxidation promoted by the presence of manganese or iron compounds in airborne particulate material, and finally reactions with ammonia and other basic compounds to form airborne sulphates.

As sulphur dioxide disperses downwind from each source, it tends to be absorbed by vegetation, or dissolved in any film of moisture or at the surface of rivers, lakes and the sea. Sulphur dioxide is also readily adsorbed onto many dry surfaces, especially those of buildings. But the main mechanism for the removal of sulphur oxides and the other sulphur compounds from the atmosphere is by precipitation in rain.

The release of these enormous quantities of SO_2 and other sulphur compounds can lead to widespread damage to buildings, to metal structures and vehicles and to many articles in everyday use. Vegetation is injured, crops are damaged and air pollution by sulphur compounds plays its part in damaging human health. For all these reasons it is now widely recognised that the emission of sulphur dioxide to the atmosphere should be subject to much more stringent control, and it is in this context that measurement has an essential role. The text which follows describes those methods of measuring ground level concentrations of sulphur dioxide that are either already in widespread use or seem likely to be in frequent use in the 1980s.

2. MEASUREMENT

Measurement of the concentrations of sulphur dioxide and the other sulphur compounds are made for any one or more of the following reasons:

(1)   identifying or assessing trends in average ground level concentrations,
(2)   evaluating particular emission control strategies,
(3)   confirming compliance with emission standards,
(4)   activating specific measures to reduce pollution emissions during adverse meteorological conditions,
(5)   evaluating risks to human health or environmental damage, or for other research purposes,
(6)   investigating complaints of excessive emissions,
(7)   validating models of the pollution dispersion process, and
(8)   collecting data to facilitate land-use planning.

In contrast to these obvious direct needs, the measured concentrations of sulphur dioxide may be used as a convenient index of the general level of industrial air pollution and also of the probable presence of other air pollutants whose actual concentration is less easy to measure directly.

Sulphur dioxide concentrations may be measured either directly in the combusion gases passing up the chimney stack before discharge, or at ground level after their dispersal and dilution in the atmosphere. Alternatively, remote measurements may be made high in the atmosphere as part of a research study of some aspect of the dispersion process. Concentrations of sulphur oxides in flue gases may be of the order of $10 \, \mathrm{gm^{-3}}$, but at the other extreme after dispersion in the atmosphere, the background level of sulphur dioxide may be only around $10 \, \mu\mathrm{g\,m^{-3}}$.

Finally, therefore, in assessing the suitability of any measurement method for its intended purpose, various other characteristics must be taken into account. They include:

(1)   the basic sensitivity,
(2)   the accuracy of the measurement (and the linearity of indicated response to different concentrations over the likely range of occurrence),
(3)   the need for a continuous indication, or the duration of the period over which a single measurement is to be averaged,
(4)   the speed of response to changing concentration,
(5)   the extent to which other substances can interfere with the accuracy of the measurement,

(6) the way in which the measured data are obtained, presented or recorded, and

(7) the convenience and cost of performing the sequence of measurements.

2.1. Static Collectors

One of the earliest methods of assessing trends in pollution by sulphur oxides, and one that is still in widespread use in the 1980s, involves the exposure of a quantity of lead dioxide paste on an inert gauze fabric wrapped round a porcelain cylinder. This constitutes the traditional lead dioxide candle, first introduced in the UK in 1932 and currently specified in reference 1. Exposed for a typical period of a month or so in a protective louvred screen, the lead dioxide paste is converted to lead sulphate at a rate that is roughly proportional to the atmospheric concentration of sulphur oxides. The result of an analytical determination of lead sulphate is then expressed as a weight in milligrams of sulphur trioxide per $100\,cm^2$ of exposed surface. This is obviously not a measurement of atmospheric concentration, but a simple index that can be used month by month to indicate trends in average pollution levels. Unfortunately the accuracy of the index is spoilt by the fact that the sulphation rate varies significantly with changing weather conditions, i.e. windspeed, temperature and humidity.

Huey[2] has greatly simplified the lead dioxide measurement. He developed a method of exposing the reactive material in an inverted petri dish that could simply be held by a bracket mounted on any convenient support. Performance tests showed that these plates were some 20% more reactive than the traditional candles. Liang *et al.*[3] subsequently evaluated the effectiveness of the lead peroxide method, in both configurations, for monitoring sulphur dioxide. They developed two alternative mathematical models to express the observed sulphation rates, and concluded that the rate could be adequately expressed by considering only the local concentration of sulphur dioxide. Rider *et al.*[4] then extended the study of sulphation rates to higher ambient concentrations and confirmed the factor derived by Huey for converting the sulphation rate to a local average concentration of sulphur dioxide.

2.2. Mechanised Bubblers

No review of sulphur dioxide measurement is complete without a note on the procedure used for the UK National Survey of Air Pollution which is also recommended for use in European Member states by the OECD.[5] The procedure is specified in reference 6.

A small suction pump is used to draw in a sample of ambient air through a one-volume solution of hydrogen peroxide (0.3% w/v) held in a glass Drechsel (bubbler) bottle at a rate of about $2\,m^3\,day^{-1}$. The air flow is measured by a simple gas meter. Before exposure, the hydrogen peroxide absorbing solution is first adjusted to have a pH value of 4·5 by adding a small quantity of acid or alkali as appropriate. Sulphur dioxide in the air sample is quickly oxidised and absorbed to increase the acidity of the solution. At the end of the 24 h measurement period, a standardised dilute alkali solution is used to readjust the pH value to 4·5. The titration measurement is carried out using either a convenient colour indicator or a pH electrode and meter to indicate the end point. The amount of alkali used is then a direct measure of the sulphur dioxide absorbed from the air sample.

The starting pH value of 4·5 is selected because it is below the pH value of the acidity formed by carbon dioxide in solution, and interference by this gas is thereby prevented. In some country districts, the presence of ammonia can reduce the apparent concentration of SO_2. If ammonia is suspected, the amount can be determined independently. It is rare for other alkaline or acid gases to interfere with the hydrogen peroxide method of measurement.

In the UK instruments the sample of ambient air is first drawn through a paper filter to collect particulate material, and this filter will also retain small droplets of acid mists so that they do not contribute to the acidity of the peroxide solution in the Drechsel bottle. The amount of sulphuric acid trapped on filter papers in this way can be estimated by using a procedure described by Commins.[7] Killick,[8] of the Warren Spring Laboratory, has outlined four other more sensitive, but non-specific methods for determining the concentration of sulphuric acid in the atmosphere on a routine basis. Unfortunately three of them have the disadvantage that they require the use of expensive equipment and trained personnel.

The need for operator supervision can be reduced by using an installation of eight sample bottles and filter papers. An automatic valve is then arranged to bring a fresh bottle into use each day sequentially through the week. With this device in use the measuring site need then be visited no more frequently than once a week.

The UK National Survey of Air Pollution is co-ordinated by staff of the Warren Spring Laboratory, Stevenage, who recently reviewed the sampling arrangements at the National Survey sites,[9] and the accuracy of the titration measurements.[10] The authors concluded that, disregarding the effects of interference by ammonia, 70 % of the individual determinations were likely to be within 15 μg m^{-3} of the correct value and over 85 % within 30 μg m^{-3}. There was evidence to show that some measurements could be grossly in error by as much as 100 μg m^{-3}, but it was not thought that there was any systematic under- or over-estimation by individual operators. Weatherley[9] drew particular attention to the need for the regular replacement of air sampling lines which should be of a suitable grade of material. This subject has been reviewed much more fully by Wohlers et al.[11] who showed that Teflon, polypropylene, PVC, glass, aluminium and stainless steel were all suitable materials for the inlet sample lines.

Having used hydrogen peroxide to collect and absorb sulphur dioxide, there are several alternative ways in which the amount of SO_2 can be determined, and the measurement of the electrical conductivity of the solution is one long-established method. The Thomas Autometer was described in 1946[12] and there have since been many variants of this convenient but non-specific instrument technique. The determination relies on an assumption that the increase in conductivity of the solution is due only to the absorption of sulphur dioxide, whereas many other substances can cause this increase and interfere with the measurement.

In 1969, Rodes et al.[13] and Palmer et al.[14] reported the results of an extensive laboratory and field evaluation of the performance characteristics of 12 commercial instruments designed for continuously recording concentrations of sulphur dioxide; their tests included eight conductivity-measuring instruments produced by six different manufacturers. After calibration, each instrument was tested for interference effects produced by nine common pollutant gases on the measurement of SO_2. Ammonia, chlorine, hydrochloric acid and nitrogen dioxide all caused serious measurement errors, but the effects of ozone, nitric oxide, hydrogen sulphide and carbon dioxide were apparently of little significance. Carbon monoxide had no effect. Ammonia was particularly troublesome for the conductivity instruments, as explained by Marshall[15] in his comprehensive survey of interference effects on the determination of SO_2 levels in the atmosphere. The initial effect of interference by ammonia is to neutralise the sulphur dioxide and produce ammonium sulphate and so reduce conductivity. Beyond that stage, additional ammonia forms ammonium hydroxide which then increases the electrical conductivity of the solution in the collecting cell.

The laboratory study by Rodes et al.[13] produced many interesting data on the stability, sensitivity, lag and response time to changing concentrations of SO_2. The collection efficiency of all the instruments was uniformly high. The field trial reported by Palmer *et al.*[14] then provided practical information on calibration drift and the correlation between instruments, as well as the maintenance requirements and associated operating costs.

In the United Kingdom, Cummings and Redfearn[16] described the operating principles of the original conductivity instruments used by the Central Electricity Generating Board, from 1965 onwards, for monitoring the dispersal patterns of sulphur dioxide around their newly built fossil fuel fired power stations. Although in use only recently, this design of instrument is now obsolete, but the conductivity principle of measurement is still available in simplified instruments designed for portable use.

Killick[8] has also outlined several other methods for determining the amount of sulphur dioxide absorbed by the hydrogen peroxide collecting solution. Since they are both sensitive to, and effectively specific for, sulphate, they can be used when ammonia is present and the concentration of sulphur dioxide is relatively low.

2.2.1. *Use of Barium Perchlorate*

In the procedure outlined by Fritz and Yamamura[5,17] titration is performed in an 80% organic solvent with dilute barium perchlorate in the presence of thorin 1-(O-arsenophenylazo)-2-naphthol-3,6-disulphonic acid used as an indicator. The end point of the titration is rather difficult to determine so it is necessary to use a lamp and photo-electric cell to detect changes in optical density of the solution. This provides a convenient galvanometer indication so that output readings may be plotted against the amount of barium salt added to the solution. The end point of the titration is then clearly indicated by extrapolation of the plotted results. Killick reports that 10 μg of sulphur dioxide can be determined in 10 ml of aqueous solution to $\pm 10\%$.

In an alternative procedure attributed to Persson,[18] an excess of barium as barium perchlorate is added to the sample in 80% organic solvent, followed by the thorin indicator. The amount of excess barium can then be determined spectrophotometrically. In this procedure Killick reports the sensitivity for sulphur dioxide as $0.3 \mu\text{g ml}^{-1}$. If a conductivity meter or bridge is available, barium trichloroacetate can be used for the titration.[5] In this procedure, the electrical conductivity is plotted against the amount of barium salt added and again the end point is clearly indicated by an abrupt change in slope of the graph.

Yet another physical characteristic can be utilised to determine the level of sulphate in the hydrogen peroxide solution. In this instance barium chloride is added under carefully controlled conditions and the level of sulphate is estimated by measuring the turbidity in a spectrophotometer. Although the measurement is both sensitive and specific for sulphate—and thus for sulphur dioxide—the range of concentrations that can be determined in this way is restricted. Turbidimetric procedures to determine sulphate levels after precipitation as barium sulphate have been dealt with by the Interbranch Chemical Advisory Committee.[19]

2.3. A Reference Method for Determining SO$_2$

In 1971, the US Environmental Protection Agency specified the pararosaniline method for determining sulphur dioxide as the reference method to be used for comparing concentrations in the atmosphere.[20] The specified procedure is essentially the same as one of the two recommended by Scaringelli *et al.*[21] following their careful evaluation of the classic procedure first described in 1956 by West and Gaeke.[22] A considerable amount of research effort was expended in the United States to develop the procedures recommended by Scaringelli *et al.*, and to eliminate minor inconsistencies and interferences by trace substances in the atmosphere. Adams[23] has reviewed the sequence of events which led to similar procedures being recommended by the Sulfur Subcommittee of the US Intersociety Committee[24] and The American Society for Testing and Materials.[25] There was extensive collaborative testing of various aspects of the specified procedures and in 1973 Blacker *et al.*[26] concluded that the remaining differences between investigators could be attributed either to their use of alternative calibration procedures or to airborne interferences. They found that the differences were substantially reduced when permeation tubes were used for calibration instead of standardised sulphite solutions.

Eventually, in 1976, the World Health Authority selected the pararosaniline procedure as one of the two preferred methods of measuring sulphur dioxide.[27] The other was the hydrogen peroxide procedure already described.

2.3.1. *The Pararosaniline Procedure*

In outline, the sulphur dioxide is absorbed to form a stable, complex mercury compound that resists oxidation by ozone and is prevented from reacting with oxides of nitrogen. The amount of SO$_2$ absorbed is then determined colorimetrically by reacting the mercury compound with formaldehyde and a specially purified pararosaniline dye at a controlled pH value. The amount of light of a particular wavelength that is absorbed by the solution is then a direct measure of the original concentration of sulphur dioxide.

The absorbing solution is 0·04 molar strength potassium tetra-chloromercurate (TCM), made up from a solution of mercuric chloride and potassium chloride in double-distilled water. A small amount of ethylenediamine tetra-acetic acid disodium salt (usually abbreviated to EDTA) is added to prevent traces of heavy metals interfering with the measurement. The TCM solution should have a pH value of 4·0 when made up and it is normally stable for six months.

Because of the mercury content, the reagent is highly poisonous and if any is spilt on the skin it should be flushed off immediately with plenty of water. For the same reason, great care is necessary to ensure that the used reagent is disposed of safely. It is recommended that it should first be neutralised with sodium carbonate and then stirred for 24 h in contact with metallic zinc or magnesium in a protective fume cupboard. After this period, a layered solid will have formed in the bottom of the container. The liquid can be decanted and the solid dried before being placed in a suitable container for safe disposal.

10 ml of the TCM absorbing solution is placed in a small all-glass midget impinger, and a sample of air is drawn through it at a constant rate between 0·2 and 1·0 litres min^{-1}. The air flow rate, the duration of the sampling period and the volume of the absorbing solution may all be varied to take account of different conditions and the particular requirements of the measurement. Sulphur dioxide concentrations between 25 and 1000 μg m^{-3} can be measured conveniently by following the specified procedures. However, the collection efficiency, normally better than 98 %, may fall off if large air volumes are used to counteract an expected low concentration of SO_2.

It is important that the TCM absorbing solution should be protected from direct sunlight to avoid losses of SO_2 and, for the same reason, high temperatures must also be avoided. At 22 °C, the daily loss of SO_2 is only about 1 %. Care must be taken to ensure that the samples do not freeze during the collection period. After collection, the samples are transferred to a volumetric flask and set aside for 20 min to allow any ozone to decompose so that it does not interfere with the measurement. Interference by oxides of nitrogen is prevented by adding 1·0 ml of freshly made 0·6 % sulphamic acid (H_2NSO_3H) to each collected sample. This is allowed to react for 10 min to destroy any nitrite ions that may be present.

The pararosaniline dye must be specially purified to meet the following stringent specifications. At a strength of 0.2%, it must:

(1) exhibit a maximum light absorbance at a wavelength of 540 nm when assayed in a buffered solution of 0.1 molar sodium acetate–acetic acid;

(2) have a light absorbance of no more than 0.17 absorbance units, when prepared according to the prescribed procedure and tested at $22°C$ in an optical path length of 1 cm;

(3) have a calibration curve with a slope of 0.03 ± 0.002 absorbance units per μg of sulphur dioxide, when the calibration procedure with a specific sulphite solution is properly standardised.

Alternatively, the stock solution of dye may be purified, prepared and assayed according to the procedure set out by Scaringelli et al.[21] Instructions are given for adjusting the strength of the dye so that it has the specified absorbance, and it is then acidified with 3-molar strength ortho-phosphoric acid. The dye solution is then stable for at least nine months.

The collected samples of sulphur dioxide in the TCM solution are now treated with 2 ml of freshly prepared 0.2% formaldehyde solution and 5 ml of the pararosaniline dye solution. The volume of liquid in the volumetric flask is then adjusted with freshly boiled and cooled distilled water and set aside for 30 min for the dye to develop. During the following 30 min, the light absorbance of each sample solution is determined at a wavelength of 548 nm in a colorimeter or spectrophotometer, again using a 1 cm optical path length. The concentration of sulphur dioxide can then be deduced directly from the calibration curve. If, as a result of an unexpectedly high concentration of SO_2 in any sample, the dye develops a greater density than expected, it may be diluted up to six-fold with blank reagent solution. This will enable the true absorbance to be determined within 10%.

Some of the disadvantages of this reference method of SO_2 measurement are self-evident from the above description. The mercury in the absorbing reagent is highly poisonous and requires constant care to ensure that it is handled safely. The analytical procedure is relatively tedious and calls for close attention to detail if the results are to be accurate. Although the collection of samples requires only simple apparatus, their analysis calls for a well equipped analytical laboratory and a competent laboratory technician. On the other hand, the significant errors caused by the more common substances that can interfere with the measurement of SO_2 concentrations have been entirely eliminated, and it is principally for this reason that the pararosaniline method is so widely recommended. The analytical procedure can be greatly simplified by the use of automated equipment and one such instrument has been described schematically by Faith and Atkisson.[28] Instruments of a similar design are available commercially and representative versions were tested in 1968–69.[13,14]

2.4. Calibration Procedures

No matter what measurement method is adopted, what instruments are used or what procedure is followed, the results of the reference measurement must be related to the actual concentration of pollutant in the atmosphere by calibration. The reference measurement is standardised when there is a one-to-one correspondence with the true concentration.

Calibration is carried out either by using accurately produced test atmospheres of different known concentrations, or by using intermediate solutions of known standard strength. Nelson[29] and Axelrod and Lodge,[30] have described the problems of producing controlled test atmospheres and the techniques of calibration. Two selected methods are described in detail in a WHO publication.[27]

In the first procedure, a standardised sulphite solution is made up by adding a known quantity of either sodium sulphite or sodium *meta*-bisulphite to a measured quantity of recently boiled and cooled distilled water of the highest purity. The solution is unstable, so the actual concentration of sulphite is determined by accurate titration procedures in which excess iodine is added and estimated by back titration with sodium thiosulphate. When the actual strength of the sulphite solution has been determined, known amounts are added to the tetra-chloromercurate (TCM) absorbing solution to produce test samples directly equivalent to the absorption of known concentrations of sulphur dioxide from the atmosphere. These solutions are then used to derive the calibration curve of the colour density produced by the pararosaniline dye.

Alternatively, a permeation tube can be used to generate a test atmosphere having a known concentration. This is then measured in the same way as samples are taken from the atmosphere. A permeation tube is simply a small tubular container made of a permeable plastic such as PTFE which is filled with sulphur dioxide gas and sealed at either end. Provided the tube is held at a constant temperature, the SO_2 gas diffuses out of it at a low but constant rate that is determined by weighing the tube accurately at intervals. As the gas permeates out through the tube walls, it is carried along by a low flow of inert gas to a mixing chamber where it is accurately diluted by SO_2-free air to the required test concentration. The construction and preparation of permeation tubes, with explicit directions for their use in calibration procedures has been set out by Scaringelli *et al.*[31]

2.5. Other Representative Methods of Measuring SO_2

Even in the 1980s, new methods of measuring the concentrations of air pollutants are still being evolved, and this is particularly true for sulphur dioxide. Here there is space for only a small selection of the many methods that have been evolved to meet special requirements. For example, instruments designed for continuous operation in large networks must have certain special features. The following description refers to the operation of one such instrument.

2.5.1. *A Coulometric Method for Estimating SO_2 Concentrations*

This instrument was developed by Philips of Eindhoven[32] primarily for long periods of unattended operation, and it has been used in the Dutch network of monitoring stations as described by Brouwer *et al.*[33] The word coulometric is used to describe the method because it involves passing a quantity of electric charge, measured in coulombs, through an electrolytic cell. A sample of ambient air is drawn into the instrument through a dust filter at a constant rate of about $150\,ml\,min^{-1}$. The filter is heated to a temperature between 100° and 120°C. This prevents sulphur dioxide from being absorbed by moisture droplets which might otherwise condense out on the filter during foggy weather. It also prevents SO_2 adsorption onto trapped insects or dust particles. The air then passes on through a three-way valve and a second filter which contains a roll of silver gauze heated to about 120°C. This filter decomposes or reacts with other gases in the air flow such as ozone or hydrogen sulphide, and so prevents them from interfering with the measurement.

The measuring cell which holds the absorbing solution consists of an inner glass tube within and interconnected to an outer glass flask so that the liquid can pass from one to the other. The absorbing medium is a solution of potassium iodide in sulphuric acid which also contains a small quantity of free bromine molecules. The whole container is maintained at a steady temperature of 37°C. The incoming sample of air is led below the liquid surface in the inner tube. In bubbling up through the liquid, sulphur dioxide in the air is oxidised by the bromine to form negatively charged sulphate ions and negatively charged bromine ions together with an equal number of protons, i.e. positively charged hydrogen ions, according to the following reaction.

$$Br_2 + SO_2 + 2H_2O \rightarrow 2Br^- + SO_4^{2-} + 4H^+$$

Four electrodes are arranged to make contact with the liquid, two in the outer container and two in the inner tube. As the concentration of free bromine is depleted, a redox potential is developed between a platinum electrode in the central tube and a silver/silver bromide reference electrode in the outer container. The difference between this voltage signal and a reference voltage is detected by an amplifier, which is arranged to drive an electric current between the second electrode in the inner tube and an auxiliary electrode. This current, which is proportional to the out-of-balance voltage, has the effect of electrolysing the potassium iodide to restore the concentration of free bromine molecules in the solution according to the following reaction:

$$2Br^- \rightarrow Br_2 + 2\,electrons$$

For each molecule of sulphur dioxide trapped by the absorbing solution, two electrons have to be supplied to replace the free bromine split up by the first reaction. An output amplifier senses this transfer of electric charge as a current and provides an appropriate analogue output signal. The output signal is thus directly and continuously proportional to the changing concentration of sulphur dioxide in the sample of air drawn from the atmosphere.

A capillary tube in the outgoing flow line acts as a critical orifice to stabilise the air flow at about $150\,ml\,min^{-1}$. Whenever the quantity of the absorbing solution falls below a predetermined level, this is detected by a level-sensing switch which energises a Peltier cooling device in the outgoing air line. Water vapour then condenses onto the cool surface and trickles back to restore the electrolyte level in the cell. A small proportion of the free bromine is lost by evaporation and this must be continually restored by a small standing current, and there is thus a small offset on the output signal.

This highlights another feature of the Philips coulometric instrument. At predetermined intervals, e.g. twice daily, or when instructed by a remote command, the three-way air flow control valve is driven sequentially through the three positions. After the first movement, the incoming air is drawn through an extra filter holding activated charcoal. This removes all the sulphur dioxide from the air and provides an output signal indicating a zero level of SO_2.

After the second movement, the same flow of SO_2-free air is mixed with a constant quantity of sulphur dioxide gas derived from a permeation source to provide a calibrating signal representing a known concentration of SO_2. This calibration concentration is measured during routine service visits by the pararosaniline method described earlier. A third movement of the three-way valve restores the instrument to normal operation.

The analogue output signal can be recorded or sampled at convenient intervals. The overall response of the instrument, which depends on the dimensions of the inner glass tube, is fairly rapid. An output change representing 63% of a true change in sulphur dioxide concentration is indicated in about $1\frac{1}{2}$ min, and 95% of the correct indication is reached in 3 min. The sensitivity is relatively high; the instrument can be adjusted to give a full scale indication to represent 299 μg m^{-3} above an offset of about one division.

This instrument is extremely convenient in use, for it requires only infrequent supervision. When provided with reagents and a supply of electricity, it will operate for periods of weeks or even months between routine service visits. Adams[23] has described similar instruments made by other manufacturers.

2.5.2. *The Flame Photometric Detector for Sulphur Compounds*

This instrument has an even faster response than the coulometric instrument just described. When pure hydrogen is burnt in a hydrogen-rich flame in air, any molecules containing sulphur which may be present are reduced, and the resulting sulphur molecules (S_2) are excited and raised from their normal or *ground state* to a higher *energy level*. On leaving the flame the excited sulphur molecules return to their ground state and emit light radiation at wavelengths characteristic for sulphur between 300 and 420 nm. Several instruments have been developed to use this physical effect for continuously indicating the concentration of sulphur compounds in air and the Meloy flame photometric detector for total sulphur is one representative version.[34]

A low-pressure supply of hydrogen for the flame may be taken from an electrolytic hydrogen generator or from a high-pressure storage bottle via suitable reducing valves. It is essential that the flow rate should be steady, so any fluctuations are evened out by passing the gas through a capillary tube wound inside a temperature controlled block. This in turn leads into a small capacitive storage chamber connected directly to the burner chamber in the burner block. The hydrogen is ignited by a glowplug and the temperature of the burner block is maintained steady between very narrow limits under the combined control of a heater and thermo-electric cooling device.

A sample of ambient air, stabilised by a critical orifice, is drawn through the burner block to maintain the hydrogen flame. A photo-multiplier tube is mounted on the side of the block, and is arranged to sense light radiation from the region above the flame through a narrow-pass-band optical filter centred on a wavelength of 394 nm. The photo-multiplier tube is shielded from a direct view of the hydrogen flame within the block, and sees only the region immediately above it. The output response of the photo-multiplier tube to changing concentrations of sulphur in the airflow is non-linear, so the signal is passed through a log-linear amplifier.

Compounds containing phosphorus, such as agricultural pesticides, interfere with the measurement, so that if their presence is suspected they must be removed by suitable filtration techniques. Air also produces a measurable response at 394 nm, and this contributes to the unwanted background noise which must be backed off from the wanted signal.

Current versions of the instrument are now sufficiently sensitive to have a linear response within 1% to changing concentrations of sulphur dioxide over the range 0–143 μg m^{-3} (0–50 parts per US billion (10^9)). Other full scale ranges are provided up to 2860 μg m^{-3} (1 ppm). The output responds rapidly to small changes in sulphur concentration and alternative electrical time constants of 1 s and 10 s can be selected to minimise spurious noise in the output signal.

When the measurement is required to be specific for one or more particular sulphur compounds, a variety of filters may be incorporated in the inflow air line to remove other unwanted substances. Scrubbers, or molecular sieves, are now available to remove more than 98% of the hydrogen sulphide so that the instrument responds mainly to sulphur oxides. Alternatively the sulphur oxides can be removed to leave the instrument responsive only to reduced compounds of sulphur. The flame photometric detector is now used extensively to measure the concentrations of individual sulphur compounds eluted, i.e. desorbed, from gas chromatograph columns. The need for a continuous supply of hydrogen is not only inconvenient, but it presents a slight but ever-present safety hazard. Where high measurement sensitivity is not required, the measurement of SO_2 concentrations by stimulating fluorescence can now be an attractive alternative procedure.

2.5.3. *Sulphur Dioxide Measurement by Stimulated Fluorescence*
In 1973, Okabe *et al.*[35] outlined the principles by which sulphur dioxide concentrations might be measured by stimulating the molecules to fluoresce with ultraviolet radiation. There are three main regions in which SO_2 molecules absorb radiation from the near ultra-violet part of the spectrum. Of these, the wavelength band from 190 to 230 nm appears to be the most suitable for the purpose of measurement. When stimulated by UV radiation sources in this band, SO_2 molecules emit fluorescent radiation over a band of longer wavelengths. Okabe[35] conducted a series of

experiments using a restricted part of the spectrum emitted by cadmium and zinc vapour lamps. A sample of pure sulphur dioxide was illuminated by these sources in turn, and the fluorescent radiation passing out of the cell through a Corning 5840 optical filter was detected by a photo-multiplier tube using photon counting techniques. Okabe was able to show that the system had a linear response up to 500 ppm SO_2 with the zinc lamp and even higher with the cadmium source.

More recently, Homolya[36] outlined the principle of a similar instrument which had just become commercially available for source monitoring, and which used short bursts of ultra-violet light from a flash tube to stimulate SO_2 fluorescence.[37] In another interesting development, Homolya[36] described the use of a lanthanum fluoride phosphor which was stimulated to emit radiation centred on the 280 nm wavelength by a small mercury lamp. This is very near to the absorption maximum wavelength for SO_2. The device was part of a prototype system for monitoring SO_2 concentrations in an emission source based on the principle of measuring the adsorption of radiation by sulphur dioxide gas using a UV-enhanced photo-diode.

The last two developments mentioned above merely illustrate some of the instrumental techniques that were being developed in the late seventies. There were many more. For example, Lindqvist[38] described the use of a galvanic method for detecting trace concentrations of sulphur dioxide in air. This depended on the anodic oxidation of SO_2 in a galvanic cell. The minimum values for the time constant and lower detection limit were 3 s and about $3 \mu g \, m^{-3}$, respectively. Trace concentrations measured by this galvanic method, in the range from $12-135 \mu g \, m^{-3}$, were said to be in good agreement with comparable measurements made by the West–Gaeke pararosaniline and flame photometric methods. In 1973, when Forrest and Newman[39] reviewed the available methods, there were approximately one hundred commercial instruments on the market for continuously monitoring sulphur dioxide. Monitoring techniques are still being evolved to meet particular needs and constraints so that at the beginning of the 1980s, the choice must be even wider.

3.   CONTROL OF SULPHUR DIOXIDE EMISSIONS AT SOURCE: AN OUTLINE

Inevitably waste gases containing sulphur compounds are evolved wherever fossil fuels are burnt in coal or oil-fired electricity generating stations, in steam-raising plant for industry and transport, in petrol or diesel engines, or in furnaces and fires in the home. Sulphur compounds are also evolved during the refining of metals and petroleum products, and from a wide variety of industrial manufacturing processes. The principal constituent sulphur compound is almost invariably sulphur dioxide and it may be accompanied by varying proportions of sulphur trioxide, sulphuric acid, sulphate or other sulphur compounds according to the nature of the particular process involved and the fuel used. When the source is relatively small, as in domestic heating installations, discharge of the waste gases to atmosphere is the only practicable method of disposal. But even when the source is vastly larger, discharge to atmosphere is still the expected norm in most countries, an approach most obviously characterised by the tall-stack dispersal policy that has been favoured by the Central Electricity Generating Board of England and Wales.

It was soon after the Second World War that a sequence of severe air pollution episodes in the UK first effectively drew public attention to the consequent adverse effects on respiratory health. With a gradual revival of prosperity over the same decade, the public became increasingly aware of the damage to buildings and structures that had been caused by half a century or more of unrestrained air pollution. Implementation of the 1956 Clean Air Act in the UK then led to sharply reduced emissions of dark smoke and a dramatic improvement in the quality of urban air. Over the same period, there was a steady and continuing rise in the total emission of sulphur dioxide, as demand for electricity was met by the construction of large new fossil-fuel fired power stations discharging waste gases at a great height. However, this trend was more than counterbalanced by a move away from coal for domestic heating to the low-sulphur fuels of oil and natural gas. Consequently the average concentrations of sulphur dioxide over urban areas also continued to decline. In the UK this was generally seen to be a satisfactory outcome of the Chief Alkali and Clean Air Inspector's subjective judgement that discharge of sulphur oxides from tall stacks constitute the *best practicable means* for rendering the wastes harmless and inoffensive. Alternative control philosophies were favoured elsewhere, and some aspects of control in Japan and the USA are instanced to illustrate the diversity of legislative approach.

In the late 1960s, the Japanese government acknowledged public pressure and instituted a complex system of ambient and emission standards for certain air pollutants, including sulphur dioxide. Super-imposed on these standards was a system of charges levied on the principle that it is the polluter, rather than the government, who should pay for the social and environmental costs associated with the dispersal of air pollution. As an example of the effect of this legislation, all Japanese emitters of SO_2 in excess of $5000\,\mathrm{m}^3\,\mathrm{h}^{-1}$ pay a penalty charge assessed in proportion to the actual quantity of SO_2 released. The tax rate is variable and depends on the amount of industrial development and air pollution in the district concerned. The proceeds of the tax are used both to aid those suffering from certain types of respiratory ailment and to finance appropriate research. Corwin[40] has described in some detail the positive and beneficial effects on the Japanese economy that have resulted from implementing this philosophy of control.

In 1971, the US Environmental Protection Agency also promulgated rigorous standards of performance for new stationary sources of air pollution that were to constrain permissible emissions of sulphur dioxide. These standards have since been revised and an up to date summary has been set out by Tabler.[41]

For existing plants discharging sulphur oxides, the emission regulations vary widely both internationally and nationally, since they come within the jurisdiction of widely different municipalities, states or national agencies. In some parts of the world, emission standards are set by reference to the characteristics of the surrounding area rather than the plant itself. In these places, the standards may depend to a varying degree on the type of process involved, the age of the equipment, the sulphur content of the fuel used, and the apparent local costs of SO_2 removal processes. In many situations, the simultaneous emission of particulate material will also be controlled and inevitably the regulations covering the two pollutants will be inter-related. In these instances, the choice of process equipment for emission control will necessarily be determined by the characteristics of both pollutants considered together.

In principle, the emission of sulphur dioxide can be controlled and reduced at source either:

(1)   by removing the sulphur oxides from the effluent stack gases before release to atmosphere, or

(2)   by modifying the combustion process so that the sulphur is retained amongst the ash and other solid wastes, or

(3)   by removing the sulphur compounds from the fuels before combustion.

A general inclination to pursue the first of these options has led to the greatest research effort over the years being applied to methods of cleaning the flue gases.

3.1. The Development of Flue-Gas Cleaning Processes

Flue-gas desulphurisation processes have now been studied actively for well over a century. Two representative accounts[42,43] provide abundant information on current systems. It may be helpful here to classify them into three groups. In the first of these, lime, limestone or other alkaline materials are used to absorb SO_2 in a wet gas washing process which generates large quantities of wet sludge. Since this sludge has to be thrown away, a large area of land must be available for its disposal. These systems have often been troubled by scale formation on surfaces, and plugging of liquid flow lines.

In the second group, the double-alkali type of process, the scaling troubles are minimised by the use of SO_2-absorbing materials that are more soluble than lime or limestone. Finally, the third group includes all those processes in which the absorbing medium is regenerated.

By outlining a few historical developments the following paragraphs will provide the context for the flue-gas desulphurisation processes which, after further development, are now believed to offer the best compromise solution to controlling SO_2 emissions at source.

All gas washing or scrubbing processes rely on bringing the polluted gas stream into close intermingling contact with the absorbing solution. The most convenient way is to allow the liquid to trickle or cascade down through a tower packed with obstructions, whilst the gas to be cleaned passes upwards in the opposite direction. Alternatively, the liquid can be broken up into fine droplets by pumping it through suitable sprays into a reactor vessel. Early research showed that when sulphur dioxide dissolves in water, a proportion of the gas reacts with it to form dilute sulphuric acid. If the water is recycled, the acidic concentration naturally increases until eventually there is no further absorption and the liquid must be discharged back into the environment via river, lake or sea. One form of pollution is merely converted into another. This problem of waste disposal faces all those who seek an acceptable throw-away technique for cleaning flue gases, and who must obviously avoid creating a second pollution problem as bad or worse than the first. Many developed countries have now established clear standards for the maximum permissible discharge of wastes both to water and to air. For plant operators in these countries, the choice then lies between selecting either a regenerable/recovery type of process, from which there is little waste to be disposed of, or a throw-away process from which the wastes must be deposited, preferably on land, in a safe non-polluting form.

Early work on gas washing processes showed that between 45 and 57 tons of water might be required to remove SO_2 completely from the flue gases produced by burning 1 ton of coal. It was then found that by adding certain metal ions in solution, principally those of iron and manganese, the rate of oxidation of the SO_2 absorbed in the water was greatly speeded up. By this means, the water requirement could be reduced by almost 98 % to about $1\frac{1}{4}$ tons.

3.2. Lime/Limestone Scrubbing

The next development was to neutralise the acidic wash water with lime which is strongly alkaline in solution. In other experiments, the cheaper materials chalk or limestone (from which lime is calcined in the traditional burning process) were ground up and used in liquid slurries instead. Chalk and limestone are poorly soluble, and it was quickly found that there were serious problems in managing gas washing processes using slurries of these materials. Solids tend to be deposited as scale on surfaces and plug up and block liquid flow lines. In addition, the partly washed plume of effluent gases becomes wet and cold, and with its buoyancy impaired it disperses only poorly. Much of the early work on gas washing techniques was done in the United Kingdom, but with the Second World War they fell out of favour and the installations were abandoned. Development was then resumed in the United States and Japan during the 1960s but, because the chemistry of the process was not then properly understood, the technique was dubbed more of an art than a science. The first real understanding came from research work sponsored mainly by the US Environmental Protection Agency. Slack and Hollinden[43] have outlined what was known of the complex chemistry in the mid-1970s.

Describing the results of the US EPA research, the authors list the important chemical species involved in the flue gas cleaning processes. These include calcium and magnesium from the lime or limestone; carbon dioxide, sulphur dioxide, sulphur trioxide, oxygen and nitrogen oxides from the waste gases, and sodium, potassium, chlorine and other elements carried over from the ash. All these chemical species then take part in a complex train of chemical reactions to produce many other new species. However, the overall reaction of sulphur dioxide with the calcium oxide or carbonate, is to produce calcium sulphite with some oxidation of this sulphite to calcium sulphate. Any magnesium oxide or carbonate in the scrubbing liquid may react in a similar way, or may be precipitated as magnesium hydroxide. Magnesium sulphate has a special role to play in helping to prevent the formation of troublesome scale.

3.3. Problems of Scale Formation in Scrubbers

There appear to be five particular problem areas in controlling the chemistry of the process. These are:

(1)   controlling the pH value of the scrubbing solution to avoid hard scale formation.

(2)   controlling the pH value to avoid the formation of soft scale which causes plugging,

(3)   controlling the liquid-to-gas ratios and the pH value to optimise the uptake of SO_2 whilst minimising the collection of CO_2,

(4)   understanding and modifying the characteristics of the sludge discharged from the system, so that it may be safely deposited as a stable landfill material, and

(5)   controlling and optimising the use of the primary reagents to minimise costs.

The control of pH is thus a prominent feature of efficient flue-gas scrubbers using lime or limestone, and their operational problems were recently reviewed by Jones *et al.*[44] They studied several full-scale plants in the USA and concluded that provided the pH sensors could be made sufficiently reliable, the system chemistry could be controlled sufficiently well to prevent scale formation.

An alternative approach to the scaling problem has been provided by the National Lime Association Lewis scrubber which has a completely unconventional horizontal layout. First described by Lewis[45] in 1974, an account of operational experience with the scrubber was recently given by Bacchetti and Burgener of the Pfizer Co.[46] The scrubber consists of a long cylindrical shell container which is mounted on trunnion bearings for slow rotation about its longitudinal axis. This slopes downwards about $\frac{1}{2}$ a degree from the horizontal, so that a lime slurry will flow by gravity from one end to the other. The whole cylinder contains a complex system of freely hanging chains which move in and out of the lime slurry as the cylinder rotates. The flue gases to be cleaned pass through the cylindrical shell in the opposite direction and, in doing so, come into close contact with the lime slurry adhering to the chains or dripping from them. By this imaginative design innovation, the scaling problems associated with conventional scrubbers are said to be overcome without modifying the system chemistry.

Disposal of the calcium sulphite sludge from any scrubber presents a serious environmental problem, since its thixotropic properties make it unstable as a landfill material, and dewatering it is a difficult and costly physical process. One solution is to mix it with fly ash from coal-fired power stations and so confer sufficient mechanical stability to the material. An alternative solution is to oxidise the calcium sulphite to sulphate which settles out more readily and is easier to filter and dewater. Goodwin[47] has described experiments which show that oxidation could be an effective aid to better disposal characteristics, and that for best results it should be carried out in two stages maintained at different pH values.

Finally in this section it is relevant to mention recent developments in the techniques for the dry absorption of SO_2 in spray dryer absorbers. Systems of this type are soon to be incorporated in at least two large power stations in the US and should be operational by 1982. In principle, a suitable absorbent slurry of lime or soda ash is atomised and directed as a fine spray into a chamber through which the waste gases must pass. The fine spray droplets provide an extensive surface area to absorb the SO_2 and, because of the heat content, the water is quickly evaporated to leave dry particles that can be collected by electrostatic precipitator or bag filter. Felsvang and Masters[48] have described a recent Danish proposal to use this technique.

3.4. Indirect Lime/Limestone Scrubbing

As another approach to the problem of scale formation, many process developers have made use of a more soluble alkali material for absorbing sulphur dioxide in the primary scrubbing systems. Sometimes referred to as double-alkali processes, the primary absorbent may be a soluble sodium salt, but other absorbents such as solutions of ammonium sulphate, aluminium sulphate and even water acidified with dilute sulphuric acid and a catalyst have all been used with some success. Slack and Hollinden[43] have described in some detail the various systems that have been tried out, mostly in Japan.

In the second stage of this type of indirect system, all the absorbing solutions are regenerated by reaction with lime or limestone in a separate reactor vessel and process loop. As with direct scrubbing systems, the end result is usually the same throw-away waste product of calcium sulphite or sulphate sludge. Although indirect scrubbing systems appear generally to have better collection efficiencies, they tend to be more costly in operation because in most cases additional process equipment is required. Other increased costs arise from the need to make up losses of the primary absorbing material which can be carried over into the waste product, and make its safe disposal more difficult.

All wet gas scrubbing systems have a major inherent disadvantage in that the washed gases are cold and wet. With their buoyancy and momentum thus reduced, the rise of the effluent plume above the top of the chimney stack is also reduced. This would scarcely matter if all the sulphur dioxide and other pollutants had been removed from the gases before discharge, but a typical scrubbing efficiency may be only 80%. With a reduced effective plume rise, dispersion in the atmosphere will be impaired and the ambient pollutant concentration at ground level will be reduced, not by 80% but by some lesser and unsatisfactory proportion.

Washing and cooling the waste gases can also lead to other problems. There may be serious corrosion from acid condensation in ducts and chimneys and on any fan used to aid gas movement. This can be overcome only by the use of more expensive materials or design. There will be a greater likelihood of acid rain from water droplets forming near to the chimney stack and absorbing residual SO_2. In cool weather, a steam plume will form more frequently, and this too may lead to public complaint. For all these reasons it became standard practice in the 1970s to reheat gases discharged from scrubber installations. But with a continued depletion of energy resources and rising costs, reheating the stack gases for improved dispersion will be doubly unattractive. It is likely to be acceptable in the future only if heat can be conserved and exchanged from some earlier stage of the firing process. The alternative is to use an SO_2 absorbing system that does not reduce the temperature of the waste gases, as for example the spray dryer absorber mentioned earlier.

Activated carbon has been used in this way as the primary absorbent in indirect systems. When sulphur dioxide is absorbed, oxidation and water condensation also occur so that if the carbon is purged with water, the end product is a dilute solution of sulphuric acid. Since it is expensive to concentrate the acid, which may have a strength of no more than 15%, it is neutralised with limestone to make saleable gypsum. This process has been used in large-scale plants both in Japan and Germany but the size of the absorbing stage is a serious disadvantage and may preclude further development.

3.5. Recovery Processers

Although it may seem obvious that sulphur, a valuable natural resource, should be recovered wherever possible, there are both economic and practical problems which make this difficult.[43] In metal smelters, where SO_2 concentrations in the waste gases are relatively large, direct recovery from the waste gas stream has been practised for many years. Sulphuric acid can be produced directly by catalytic oxidation, or alternatively elemental sulphur recovered by a reduction process. For waste gases having lower

SO$_2$ concentrations, several systems offering good prospects of practical success are still being studied and developed, but it appears to be too early yet to pick the winners.

One representative system—the Wellman Lord SO$_2$ recovery process, which is currently receiving considerable attention, was recently described by Pedroso and Press.[49] Already 26 large installations are operating commercially in the US and Japan. After appropriate pre-treatment to remove particulate material, the flue gases are scrubbed with a clear solution of sodium sulphite in a sequence of stages to reduce the sulphur dioxide concentration down to any desired level. The sulphite is thus converted to sodium bisulphite, and this is then decomposed and regenerated to sodium sulphite for reuse by heating with low pressure exhaust steam. Water vapour is condensed out to produce an SO$_2$-rich gas flow that can be further treated to recover sulphuric acid or elemental sulphur.

The Monsanto Cat-Ox process is an example of a dry catalytic oxidation process that has already been applied to a large power station. Based on the use of vanadium pentoxide as a catalyst, SO$_2$ is converted directly to SO$_3$ in the waste gas stream for downstream recovery as sulphuric acid. Although the size of the effort required to make the system work was not fully appreciated at the outset, and the system was shut down in 1974, Murthy *et al.*[50] claim that the process appears to be both technically sound and workable if sufficient funds and effort are committed to the project.

Investigations continue into many other cleaning processes. Various alkaline absorbents based on ammonium, sodium, potassium, lithium, hydrogen and aluminium have all been used,[43] although the first two have had more attention than the others. Regeneration of the alkali from the sulphite which is formed is then carried out by a chemical reaction with oxygen, acid or reducing agent. Alkaline earths have been studied for SO$_2$ absorption at the pilot plant level. Metal oxides have been investigated, especially manganese oxide which takes up SO$_2$ faster than any other sorbent, whilst a process based on copper oxide has been subject to large scale testing in Japan.

3.6. Fuel Desulphurisation

Here there is space only to note that the removal of sulphur from oil and coal fuels before combustion has received considerable attention. Numerous methods for coal have been proposed, and many tested. Although a small proportion of the sulphur compounds in coal can be removed by simple washing, it is much more difficult and expensive to remove the remainder. The technology for removing sulphur from oil fuel is at a rather more advanced stage than the technology for removing sulphur from coal, but it too is a relatively expensive process. As the oil must be treated with hydrogen at high temperatures and pressures in the presence of a catalyst, the desulphurisation process is one to be integrated into refinery operations.

3.7. Sulphur Removal in Fluidised Bed Reactors and Furnaces

Finally, methods for controlling the emission of sulphur dioxide at source by absorbent fluidised bed reactors, and fluidised bed combustion furnaces, are still being actively researched. Coal gasification systems based on fluidised bed reactors are now being developed for electrical power generation.[51] In principle, a low calorific fuel gas is produced at high pressure, from which most of the sulphur has already been removed at high temperature with calcium-based materials, i.e. limestone or dolomite, in a fluidised bed. In 1978, Keairns *et al.*[51] described the systems then being developed at the pilot plant stage. The authors showed that, to ensure compatibility, fluidised bed reactors should be properly integrated both with the power plant design and the environmental need. The investigators were developing relevant design and operating parameters and identifying the potential limitations of the alternative designs. The critical requirement for achieving usable commercial systems include the selection of suitable activated absorbents, and the efficient control of their usage, attrition, regeneration and disposal.

In fluidised bed combustion systems the fuel, which may be coal, lignite or oil, is maintained in a state of turbulent motion by jets of air directed upwards. With the whole of the fuel exposed to air, combustion is extremely rapid. If finely divided materials like dolomite, limestone or chalk are introduced into the bed under suitable conditions, rather more than 75 % of the sulphur in the fuel will be retained in the furnace slag. Murthy *et al.*[52] have set down how the objectives for environmental control by fluidised bed combustion techniques are to be assessed, but Barnes[53] has concluded that although pilot plant trials are encouraging, full-sized commercial units for large power stations are unlikely to be available before the 1990s.

4.   CONCLUSIONS

The effort currently being expended world-wide on the control of air pollution is now extremely large, with flue-gas desulphurisation systems apparently offering the best immediate prospect of meeting present emission standards. By 1975, over 1000 installations had already been made in Japan where annualised costs were reported to be running at about 2% of the gross national product.[40] According to Barnes,[53] 58 of the Japanese installations were large-scale plants, whilst there were another 26 major units in the United States and six more in Europe.

For some years now the environmental cost of pollution by sulphur oxides has been held to justify active development of flue-gas cleaning systems in both the United States and Japan. In contrast, the governments of many European countries have been slow to recognise the environmental cost of steadily increasing SO_2 emissions, for it was not until 1979 that the UN ECE Convention on Long-Range Transboundary Air Pollution was signed. When ratified and given effect, the convention should provide an equitable mechanism and incentive for all signatory states to introduce a more effective control and reduction of SO_2 emissions at source. Implicit in all these developments is the need to be able to make accurate and representative measurements of ambient concentrations, and this chapter has set out the recommended procedures.

REFERENCES

1. British Standards Institution. *Methods for the measurement of air pollution: the lead dioxide method*, BS 1747: Pt. 4, London, 1969.
2. HUEY, N. A. *J. Air Pollut. Contr. Ass.*, 1968, **18**, 610.
3. LIANG, S. F., STERNLING, C. U. and GALLOWAY, T. R. *J. Air Pollut. Contr. Ass.*, 1973, **23**, 605.
4. RIDER, P. E., RIDER, C. C. and CORNING, R. N. *J. Air Pollut. Contr. Ass.*, 1977, **27**, 1011.
5. Organisation for Economic Co-operation and Development. *Methods of measuring air pollution*, Paris, 1964.
6. British Standards Institution. *Methods for the measurement of air pollution: determination of sulphur dioxide*, BS 1747: Pt. 3, London, 1969.
7. COMMINS, B. T. *Analyst*, 1963, **88**, 364.
8. KILLICK, C. M. *The monitoring of gases containing sulphur*, Warren Spring Laboratory, Stevenage, UK, 1975.
9. WEATHERLEY, M-L. *The national survey of smoke and sulphur dioxide—quality control and the air sampling arrangements*, LR 308(AP), Warren Spring Laboratory, Stevenage, UK, 1979.
10. WEATHERLEY, M-L., APPLETON, J., CHARNOCK, J. and COATES, J. *The national survey of smoke and sulphur dioxide—quality control tests on the analysis of samples*, LR 307(AP), Warren Spring Laboratory, Stevenage, UK, 1979.
11. WOHLERS, H. C., NEWSTEIN, H. and DAUNIS, D. *J. Air Pollut. Contr. Ass.*, 1967, **17**, 753.

12. THOMAS, M. D., IVIE, J. O. and FITT, T. C. *Ind. Eng. Chem., Anal. Ed.*, 1946, **18**, 383.
13. RODES, C. E., PALMER, H. F., ELFERS, L. A. and NORRIS, C. H. *J. Air Pollut. Contr. Ass.*, 1969, **19**, 575.
14. PALMER, H. F., RODES, C. E. and NELSON, C. J. *J. Air Pollut. Contr. Ass.*, 1969, **19**, 778.
15. MARSHALL, G. B. *Clean Air*, 1975, **5**, 15.
16. CUMMINGS, W. G. and REDFEARN, M. W. *J. Inst. Fuel*, 1957, **30**, 628.
17. FRITZ, J. S. and YAMAMURA, S. S. *Anal. Chem.*, 1955, **27**, 1461.
18. PERSSON, G. A. *Int. J. Air Wat. Pollut.*, 1966, **10**, 845.
19. Interbranch Chemical Advisory Committee. *US Pub. Health Serv.*, Publ. 999-AP-11, 1965.
20. *US Federal Register,* 30 Apr. 1971, **36**(84), 8186.
21. SCARINGELLI, F. P., SALTZMAN, B. E. and FREY, S. A. *Anal. Chem.*, 1967, **39**, 1709.
22. WEST, P. W. and GAEKE, G. C. *Anal. Chem.*, 1956, **28**, 1816.
23. ADAMS, D. F. Sulfur compounds, in *Air Pollution*, 3rd edn, Stern, A. C. (Ed.), Academic Press, London and New York, 1976, pp. 111, 214.
24. ADAMS, D. F., CORN, M., HARDING, C. I., PATE, J. P., PLUMLEY, A. L., SCARINGELLI, F. P. and URONE, P. Methods of air sampling and analysis, (Tentative method of analysis of sulfur dioxide content of the atmosphere (colorimetric)), *Amer. Pub. Health Ass. Washington, DC*, 1972, No. 42401-01-69T, p. 447.
25. *ASTM Standards—Water; Atmospheric Analysis*, Amer. Soc. Test. Mater., Desig. D2914-70T, Pt. 23, Philadelphia, Penn., 1972.
26. BLACKER, J. H., CONFER, R. G. and BRIEF, R. S. *J. Air Pollut. Contr. Ass.*, 1973, **23**, 525.
27. WHO. *Selected methods of measuring air pollutants*, World Health Organisation Offset Publication No. 24, Geneva, 1976.
28. FAITH, W. L. and ATKISSON, A. A. *Air Pollution*, 2nd edn, Wiley-Interscience, New York, 1972.
29. NELSON, G. O. *Controlled Test Atmospheres*, Ann Arbor Science Publ., Michigan, 1971.
30. AXELROD, H. D. and LODGE, J. P. Sampling and calibration of gaseous pollutants, in *Air Pollution*, 3rd edn, Stern, A. C. (Ed.), Academic Press, London and New York, 1976, pp. 111, 145.
31. SCARINGELLI, F. P., O'KEEFFE, A. E., ROSENBERG, E. and BELL, J. P. *Anal. Chem.*, 1970, **42**, 871.
32. Philips Industries, Eindhoven, The Netherlands.
33. BROUWER, H. J., DE VEER, S. M. and ZEEDIJK, H. *Philips Tech. Rev.*, 1971, **32**, 33.
34. Meloy Laboratories Inc., 6631 Iron Place, Springfield, Virginia, 22151.
35. OKABE, H., SPLITSTONE, P. L. and BALL, J. *J. Air Pollut. Contr. Ass.*, 1973, **23**, 514.
36. HOMOLYA, J. B. *J. Air Pollut. Contr. Ass.*, 1975, **25**, 809.
37. Thermo Electron Corporation, 108 South Street, Hopkinson, Ma. 01748.
38. LINDQVIST, F. *J. Air Pollut. Contr. Ass.*, 1978, **28**, 138.
39. FORREST, J. and NEWMAN, L. *J. Air Pollut. Contr. Ass.*, 1973, **23**, 761.

40. Corwin, T. K. *Environ. Sci. Tech.*, 1980, **14**, 154.
41. Tabler, S. K. *J. Air Pollut. Contr. Ass.*, 1979, **29**, 803.
42. Anon. A history of flue gas desulfurization systems since 1850 (Condensed version of Fed. Power Comiss. Report), *J. Air Pollut. Contr. Ass.*, 1979, **27**, 948.
43. Slack, A. U. and Hollinden, G. A. *Sulfur Dioxide Removal from Waste Gases*, 2nd edn, Noyes Data Corp., New Jersey, 1975.
44. Jones, D. G., Hargrove, O. W. and Morasky, T. M. *J. Air Pollut. Contr. Ass.*, 1979, **28**, 1099.
45. Lewis, C. J. A new concept of lime scrubbing of SO_2-gas, *3rd Int. Symp. on Lime*, Berlin, 1974.
46. Bacchetti, J. A. and Burgener, I. L. Performance of environmentally approved national lime assoc. scrubber for SO_2, *4th Int. Lime Congress*, Hershey, Pa., USA, 1978.
47. Goodwin, R. W. *J. Air Pollut. Contr. Ass.*, 1978, **28**, 35.
48. Felsvang, K. and Masters, K. Flue gas desulphurization of coalfired power plant by dry absorption in spray dryers (absorbers), *The Control of Sulphur and Other Gaseous Emissions: 3rd Int. Symp. Inst. Chem. Eng.*, Salford, UK, 1979.
49. Pedroso, R. I. and Press, K. M. Sulphur recovered from flue gas at large coal fired power plants, *The Control of Sulphur and other Gaseous Emissions: 3rd Int. Symp. Inst. Chem. Eng.*, Salford, UK, 1979.
50. Murthy, K. S., Rosenberg, H. S. and Engdahl, R. B. *J. Air Pollut. Contr. Ass.*, 1976, **26**, 851.
51. Keairns, D. L., Newby, R. A., O'Neill, E. P. and Archer, D. H. *J. Air Pollut. Contr. Ass.*, 1978, **28**, 328.
52. Murthy, K. S., Nack, H. and Henschel, D. B. *J. Air Pollut. Contr. Ass.*, 1978, **28**, 213.
53. Barnes, R. A. *J. Air Pollut. Contr. Ass.*, 1979, **29**, 1231.

Chapter 5

ASBESTOSIS AND OTHER DUST RELATED DISEASES: DIAGNOSIS, PREVENTION AND CONTROL

J. M. HARRINGTON,† M.Sc., M.D., M.R.C.P., M.F.O.M.

Formerly, Senior Lecturer in Occupational Medicine,
London School of Hygiene and Tropical Medicine
and Honorary Consultant, Occupational Medicine,
University College Hospital, London, UK

SUMMARY

Asbestos is one of the naturally occurring minerals which can produce fibrotic lung disease following the inhalation of dust. Disease attributable to coal and silica dust may be more important in occupational health but the ubiquitous nature of asbestos and its additional role of producing tumours of the lung and pleura suggest that it is the most hazardous of the group. New control limits for asbestos dust are being promulgated in the United Kingdom but despite considerable research for several generations, many questions remain unanswered concerning the relative risks to health of different asbestos fibre types. Current knowledge regarding technological control and environmental monitoring are just capable of ensuring compliance with the new limits. Substitution of asbestos with other fibres is feasible for some uses but these substitutes themselves may not be without risk to human health.

† Present address: Department of Medicine, Birmingham University, Birmingham, UK (see List of Contributors).

    J. M. HARRINGTON

1. INTRODUCTION

The volume of published material on the dust related diseases seems to increase each year. Though this increase seems to approach exponential proportions when considering asbestos, the numbers of new cases of asbestos related disease belies this. What appears to be happening is that the environmental impact of asbestos has become appreciated and the assertion that asbestos can cause cancer has added an emotive dimension to the subject. This chapter will concentrate on the health effects of asbestos but can serve only as a stimulus to further study for the interested reader.

In occupational medicine, asbestos related disease has less numerical importance than, say, coal workers' pneumoconiosis. Coal dust, however, is hardly a major environmental pollutant whereas asbestos fibres are ubiquitous in modern industrial communities. It is in this contrasting context that the present chapter is drafted.

It is necessary to view asbestos related disease as part of the overall picture of occupational exposure to dusts and then extrapolate these findings to broader environmental contamination. Thus, the chapter is divided into several sections. The first section deals with dust related diseases—the pneumoconioses—other than asbestosis. Brief descriptions are given of the more important dusts, their measurements and their health effects. This account provides a summary of the ways dusts can damage the lungs and of the means available for the diagnosis, treatment and compensation of workers thus affected. The central section focuses on the asbestos fibre including its geology, measurement, and health effects. As most dust related diseases are not reversible and rarely curable, much emphasis must be placed on the prevention and control of human exposure. The advent of new proposed legislation for asbestos in the United Kingdom provides a suitable basis for discussing current control measures and the outlook for the future.

2. GENERAL ASPECTS OF DUST RELATED DISEASE

The term 'pneumoconiosis' was coined over a century ago but is much misused. The literal derivation from the original Greek means 'dusty lung' but modern usage tends to include those conditions (and dusts) that produce no harm. It is perhaps more appropriate to consider the term pneumoconiosis as meaning *the presence of inhaled dust in the lungs and their non-malignant reaction to it.*

2.1. Scope and Types of Dust

Dusts may be considered to be solid particles dispersed in the air and, therefore, capable of being inhaled. For the purposes of human effects, the target organ is really the air passages from windpipe (trachea) right down to the furthest air space (alveolus) of the lung. This anatomical unit can react in a variety of ways to the inhalation of dust. The effect may be transient or chronic, mild or life threatening. In practice, the most significant effect of dusts in the lungs is the excessive production of an elastic-like material called collagen which, whilst healing the scars resulting from the dust damage, can lead to compensatory dilation of air sacs (emphysema). This

TABLE 1

A CLASSIFICATION OF DUSTS AND THEIR EFFECTS OF OCCUPATIONAL EXPOSURE

| | *Inorganic* | | *Organic* | |
Benign	*Inflammatory*	*Fibrotic*	*'Toxic'*	*Fibrotic*
Iron	Vanadium	Silica	Mouldy hay	Mouldy hay
Tin	Manganese	Silicates	Cotton	
Barium	Beryllium	(including asbestos)	Fungi	Cork
	Cadmium	Coal (late)	Red wood	
	Aluminium	Beryllium	Cork	
	Platinum		Isocyanates	

seriously disrupts the lung's ability to perform its main function—namely the exchange of oxygen and carbon dioxide across the air–alveolus–blood barrier. Other effects may also be important, however, and these include inflammatory reactions and allergic phenomena. Add to this a group of dusts which appear to be inert, but can have dramatic effects on the X-ray appearances of the lungs, and you have the gamut of effects. These are summarised in Table 1.

It must be emphasised, however, that these neat classifications break down in practice. For example, iron dust has been alleged to cause lung damage and even be a contributory factor in occupationally induced lung cancer, whilst the ways in which cotton dust causes byssinosis are ill understood and most unlikely to be as simple as an allergic reaction. Some, such as coal dust, may be benign in most people exposed to moderate quantities but can kill a certain number of workers through the development of progressive massive fibrosis. The list of organic dusts and fumes causing occupational asthma is getting extremely long—only a few are included here.

2.2. The Fate of Inhaled Dust

Dust particles are small and can be inhaled by anyone coming into the vicinity of dust laden air. The fate of these inhaled particles depends on a variety of factors such as the aerodynamic properties of the particles and the ability of the creature inhaling it to rid itself of the particle. More detailed accounts written for the non-medical scientist are available.[1]

2.2.1. *Particle Properties*

The size and weight of the particle obviously plays a major part in determining its ability to be inhaled. For our purposes, rock is the starting point of most such dusts and the processes of mining and milling change the rock from large lumps to manageable portions. The more a rock is broken down, the smaller are the resultant particles and the more capable such fragments are of becoming airborne—the essential pre-condition for inhalation.

Some minerals, such as coal or quartz, can be ground down to particles which approximate to a sphere; others such as asbestos are fibrous and may have a length which exceeds its diameter by a factor of three to one or more (frequently ten to one). Furthermore, these units may aggregate and thereby change their aerodynamic properties. All airborne particles have a small independent motion of their own but they all tend to settle out under the influence of gravity. The terminal velocity of these particles is proportional to the square of their density. The weight, along with the shape and surface characteristics, influences the fall out and, therefore, determines how far such particles will penetrate into the deeper recesses of the lungs. The whole subject is highly complex and what follows in relation to the body's reactions assumes the particles are roughly spherical. Long thin fibres—such as asbestos—will behave in a different and more complicated manner, dependent upon their diameter.

2.2.2. *The Airway's Response to Inhaled Particles*

If a particle is small enough to be airborne and close enough to the worker's nose or mouth, it is likely to be inhaled with the next breath. The larger particles greater than 10 μm in diameter, will be trapped by the hairs of the nose and eventually sneezed or blown out again with the next—perhaps literally, without touching the sides! The rest—with diameters between 1 and 10 μm—suffer a variety of fates. Some sediment out, others impact on the surfaces of the air passages whilst others succeed in penetrating to the lung itself. It is those particles which reach the air sacs and remain that cause the trouble. Further up the path from lungs to windpipe, the bronchial passages are lined with tiny hair-like structures called cilia. In addition, these ciliated surfaces are coated with mucus. The continual wafting of the cilia upwards away from the lungs helps move the mucus upwards too. Any particles trapped on this moving layer, the so called muco-ciliary escalator, will be passed up the airways to be coughed up or swallowed. Although this means of particle removal is highly efficient, repeated assault by irritant or noxious gases, fumes or particles leads to increased mucus and defective ciliary action.

Long fibres may escape impaction or sedimentation in the upper airways: they may reach the distant divisions of the airways or the alveoli themselves. Curly chrysotile asbestos fibres are less effective penetrators than the straight amphiboles such as crocidolite.

Having reached the lung proper, the body still has protective devices it can call upon to defend itself. Scavenger cells called macrophages will attempt to 'swallow' the particles and either break them up or at least sequestrate them from the lung tissue. In addition the lung can deposit collagen fibre around the intruding particle to effect the same end. Unfortunately some particles excite a particularly florid collagen deposition, and this may prove counterproductive if the inhaled load is large and widespread. In these circumstances, massive collagen deposition may damage the integrity of the lung architecture and thereby disrupt its function. Thickened air sac walls are more impervious to gas exchange and also cause a diminution of normal lung elasticity. The lungs thus fail to transport oxygen into, and carbon dioxide out of the blood and the increased stiffness of the lung tissue hampers respiration. Silica particles and asbestos fibres are particularly adept at producing these serious fibrotic changes.[2]

2.3. The Measurement of Airborne Dust

In industry, it is important to know if an inhalable dust has been generated, and it is equally important to control it. Some dusts are more capable than others of producing human disease and clinical and epidemiological studies over the years have enabled guidelines to be established on what is an 'allowable' concentration of a given dust. These threshold limit values (TLV) or maximum allowable concentrations (MAC)—or, more accurately, control limit concepts—are estimates of dust concentrations which should not be exceeded if the majority of the exposed workers are to remain healthy. Most TLVs are time weighted averages for an 8 h day, 40 h week, though the actual measurements in the workplace may be collected over time intervals measured in minutes. Some airborne materials, particularly gases, are so hazardous that even short exposures may be dangerous. Ceiling values for the TLV may thus be stated as short term exposure limits (STEL), which are on no account to be exceeded even for a short time—usually 15 min. It is important to emphasise that these somewhat arbitrary limits are not magical dividing lines between safety and hazard. They are promulgated as maxima, which should be higher than real exposure and constant efforts should be made to lower such real exposures whatever the TLV.

Measurement of dust levels may be background, source, or breathing zone. They may measure total dust or respirable dust (dust of certain diameter), and be short term 'grab' samples, or long term. The choice of method depends on the nature of the dust, the TLV and the circumstances of exposure. A detailed exposition of sampling strategies is beyond the scope of this book, but basic accounts are available elsewhere.[3] Suffice to say, most of the sampling instruments consist of a pump which draws the sampled air across a filter device. The particles trapped on the filter may be weighed, analysed and viewed microscopically. Such sampling apparatus may also incorporate devices to remove unwanted particles of non-respirable size before the air reaches the filter used for analysis. Dust may also be precipitated out by thermal or electrostatic means and these properties are exploited in some samplers.

2.4. The Health Effects of Dust Inhalation

Certain dusts can be injurious to health; the examining physician has to assess the degree of that impairment and may need to re-examine the patient at regular intervals.

In addition to the doctor's usual history taking and clinical examination, certain special investigations are very useful. The main ones are lung function tests[4] and chest radiography. It is important to emphasise however, the necessity of acquiring a detailed occupational, residential and hobby history from the patient, of studying environmental dust measurements made, and being conversant with the circumstances of exposure. Lung function abnormalities and abnormal chest X-rays are not diagnostic of occupational lung diseases on their own.

2.4.1. *Patterns of Disordered Lung Function*

In essence, the lung exchanges blood gases with respired gases so that the body acquires more oxygen and rids itself of unwanted carbon dioxide. This exchange is achieved by ensuring that the air reaches thin, healthy alveoli which are efficiently perfused by blood. Dust diseases can limit the access of air to the lungs and damage the delicate wall of the alveolus. Tests of these functions fall into two groups: measures of lung obstruction or restriction and measures of blood gas concentrations.

Let us dispose of the latter first: the sampling of arterial and venous blood and the measurement of dissolved oxygen and carbon dioxide can be used as measures of the effectiveness of lung function. Although normal values assume 'normality of function' from mouth to lung blood, blood gas measurements are useful in combination with lung function tests. There are many lung function tests but the simpler ones frequently suffice and also have the advantage of being cheap, repeatable and (usually) portable so that they can be done at the workplace at regular intervals. The spirometer or similar device is commonly used for such purposes (Fig. 1). The device measures the flow of air in and out of the mouth under maximal breathing effort. The subject usually takes a deep breath in and then blows the air out again as fast and completely as possible. A typical tracing so recorded is

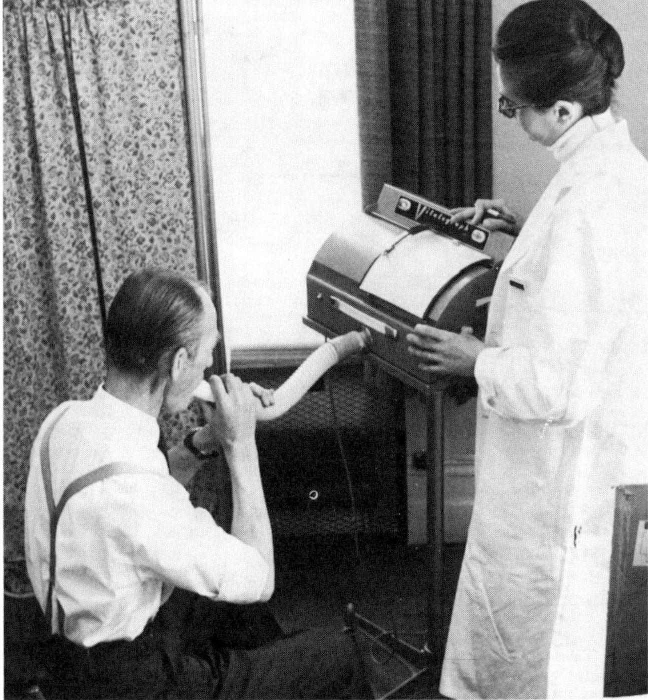

FIG. 1.   A Vitalograph spirometer.

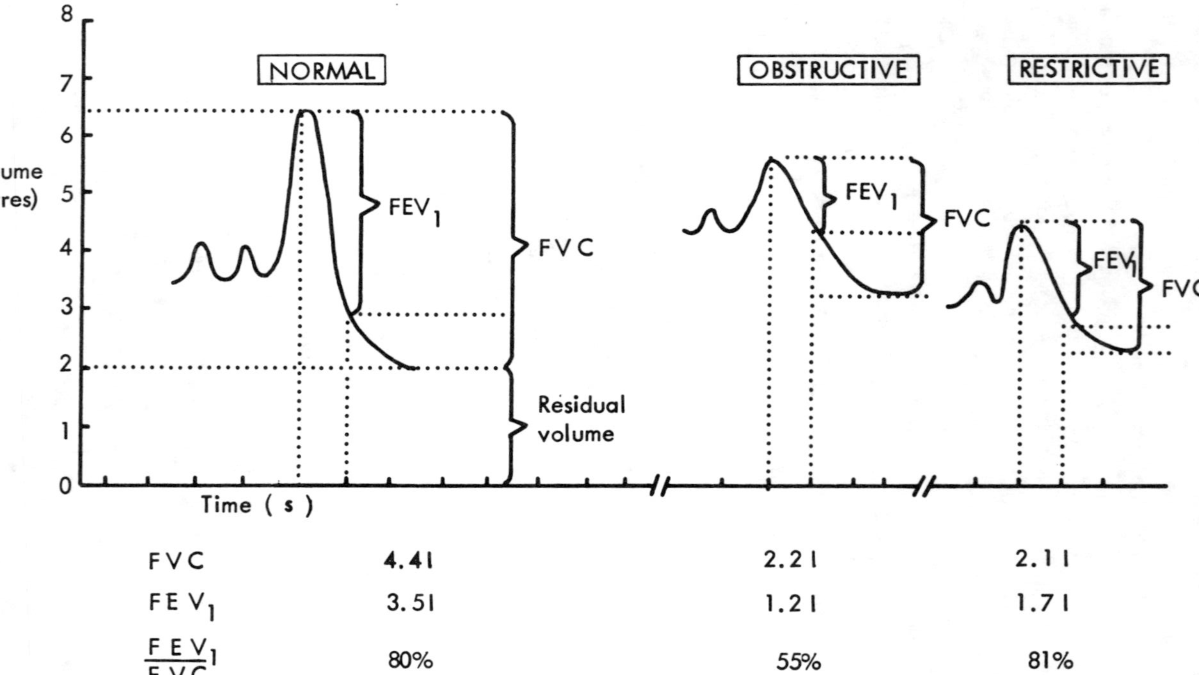

FIG. 2. Spirograms illustrating the differences in forced expiratory volume in one second (FEV$_1$) and forced vital capacity (FVC) in health, airways obstruction and restrictive defects (such as diffuse lung fibrosis and severe spinal deformity). Inspiration is upwards, expiration downwards. Although vital capacity is reduced in both obstructive and restrictive lung disease, the preparative expired in one second shows considerable differences.

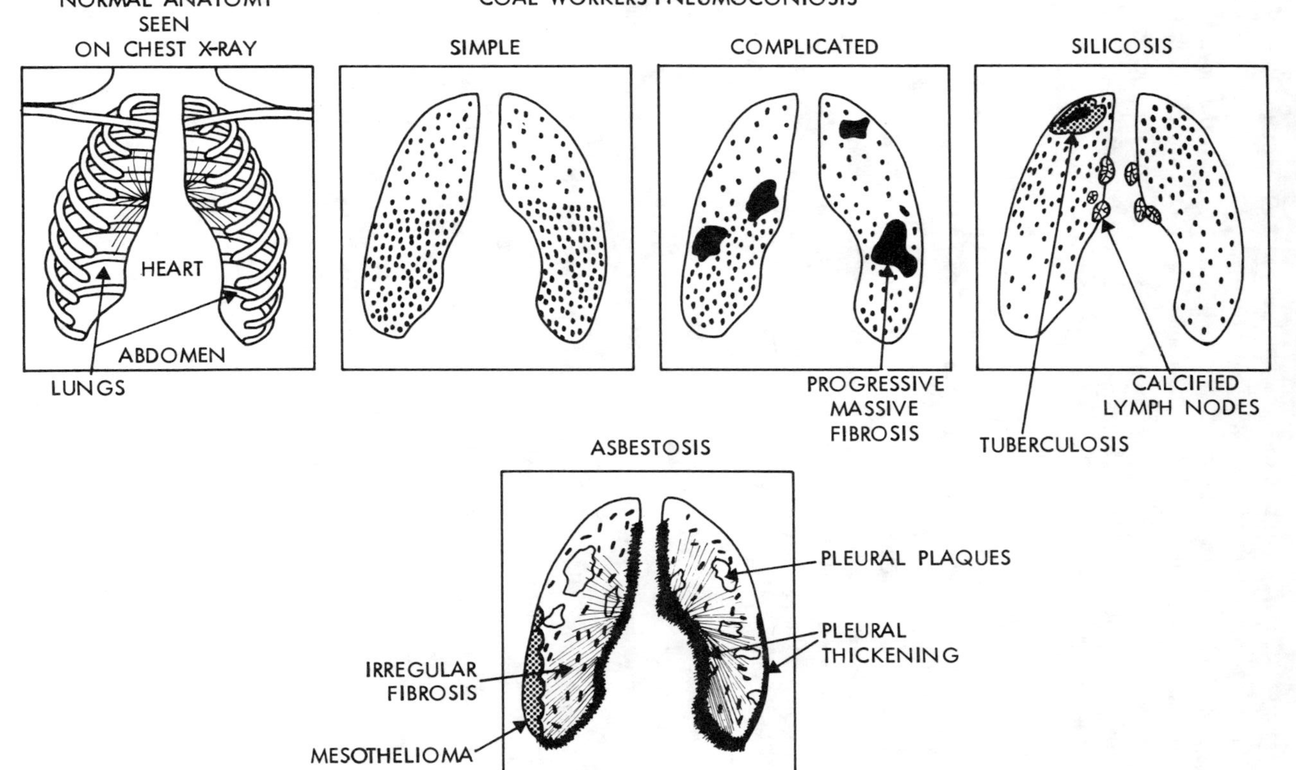

Fig. 3. Schematic representation of the chest X-ray appearances of certain dust diseases.

illustrated in Fig. 2. Failure to blow the air out fast enough implies *obstruction* to air passages, even though the total volume expired may not be particularly small. Blowing out a smaller volume, even at the normal rate, implies *restriction* of air flow in the lungs (Fig. 2). Obstructive disease is usually due to narrowing of the air passages (e.g. asthma, bronchitis/ emphysema) whilst restrictive disease is usually due to stiff lungs (e.g. asbestosis) or defective chest muscles (e.g. polio).

2.4.2. *Chest Radiography and Dust Diseases*

Most dusts encountered in occupational circumstances are derived from dense material which leads to radio-opacities. Deposition of such dusts in the lungs will show up on X-rays of the chest as white dots or blotches. Some dusts, such as coal, produce small rounded discrete shadows whilst asbestos —which produces a greater degree of fibrosis—leads to less well defined shadows which may not be rounded. Furthermore, some dusts produce additional features: silica may cause calcium deposition in the chest lymph nodes and also predisposes to tuberculosis of the lungs; asbestosis may be accompanied by thickening of the linings of the chest cavity or lung covering (pleura), calcium deposits on the thickened pleura, lung cancer or pleural cancer.

Diagrammatic representations of some of these appearances are shown in Fig. 3.

Experience over the years has shown that there is some correlation between 'dust dose' and the extent and profusion of the spots in the lungs seen on a chest X-ray. International agreement has resulted in a standardised method for taking chest X-rays and of subsequently grading of the degree of lung mottling.[5] This not only facilitates comparison between populations of exposed workers but also provides a means of following an individual worker's pneumoconiosis through serial X-rays over the years. Such films form part of the basis for establishing compensation for the afflicted worker.

3. SPECIFIC DUST RELATED DISEASES EXCLUDING ASBESTOSIS

3.1. Coal Workers' Pneumoconiosis

In the early stages of exposure to coal dust, the microphages succeed in transporting the engulfed particles away from the lungs towards the muco-ciliary escalator. If exposure continues, the dust laden macrophages become so numerous that they clog the system near some of the smaller air passages. Some fibrosis occurs around these aggregates leading to the discrete foci seen on the chest radiograph.

Nowadays coal miners seldom progress beyond this symptomless stage. Some, however, with continued exposure, and for reasons not clearly understood, progress and the aggregates of dust laden cells get larger. Fibrosis accelerates and focal dilatation of air sacs (emphysema) starts. The aggregates coalesce and may break down in the centre leaving a pool of inky black fluid which may get coughed up. When such a stage has been reached, the process is irreversible. The emphysema gets worse, breathlessness supervenes and eventually the heart fails. At current dust levels in British coal mines ($8 \, \mathrm{mg \, m^{-3}}$ measured in the outflow air from the mine with a gravimetric sampler) there is a risk of a 3% attack rate for progressive massive fibrosis in a 30 year mining career.[6]

Other complications include: rheumatoid lung, tuberculosis and other chest infections and chronic bronchitis. The radiographic appearances are represented diagramatically in Fig. 3. The rounded opacities increase in number and lung spread. Their size also increases. There is no specific treatment that will cause regression of the pneumoconiotic changes.

3.2. Silicosis

Although there is a risk of silicosis in some coal mines, the disease is largely restricted to workers exposed to free silica (SiO_2). It is an occupational hazard of quarrymen as well as of dressers of sandstone, slate and granite. Geological circumstances dictate that mining for iron, tin, copper, gold and other minerals can lead to silicosis. The risk of silicosis in metal grinding, sand blasting and the potteries has been reduced by replacing silicaceous materials with safer substitutes.

Like coal pneumoconiosis, silicosis may be simple or complicated. The fibrous reaction to silica in the lungs is more florid and the radiographic appearances show denser opacities. The lung tissue tends, therefore, to get more distorted in the face of the silicotic process. Advanced disease is irreversible leading to respiratory incapacity and/or heart failure. There is a predisposition to tuberculosis.

3.3. Other Dust Diseases

Some idea of the relative importance of the pneumoconioses can be gauged from the compensation figures compiled by the Department of Health and Social Security (Table 2).

A disease worth mentioning here is *byssinosis*. Byssinosis is a respiratory

TABLE 2
INDUSTRIAL CHEST DISEASES: CASES NEWLY DIAGNOSED 1973–1977

Disease	*1973*	*1974*	*1975*	*1976*	*1977*
Pneumoconiosis:					
coal mining	515	539	683	575	476
other mining and quarrying	31	24	41	76	—
pottery	16	15	24	17	—
Asbestosis	143	139	161	189	128
related diseases	134	192	190	236	—
Other diseases	87	71	72	78	—
Byssinosis	32	126	156	102	78
Farmer's lung	3	14	15	21	3

Adapted from Social Security Statistics, 1976, HMSO, 1978 and CMO's Report DHSS, 1980.

disease which occurs in workers who have been exposed to the dust from cotton or flax. The earlier stages of the process of converting bolls of cotton into thread are the more hazardous. Symptoms (tightness in the chest) usually start on Mondays or following a holiday. In the early stages, the worker is symptomless for the rest of the week. Continued exposure leads to a progressive condition with tightness of the chest and shortness of breath occurring on more and more days of the week until the worker is never free of it. Airways obstruction is prominent and the later stages of the disease are irreversible. The diagnosis is made on the history and the signs of obstructive airways disease coming on during the shift. The chest X-ray is unhelpful.

Other organic dust diseases which should be noted include *farmer's lung* —an acute influenza-like illness caused by allergy to a fungus in mouldy hay. Frequent acute attacks eventually give way to an insidious chronic disease characterised by progressive restrictive lung disease, shortness of breath, loss of weight and increasing respiratory incapacity. The chest X-ray in the acute phase may show fluffy opacities which resolve. Later, non-specific irregular opacities or a honeycomb appearance supervene. Similar diseases can be caused by mouldy cork (suberosis), mouldy sugar cane (bagassosis), bird droppings (bird fancier's lung) and a host of other agents —some rejoicing in titles such as paprika-splitters' lung and maple bark stripper's lung!

In practical terms, however, coal, silica, asbestos and cotton are the most important occupationally, and asbestos is the most important environmentally.

3.4. Compensation for Pneumoconiosis

Before turning to asbestosis it is worth noting that compensation of occupationally acquired dust diseases may be claimed. At present, in Britain, the following are prescribed for compensation under the Social Security (Industrial Injuries) (Prescribed Diseases) Regulations, 1975.

> Pneumoconiosis associated with: mining coal and other minerals; mining, quarrying and dressing slate, granite and sandstone; steel dressing; exposure to asbestos dust; iron and steel foundry work; pottery industry work; and refractory brick making.

In addition, claims may be made for work with cotton and mouldy hay.[7]

4.   ASBESTOS AND ASBESTOS RELATED DISEASE

Asbestos is a widely used mineral fibre which has been shown during the past 50 years to cause a variety of diseases ranging from fibrotic lung disease (asbestosis) to malignant tumours. In contrast to the dust diseases described above, occupational exposure is not an invariable prerequisite for asbestos related disease. The environmental impact of the material, therefore, exceeds that of coal, silica, cotton and the organic dusts.

4.1. Mineralogy

Asbestos is a collective term embracing a group of mineral silicates of varying form and chemical composition. In broad terms asbestos can be divided into two types: *chrysotile* and the *amphiboles* (Fig. 4).

The most important of these in industry is chrysotile (white asbestos) accounting for more than 90% of world production. Crocidolite (blue

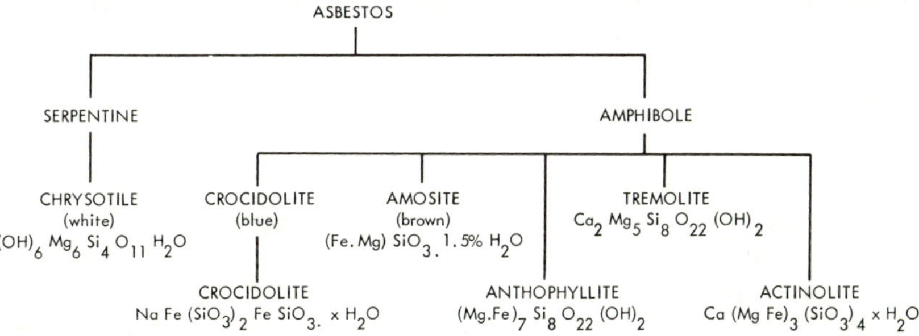

FIG. 4.   Classification and chemical composition of the main types of asbestos.

asbestos) is decreasing in use in the UK, whilst amosite (brown asbestos) may be increasing; anthophyllite, tremolite and actinolite are of minor importance.

Most Western asbestos comes from the vast chrysotile mines in Quebec with lesser quantities emanating from similar size deposits in the USSR. The only source of crocidolite is in South Africa.

Although the term asbestos is usually restricted to the above types, it is important to remember that such fibrous silicates form only a small part of a geological continuum which includes clays, mica, pyroxenes, tremolite and talc. More will be said in Section 5. regarding the risk, if any, of these forms of silicate.

4.2. Properties and Measurement

Asbestos has been used in industry for a century, but the growth in use has been exponential since World War I. The reason for its popularity is its tensile strength and its relative indestructibility. All forms are resistant to temperatures up to 800–1000 °C, and, with the exception of chrysotile, all forms of asbestos are highly resistant to acids and chemicals.

The fibrous nature of the mineral 'ore' also affords an opportunity to weave the material into textiles, whilst the shorter, finer, fibres can be used as binding agents in paint, tiles, paper and cement. The latter use thereby enhancing its value in such building materials by improving their heat and corrosion resistance. Asbestos particles are crystals of consistent shape. They, therefore, tend to split longitudinally into finer fibres and, once embedded in animal tissue, may remain there indefinitely.

The aerodynamic properties of these long fibres implies that the narrower their width the longer they will stay airborne. Electron microscopy reveals that chrysotile fibres are wavy and amphibole fibres are straight and needle-like (Fig. 5). Inhalation of equal masses of each leads to greater lung deposition of the straight amphiboles. However, these animal experiments also show that of the fibres that reach the lungs, both wavy and straight seem equally dangerous.[8]

These series of experiments—notably conducted by Timbrell and Davis —suggest that fibres longer than 200 μm and wider than 3 μm tend to be stopped in the nose (assuming mouth breathing is insignificant). Fibres shorter than 10 μm do get to the lungs but are small enough for macrophage cells to swallow and eject via the ciliary mechanism. Cancer producing effects in animals seem greatest with fibres of 0·5–2·5 μm diameter and 10–80 μm in length.[9] Whether this is relevant to human cancer is not clear but it should be noted that 0·5 μm represents the approximate limit of

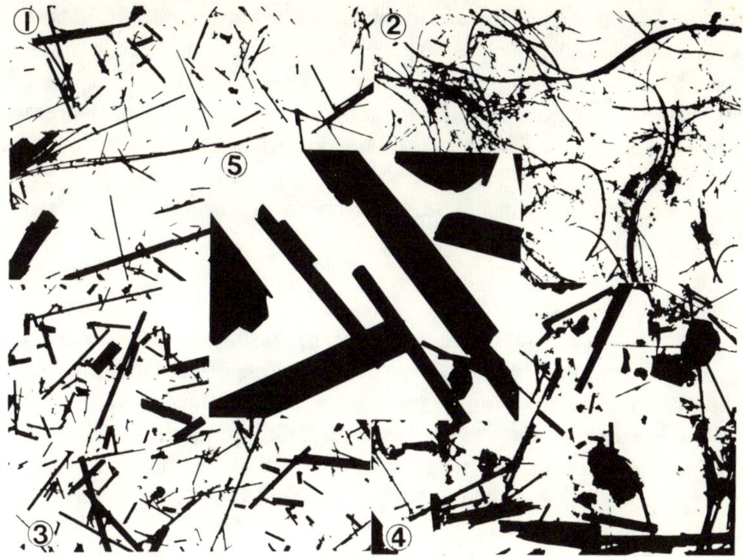

FIG. 5. Electromicrographs of four types of asbestos fibre: (1) crocidolite, (2) chrysotile, (3) amosite, (4) anthophyllite and, for comparison, (5) glass fibre.

resolution of the light microscope in respect of fibre diameter. The implication being that electron microscopic analysis of the fibre content of air is often required to establish not only an accurate dose but also the relative proportions of fibre lengths and types present in the air.

Early measurement work yielded results in the form of total particulate concentrations and a variety of sampling devices have been in vogue. Much work has been done to compare the results of dust measurements using membrane filters and midget impinger methods.[10] The correlations between the two methods are not good. It would appear that in order to predict levels of dustiness in fibres per cubic centimetre from measures of total particles per unit volume, it is first necessary to establish the correlation of the two parameters for each individual site and process considered, as the use of a single conversion factor cannot be justified.

In addition to these problems, as with all airborne particles, there is a difference in results between personal sampling methods and static samplers (the rates being anything from 0·5 to 17). Usually the personal sample results exceed static sample measures. In their final report to the Health and Safety Commission in 1979, the Advisory Committee on Asbestos recommended that a Central Reference Laboratory should be set up to produce *the* standard method for sample evaluation. In the meantime, they recommend that, 'for the purpose of assuring compliance with control limits, industry, enforcing authorities and others, should use personal sampling employing the membrane filter method'.[11] † Such measurements should be taken over a 4 h period and the control limits for asbestos should be: crocidolite, 0·2 fibres ml^{-1}; chrysotile, 1 fibre ml^{-1}; amosite, 0·5 fibres ml^{-1}. These new limits are expected to come into effect on 1st December 1980.

4.3. Work Place Exposure

The ubiquitous use of asbestos and asbestos products means that a wide range of occupational groups are potentially exposed. Obviously, those workers who mine and mill asbestos are at risk though neither job is performed in Britain and, furthermore, as mining is often open cast, the dust exposure is not necessarily as great as might occur in closed mines. The transportation of fibre by road, rail and sea adds transport workers and stevedores to the list of exposed persons.

The raw fibre is then processed to produce textiles, insulation materials, asbestos cement and other building materials. Such process workers are at risk but so are the people who use the finished product: insulators, laggers, brake repairers, fitters, roofers, plumbers and construction workers. Other groups include demolition workers and the men who dump waste materials from such demolition.

Secondary occupational exposure to asbestos may affect persons who work in the vicinity of men handling asbestos (e.g. the office next to the asbestos factory) and similar exposures may occur when farmers disturb soil containing old dumps of waste asbestos. The families of asbestos workers may be significantly exposed if the worker brings asbestos fibre home on his clothes. Clinically proven cases of asbestos related disease have also been reported in persons handling asbestos products in leisure time activities such as do-it-yourself construction work and even by living near areas where waste asbestos has been dumped.

---

† The membrane filter has now largely superseded other methods of asbestos fibre collection and become standard in the United States and Britain (British Occupational Hygiene Society—Committee on Hygiene Standards. Hygiene Standards for chrysotile asbestos dust: *Ann. Occ. Hyg.*, **11**, 47–69 (1968).) The method requires the sampled air to pass through a millipore filter AA of suitable pore size (e.g. 0·8 μm). This retains all the larger diameter fibres and entraps many down to 0·1 μm diameter. The membrane is then cleared with solvent and the fibres viewed by phase contrast light microscopy through a graticule eyepiece. Individual fibre type identification requires electron microscopy.

4.4. Environmental Exposure

Occupational exposure to any dangerous material is usually orders of magnitude greater than environmental risk. Nevertheless, such environmental exposure to asbestos can occur to a significant degree. Few studies have quantified the effect of such contact but the potential is there for asbestos related disease in the general community. For example, city dwellers have been shown to harbour asbestos fibres in their lungs despite the absence of a clear cut history of occupational exposure.[12] This risk of inhalation comes from a variety of sources including asbestos building materials, brake linings, and airborne spread from industrial process and manufacturing plants. Water may be contaminated with excess asbestos dumped near domestic water sources or asbestos may be leached from asbestos cement water pipes. A measurable effect in terms of human disease has not, so far, been detected.[13] Similar unquantified risks exist in food and beverages, though the evidence is scanty and likely to result in the ingestion of very small quantities.

It is worth emphasising that asbestos may be found almost anywhere in developed countries so that it is likely that most people have had some contact with the material at some time or other. As dose–response relationships between asbestos and disease have been demonstrated it seems unlikely that most such environmental contaminations are a significant health risk (see Section 4.5.3.). The hazard has, perhaps, been sensationalised in view of the known serious sequelae to heavily exposed occupational groups, though further epidemiological studies are required before it could be asserted that such contact is harmful.

4.5. Health Effects of Asbestos Exposure

Virtually all the evidence given of health effects in this section is derived from studies of occupationally exposed populations. However, in some cases exposures leading to tumours have been relatively short and some reports provide reasonable evidence to suggest that mesotheliomas resulted from non-occupational exposure.

Asbestos related disease falls into two broad categories: asbestotic effects (pneumoconiosis) and neoplastic effects (tumours).[14] The non-medical reader is well advised to remember that proof of causation is rarely absolute in medicine. Much of the work cited below has a strong epidemiological content and 'proof' of causation depends, in these circumstances, on the weight of evidence rather than on incontrovertible fact.

4.5.1. *Asbestotic Effects*

Asbestosis may be defined as fibrosis of the lungs caused by asbestos dusts.

The lung disease in this context is usually associated with fibrosis of the lining membranes of the inner chest wall and outer surface of the lung (the pleura).

Inhaled asbestos fibres that reach the terminal air passages or the air sacs themselves are subjected to sequestration and removal by the lung's defence mechanisms. Macrophages and red blood cells aggregate around the fibre and a network of reticulin fibres produced by the body enmesh the whole. The cells degenerate, collagen fibre replaces the thin reticulin and the nearest air sacs may thus be obliterated. Cells which produce fibrous tissue (fibroblasts) join the conglomerate and fibrosis develops. In addition some asbestos fibres, coated with some of the above ingredients may be moved out of the area or coughed up. These 'asbestos bodies' are signs of asbestos exposure but not indicative of asbestosis. Calcium deposits in areas of pleural thickening (pleural plaques) have similar connotations.

Continual prolonged exposure increases the lung thickening, and the pleural surfaces may thicken as well. The lungs thus become stiff and the thickened pleura may be likened to slow encasement of the chest in armour. Respiratory function is impaired and shortness of breath ensues.

In uncomplicated asbestosis, shortness of breath is the main symptom. Cough is not uncommon but usually only occurs in asbestos workers who are also smokers. The development of chest pain (as opposed to chest tightness) is an ominous event as it may presage the development of a pleural tumour (mesothelioma). Stethoscope examination of the patient's chest reveals a fine crackle at the bases of the lungs. Later, other signs may be added such as finger clubbing and blueness of the skin due to low blood oxygen. Lung function tests show evidence of restrictive lung disease and impaired gas transfer across the alveoli. The chest X-ray usually shows diffuse shadowing most evident at the bases with or without pleural thickening or plaque formation. The outline of the heart and the diaphragm become fuzzy (Fig. 6).

Fluid may appear in the pleural cavity between the lung and the chest wall and this further impedes normal respiratory function.

The development and severity of asbestosis is related more to continual rather than intermittent or brief exposure to asbestos. Individual susceptibility is widely different. In general, however, the disease once clinically obvious, tends to be progressive despite removal of the patient from subsequent exposure. There is no specific treatment.

4.5.2. *Neoplastic Effects*
The publication, twenty five years ago, of a paper describing an increased

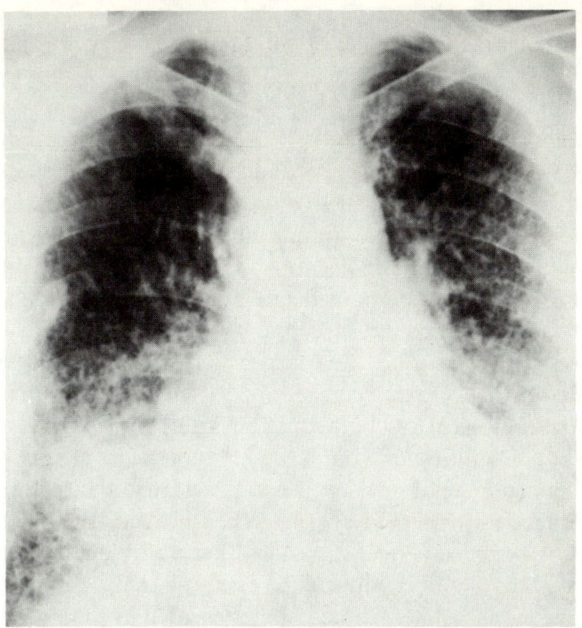

FIG. 6.   Chest X-ray showing advanced asbestosis.

risk of lung cancer in asbestos workers[15] has been followed by many similar reports. The evidence of this relationship between tumour and fibre type is dealt with in Section 4.5.3. Suffice it to say that lung cancers are more common in asbestos workers than other comparable groups and the risk has been shown to be related to fibre type and the degree of exposure, with cigarette smokers at especial risk. The precise cause of the tumour is unknown.

The pleural tumour, mesothelioma, is an unusual cancer and most cases seem to occur in persons who have been exposed to asbestos. The mesothelioma was not widely recognised before 1950. Most cases have been associated with crocidolite or amosite asbestos and the latent period between exposure and appearance of the tumour may range from 20 to well over 40 years.[16] It usually presents as a collection of fluid in the pleural or abdominal cavity with or without pain. The nodular tumour is eventually visible on chest X-ray but the course of the disease is inexorably downhill and invariably fatal—most patients dying within two years of first symptoms.

Asbestos exposure has also been implicated as a cause of tumours of the gastro-intestinal tract, and also, possibly, of the ovary and larynx.

4.5.3. *Epidemiology*

Epidemiology is concerned with the occurrence of disease and its causes. This science has been prominent in addressing certain issues related to asbestos: namely whether asbestos exposure causes certain diseases, whether all fibre types are equally implicated and whether any other factors, personal or environmental, significantly modify the link between cause and effect. A thorough review of the evidence is outside the scope of this chapter but has been lucidly accomplished recently.[17]

Asbestosis has been studied in large populations of exposed workers in a number of countries. Despite considerable attempts of late to standardise the clinical, radiological and lung function criteria for diagnosis, problems remain. The difficulties of comparability are even greater when one considers environmental measurement. Past records of exposure are frequently inaccurate or even absent. When present, the data are rarely comparable with measurements taken in other workplaces. Dose–response relationships are, therefore, difficult to establish. Even taking a relatively crude measure of asbestosis, i.e. cases compensated by the Pneumoconiosis Medical Panel in Britain, nine new cases occurred (0.5% annual incidence) in persons with a cumulative dose of less than 100 fibres-years ml^{-1} (concentration of asbestos × length of exposure).[8] Using more liberal criteria of 'possible asbestosis', a detectable rate of incidence of new cases is found to occur at exposure of less than 50 fibres-years ml^{-1}. However, the overall impression gained is that there is something approaching a linear relationship between cumulative dose and development of fibrotic lung disease. Authorities differ on what constitutes an 'acceptable' level of exposure. For example, the proposed new standards for chrysotile of 1 fibre ml^{-1} would mean that 'possible' asbestosis would be detectable in one in twenty workers exposed at this level for a lifetime.

Crocidolite appears to be more likely to cause fibrosis than chrysotile. Evidence regarding amosite may put it in the same risk category as crocidolite. These varying risks are reflected in the 1980 proposed criteria.

So far as lung cancer is concerned, there can now be little doubt of a relationship between the incidence of the tumour and asbestos exposure. The risk is *not*, as previously thought, confined to smokers. The relative potency of the different fibre types to produce cancer is less clear. The few comparable studies that exist suggest the crocidolite is appreciably more potent than chrysotile in causing lung cancer. However, most occupational exposures are mixed fibre type and therefore preclude such comparisons. Cigarette smoking appears to be a further risk factor, though it is not clear how the interaction between asbestos and cigarettes is afforded.

The first account of a cluster of cases of mesothelioma occurred in association with a crocidolite mining area in South Africa.[18] This report stimulated research into the possibly unique physico-chemical characteristics of crocidolite asbestos. Recent work has suggested that other asbestos types can cause mesothelioma if the dimensions of the fibre are appropriate. This raises the issue of how safe the asbestos substitutes are. Certain conclusions about mesothelioma can be drawn: (1) they seem to be unevenly distributed geographically, with a high concentration near dockyards and certain large asbestos plants; (2) airborne crocidolite seems more likely to produce these tumours in man than chrysotile, though animal studies show no such fibre preference; (3) the status of amosite is uncertain.

The increased incidence of gastro-intestinal tumours reported in some industrial populations is not surprising in view of the fact that if an airborne substance is inhaled, it is also capable of being swallowed. Debate continues about the significance of laryngeal cancer in association with asbestos exposure.

In summary, it may be said that there is strong evidence to suggest that crocidolite asbestos can cause mesothelioma, lung cancer and asbestosis. Crocidolite may well be more potent in producing all these diseases than chrysotile. Pure amosite exposure is rare and this has hindered comparative studies. This fibre does seem to cause asbestosis, lung cancer and mesothelioma and may be as potent in mesothelioma production as crocidolite. In view of the fact that amosite use in Britain has risen sevenfold since World War II, such conclusions, however tentative, give rise for concern. Chrysotile studies have enabled dose–response relationships to be established and thereby a hygiene standard for this fibre can be promulgated with less uncertainty. The possibility that amosite and crocidolite are more dangerous than chrysotile necessitates the establishment of more stringent control. Rough calculations of the risk to the general public of the highest recorded concentrations of asbestos in ambient out of doors air ($10 \, \mathrm{ng \, m^{-3}}$) suggest that the risk of lung cancer is negligible.[8]

4.6. Prevention and Control

The establishment of a health hazard associated with a particular material necessitates consideration of ways of preventing further exposure.

Prevention and control involves three considerations.

1. The formulation, promulgation and enforcement of some control standard which research suggests to be adequate in eliminating (or limiting) the health risk.

2. The feasibility and availability of methods of control in the workplace or the community which will ensure that the standards are not exceeded. These include segregation of the material from the worker by plant and personal protection. Implied in all these manoeuvres is the necessary expertise to monitor the dust levels in the environment and assess the effects on the workers' health.

3. Consideration of the ethical and economic implications of control. This may necessitate substitution of the material with safer alternatives. If exposure continues, *at whatever level*, some quantification of the risk to health should be calculated and a valued judgement made as to its acceptability.

4.6.1. *The Asbestos Control Limits*

The establishment of control limits for any substance is never an easy task. Many TLVs have been promulgated on meagre evidence and the story that some are snatched from the air of the proverbial smoke filled room of experts is not necessarily a fiction. The body of knowledge concerning asbestos related disease is considerable and should, therefore, lead to a control limit which enjoys some degree of confidence. Sadly, however, considerable debate surrounds the validity of even the latest proposals.[11]

For example, there is great variability between personal sampler and static sampler measures of the same working environment. Moreover, sampling is done for periods of the working shift which may not be wholly accurate in assessing the workers' exposure for 8 h a day, 40 h a week, for a lifetime. The recent advisory panel took considerable note of the calculations of lifetime risk using chest crepitations heard with the stethoscope and correlated with cumulative dose estimates. Other workers have recalculated these proposed control limits and suggest that the risk of asbestosis in a working life has been greatly underestimated—to such an extent as to make control limits impossible to enforce or even measure. At the other end of the spectrum is the industry which contends that even the 1980 control limits would be financially crippling in terms of the technology required to suppress dust.

Considering that more is known about asbestos and its health hazards than many other substances also governed by threshold limit values, the whole issue is rather depressing. To labour the point, there is still debate regarding the relative hazards of the different fibres—some contending that chrysotile is as hazardous as crocidolite and amosite; and even if today's control limits were universally acceptable and effective, the toll of asbestos related disease and death will continue as the previously exposed workers succumb to the effects of exposure acquired during the past decade or two.

4.6.2. *Control Measures*

The simplest measure in theory is substitution. However this device faces two drawbacks: the user needs assurance that the substitute is as effective as the original material and the preventive medicine specialist wants assurance that the substitute is, truly, safer. (These considerations ignore the costs of such measures.) Asbestos has unique properties of fire resistance and mechanical stability which are not readily found in other materials. The facts of the matter are that replacement of asbestos in the wide range of products in which it currently resides, requires a number of different substitutes capable of fulfilling some of its properties, but not all. For example, glass fibre is a suitable heat insulator but is useless as a friction material, neither is it as resistant to corrosion. The substitutes may be biologically hazardous themselves: silicaceous substitutes are capable of producing lung fibrosis, hair felts may harbour anthrax bacilli, polyurethanes can cause asthma and, worst of all, glass fibre seems to cause mesothelioma in certain laboratory experiments on animals. In short, there is no one safe substitute for asbestos.

If asbestos is to continue to be used, dust generated in production and manufacture must not reach the workers' lungs. The best method of control is suppression of the dust at source. Milling, screening and blending can (and should) be done within totally enclosed spaces. Fibres may be transported by enclosed carriers, pneumatic systems and bagged into impervious containers. Enclosures can be exhausted and this is particularly necessary when manipulation of the asbestos or its products requires human intervention—for example, sawing asbestos pipe. Such exhausted dust laden air is then collected by wetting the dust or precipitating by thermal or electrostatic devices before being bagged.

Such measures, however efficient, may still generate enough dust to require personal protective clothing for the worker. This is particularly so when asbestos is sprayed or when old asbestos is removed—as in delagging pipes or in demolition work. A range of respirators are available which incorporate filter devices capable of trapping the asbestos. Masks used for such work must be 'approved'—in Britain this means a design made to BS specifications.

Conveyance of asbestos on clothing has proved hazardous in the past and protective clothing such as suits, gloves and footwear may be required.

After work these must be efficiently 'decontaminated' before the worker leaves the area.

It is unnecessary at this juncture to emphasise that all these control measures must be shown to be effective by regular environmental dust monitoring for appropriate time periods, with approved samplers and acceptable analytical procedures. Monitoring the health of the workforce includes exclusion from such works of especially vulnerable people at the pre-employment screen. Periodic assessments follow but although they are used to remove the disabled from further exposure, the crude measures of detecting ill health currently available are unlikely to discover cases of asbestos related disease early enough to arrest its progress.

Finally, broad based education of the workforce regarding the hazards of the work and the precautions necessary helps to engender the appropriate degree of vigilance and concern so that plant control measures are maintained correctly and personal protection is worn appropriately.

4.6.3. *The Ethics and Economics of Control*

Improvement in the control of asbestos dust generation costs money. Every time the control limit is lowered, the manufacturer has to improve or replace existing dust suppression devices, exhaust systems, transportation containers or personal protective equipment. The proposed lowering of the limit for chrysotile from 2 fibres/ml to 1 fibre/ml will, apparently, cost the manufacturers between £300 000 and £1 000 000 in altered dust control equipment and put 3–5% on the cost of the product.[11]

Such measures could lead to a lowered share of the world market, diminished profits, a contracting industry and fewer jobs. However, even these levels of control are estimated to produce excess mortality from asbestos related disease of between 0·2 and 5% for a working lifetime (some put the risk even higher).

Ethical considerations then come into play: is a shortened lifespan acceptable in return for employment? Is a 5% excess mortality an acceptable price for society to pay for the obvious benefits of asbestos? The answers to these questions may be different depending on whether the responder is an asbestos worker, an inhabitant of a tower block whose building is insulated against fire, a man in the street or a Treasury minister. There is no one right answer. Each new standard promulgated requires each aspect to be considered. The final figure expressed as fibres ml^{-1} should be a compromise between the somewhat conflicting issues of occupational health, jobs, money and community safety.

Such conflicts perhaps explain some of the differences noted between the control limits adopted by different countries. No one is right, but the overall aim must be a consistent lowering of the exposure maxima preferably to the limit of available monitoring capability and technological expertise. Total banning of the material is rarely practicable though it is clearly the absolute answer.

5.   MAN MADE MINERAL FIBRES

The increasing use of man made mineral fibres (MMMF) and other, natural, fibres as substitutes for asbestos necessitates a short note here regarding their health effects.[19] Their use as an insulating material is due to their similar fibrous morphology to asbestos. However, some researchers contend that the physical characteristics of asbestos are the main factors controlling its health implications, therefore fibrous zeolites and MMMF may be equally hazardous to health.[20] At present this assertion is largely unsubstantiated in humans. Animal experiments have shown that mesothelioma formation can occur after injection of a variety of non-asbestos fibres *directly* into the pleura but inhalation of the same fibres seems, to date, to be without effect.

Nevertheless, pleural plaques and mesothelioma have been reported in human populations which have no known exposure to asbestos. Clusters of cases of mesothelioma have been noted in Turkey.[21] No asbestos has been found in the area but fibrous zeolites derived from volcanic rock are present in abundance. Its morphological similarity to asbestos supports the 'physical' theory of the cause of mesothelioma. Pleural plaques have been noted in villages in a mountainous area of North-West Greece, again in the absence of recognisable asbestos, but the possibility of other naturally occurring fibrous rocks has not been excluded.

In summary, although other naturally occurring fibrous silicates and MMMF have not been shown to cause occupationally induced human disease, the environmental clusters of lung pathology in Greece and Turkey suggest that a policy of prudence should be pursued in which asbestos should only be substituted for materials with an established record of safety. The history of occupational safety and health is replete with examples of jumping out of the frying pan into the fire.

6.   CONCLUSIONS

Dusts generated in the course of work with coal, silica, asbestos and some organic materials, are capable of inducing serious and sometimes fatal disease in those occupationally or environmentally exposed to them. Asbestos is particularly dangerous in view of its association with cancer and the fact that it is environmentally more widespread. Measures to control exposure include dust control limits, and the possibility of substituting the material with safer alternatives. Despite considerable research spanning fifty years, some aspects of the cause and progression of these dust diseases remain unsolved. However, current and proposed control measures should minimise future exposure, although the full impact of past exposure cannot yet be quantified.

REFERENCES

1. HARRINGTON, J. M. and WALDRON, H. A. The structure and function of the lung, in *Occupational Hygiene*, Waldron, H. A. and Harrington, J. M. (Eds.), Blackwells Scientific Publications, Oxford, 1980, (in press).
2. PARKES, W. R. *Occupational Lung Disorders*, Butterworths, London, 1974.
3. LEE, G. L. Sampling, in *Occupational Hygiene*, Waldron, H. A. and Harrington, J. M. (Eds.), Blackwells Scientific Publications, Oxford, 1980, (in press).
4. COTES, J. E. *Lung Function*, 3rd Edn, Blackwells Scientific Publications, Oxford, 1978.
5. International Labour Office. ILO/UC international classification of radiographs of the pneumoconioses (1971), *Occup. Saf. Hlth. Series*, No. 22, ILO, Geneva, 1972.
6. McCLINTOCK, J. S., RAE, S. and JACOBSON, M. The attack rate of progressive massive fibrosis in British coal miners, in *Inhaled Particles*, Vol. 3, Walton, W. H. (Ed.), Unwin, Woking, 1971, 933–50.
7. Department of Health and Social Security. *Pneumoconiosis and related occupational diseases*, NI 226, HMSO, London, Dec. 1979.
8. ACHESON, E. D. and GARDNER, M. J. The ill effects of asbestos on health, in *Asbestos* Vol. 2, Final Report of the Advisory Committee, Health and Safety Commission, HMSO, London, 1979.
9. STANTON, M. F. Some etiological considerations of fibre carcinogenesis, in *Biological Effects of Asbestos*, Bogovski, P., Gibson, J. S., Timbrell, V. and Wagner, J. C. (Eds.), IARC Sci. Publ., Lyon, 1973.
10. STEEL, J. Asbestos control limits, in *Asbestos* Vol. 2, Final Report of the Advisory Committee, Health and Safety Commission, HMSO, London, 1979.
11. Health and Safety Commission. Final Report of the Advisory Committee on Asbestos, Vol. 1, HMSO, London, 1979.
12. OLDHAM, P. D. Asbestos in lung tissue, in *Biological Effects of Asbestos*, Bogovski, P., Gibson, J. S., Timbrell, V. and Wagner, J. C. (Eds.), IARC Sci. Publ., Lyon, 1973.
13. HARRINGTON, J. M., GRAUN, G. F., MEIGS, J. W., LANDRIGAN, P. J., FLANNERY, J. T. and WOODHULL, R. S. An investigation of the use of asbestos

cement pipe for public water supply and the incidence of gastro-intestinal cancer in Connecticut 1935–1973, *Amer. J. Epidem.*, 1978, **107**, 96–103.

14. SELIKOFF, I. J. and LEE, D. H. K. *Asbestos and Disease*, Academic Press, New York, 1978.

15. DOLL, R. Mortality from lung cancer in asbestos workers, *Brit. J. Ind. Med.*, 1955, **12**, 81–6.

16. McDONALD, J. C. and LIDDELL, F. D. K. Mortality in Canadian miners and millers exposed to chrysotile, *Ann. N.Y. Acad. Sci.*, 1979, **330**, 1–10.

17. McDONALD, J. C. Asbestos-related disease: an epidemiological review, in *Biological Effects of Mineral Fibres*, IARC, Lyon, 1980.

18. WAGNER, J. C., SLEGGS, C. A. and MARCHARD, P. Diffuse pleural mesothelioma and asbestos exposure in North Western Cape Province, *Brit. J. Ind. Med.*, 1960, **17**, 260–71.

19. HILL, J. W. Man made mineral fibres—an evaluation of current knowledge, in *Current Approaches to Occupational Medicine*, Ward Gardner, A. (Ed.), Wright, Bristol, 1979.

20. STANTON, M. F. and WRENCH, C. Mechanisms of mesothelioma induction with asbestos and fibrous glass, *J. Natl. Canc. Inst.*, 1972, **48**, 797–821.

21. BARIS, Y. L. *Environmental Asbestos Related Diseases in Turkey*, Hacettepe University School of Medicine, Ankara, Turkey, 1975.

Chapter 6

WATER QUALITY MONITORING AND CONTROL

R. Briggs
D.Tech., C.Eng., F.I.E.E., F.Inst.M.C., M.Inst.W.P.C.
*Consultant Research Associate, Water Research Centre,
Stevenage Laboratory, Hertfordshire, UK*

SUMMARY

The state of the art in 1980, based largely on progress in the United Kingdom, of instruments and systems for monitoring and control of water quality is discussed, including some aspects of systems deployed in the operation of water and wastewater treatment and transport systems.

Progress with water quality and hydrometric monitoring networks in some Regional Water Authority Areas is given and philosophies for further developments discussed. Since the viability of any on-line monitoring and control system depends ultimately on the availability of robust, inexpensive and reliable sensors, developments in this area are discussed and so too are developments in systems engineering which provide better reliability when utilising existing sensors.

Also discussed are certain aspects of sampling for off-line analysis since, at the present time, networks for monitoring and control will largely depend on sampling and off-line analysis, particularly when the information is not required for immediate control action.

Finally, an indication is given of the impact on both sensors and systems developments of recent advances in the semi-conductor field.

1. INTRODUCTION

The reorganisation of the Water Industry in England and Wales in 1974 brought together, on a catchment basis, responsibility under a unified management for all aspects of the hydrological cycle including pollution control, conservation, distribution and reclamation. In order to discharge this responsibility the industry deploys at least 70 000 people and has a major capital investment programme amounting to at least £400 million per year in 1974.

It is vital, therefore, that management is effective at all levels and a major factor in achieving this is the timely availability of accurate water quality and flow data. These data can be obtained in a variety of ways but there are clearly advantages in recording continuously variables of most significance, particularly those which are labile and which vary rapidly spatially and/or temporally, and to deploy a system of storage, reduction and dissemination which allows their effective use for planning for future needs, for pollution surveillance and for control of treatment plants.

As a result there has, in recent years, been a significant increase in the deployment of instrumentation and control systems by the UK water industry and, based on the results of a recent questionnaire carried out on behalf of the DOE/NWC Working Party on Control Systems for the Water Industry,[1] it is clear that the rates of deployment of instruments and control systems are increasing also. The 10 Regional Water Authorities and Independent Water Companies are collectively intending to spend of the order of £50 million in this area over the next three to five years.

Already the value and use of telemetry has become widely accepted in water distribution and in water and wastewater treatment; automation of the more straightforward tasks such as flow control, control of filter backwashing, and operation of valves and penstocks has become commonplace. The use of central computers for simple control and data-logging purposes has also increased and the advances in the development of cheap mini-computers and microprocessors are likely to accelerate this. Process optimisation is, however, less common. In the case of water treatment, the major difficulties are the complex nature of the coagulation and flocculation processes and the lack at present of really reliable systems for monitoring colour and turbidity. In the case of wastewater treatment, not only are there difficulties in instrumentation, but in many cases the resultant cost/benefit has not yet been clearly established.

The present situation will, therefore, be briefly reviewed, and recent developments, particularly at the Water Research Centre, discussed.

2. DISTRIBUTION

2.1. In the United Kingdom

Pepper and Banks[2] have described a system currently operated by the Sunderland and South Shields Water Company in which the performance of a number of groundwater pumping stations, service reservoirs, major upland supplies, distribution transfer points, and distribution system pressures is monitored; the data are telemetred to a central control station. The major benefits reported to be derived from use of this system are as follows.

1. The ability to tune up and keep a close control over the distribution system, including the ability to assess demand patterns more confidently and, in consequence, to save energy by elimination of unnecessary pumping.
2. The provision of a more consistent service to the consumer in terms of water pressure and the more speedy repair of bursts.
3. The physical assets of the undertaking can be more effectively used. Service reservoir capacities are utilised fully, stocks are balanced over the system and bulk transfer of water is more easily arranged.
4. Manpower is more effectively deployed.

The East Worcester Water Works Company too have in recent years developed a telecontrol system,[3] at a cost of £165 000 (1973 prices), to permit the company's supply and distribution works, spread over an area of 300 square miles in Worcestershire and Warwickshire, to be supervised and controlled centrally (using an on-line computer) from the Sugarbrook Pumping Station. The system employs both land-line and radio links to supervise the company's six main source stations which derive supplies from boreholes, five spring sources, 15 boosters, 21 reservoirs and six water towers. In addition, it is capable of considerable extension to allow for future developments, including additional water towers and boreholes, control of ultra-violet sterilisation of certain Cotswold spring sources and fluoridation, utilising automatic analysers and dosing control. Already the ability to detect pressure drops in mains has resulted in a considerable reduction in losses due to leakage. A co-operative project involving the Water Company, the Severn-Trent Water Authority, the Water Research Centre and the Department of Control Engineering at Cambridge University is underway, the theme being minimisation of energy costs. Already automatic detection of waste is practicable and the scheme is well on the way to establishing complete on-line computer control.

2.2. In the USA and Elsewhere

It has been stated by Guarino and Radziul[4] that the most exercised practice in the water works field in the US is the instrumentation and automation of the various elements of distribution systems, transmission conduits and aqueducts by the use of supervisory central control stations. These stations (about 100) receive data from remote field sites via land-line or microwave radio links and also retransmit control signals, based on the information received, to operate these remote and unattended facilities. Some stations have computer capabilities and, as a result, can monitor and regulate demands for electrical power and so achieve significant reductions in energy utilisation. As yet no attempt has been made to operate these facilities under closed-loop control, although the technology exists to achieve this. It appeared at the time of the review (1977) that the funding and manpower resources required for field studies and for the development of the logistics of water distribution system control, and the required control algorithms for this purpose were beyond the scope and resources of all but the largest water works. It will be interesting, however, to see if recent developments in micro-processor technology alter the situation in the near future.

Work on the development and testing of prototype water quality sensors for monitoring certain water quality indicators in water distribution, has also been reported.[5]

Developments in instrumentation and automation in water treatment and distribution in Europe, Japan and elsewhere have, in general, followed similar lines to those in the UK and the USA. Progress in Northern Europe and Japan has been summarised by Hultman[6] and Hiraoka and Nogita,[7] respectively.

3. WATER TREATMENT

3.1. In the United Kingdom

Griffiths[8] presented in 1970 a comprehensive review of water-treatment plant control and instrumentation in the United Kingdom and reported that, although Lewis[9] had developed an empirical equation which could be used to predict the required coagulant dose at the Strenshaw works, accurate coagulation dose control for sedimentation plant was extremely difficult. Practicable control of coagulation, flocculation and sedimentation has been recently discussed in detail by Melbourne and Butcher and relevant work at the Water Research Centre has been described.[10] Control of most of the other aspects of water treatment such as flow, filter backwashing, chlorination, and dechlorination can be fully automated and over the years adoption of instrumentation and automation has steadily increased. Operation of the first rapid gravity filter to be controlled by head loss and automatically backwashed began in 1949. In 1952 the Broadside works in Scotland was equipped with centralised flow control and automatic backwash facilities on the filters, and in 1956 the Pitsford softening plant at Northampton was commissioned with extensive automation for preparation and handling of chemicals, and disposal of sludge. Chemical doses were, however, controlled manually. The first fully automated plant in the United Kingdom was the Elvington softening works supplying Sheffield; this was commissioned in 1960. Control of flow, filter backwashing, chlorination and dechlorination was fully automatic, but chemical additions were largely controlled on the basis of flow. However, trimming quantities of lime and soda ash were added under the control of signals from raw water, alkalinity and total hardness monitors. A computer was installed, initially to log essential water quality parameters and subsequently for complete automation of the chemical treatment, based on quality rather than flow.

Because no general solution to the problem of coagulation plant control has yet been found, empirical control procedures (largely of a manual nature) have been developed in many cases to suit particular plant design and raw water characteristics.[11–15]

The recent developments, described in subsequent sections, of instruments and systems for monitoring the quality of raw waters are likely, however, to result in the use of feed-forward control systems in the not too distant future, possibly using empirical models such as that of Lewis[9] to automate the coagulation and flocculation processes.

3.2. In the USA

The status in the USA of instrumentation and automation for water treatment plants as indicated by Guarino and Radziul[4] is summarised below. The literature contains about 30 references to the automation of water treatment plants in the United States. Most of these installations, however, are supervisory and devoted to monitoring local analogue loops with alarm indication, data logging being the most prominent feature, little attempt having been made at the time of the review (1977) to derive optimising process control algorithms or strategies. Control of the total water treatment system based on automating the measurement of indicator variables and the use of feed-forward and feedback techniques has been discussed by Radziul and Suffet.[16] Their work contains a generalised appraisal of general instrumentation and associated control loops which is still valid today. It is of note that out of some 61 variables identified as being important for water treatment, only 26 were thought to be suitable for measurement instrumentally, and, of those, only 10 could readily be automated for on-line applications provided some agency or party were given sufficient incentive. An important point made was that 10 of the more important variables appeared at that time to be limited to a strictly manual method of analysis for the foreseeable future. However, it was also suggested the output for the few available on-line sensors might be fed to a suitable 'black box' mathematical model which could then be used for process control. Finally it was noted that recent legislation might result in the requirement to remove or limit the level of certain trace organic substances from drinking water and this, in turn, would result in a requirement for new analytical techniques and on-line instruments.

4.   WASTEWATER TREATMENT

4.1. In the United Kingdom

As indicated earlier, less progress has been made in the automation of wastewater treatment plants than has been made in the automation of distribution systems and some aspects of water treatment. Only two major works in the UK, namely, Whitlingham and Carbarns have had much long-term experience in the use of centralised computing facilities for operational control and have not, as yet, progressed very far with the optimisation of unit processes, except perhaps control of the concentration of dissolved oxygen in aeration lanes. However, other possibilities for automating this process have been discussed in detail by Briggs and Jones[17] who concluded that the use of telemetry for data gathering, the use of mathematical models (supplied with data obtained both on and off-line) to aid in day-to-day operations and in longer term management decision processes and the use of a minimum of on-line control loops with centralised set-point adjustment could result in considerable benefit at modest cost.

4.2. The Whitlingham Sewage Treatment Works of the Anglian Water Authority, Norwich Sewage Division[18–26]

The Whitlingham Works of the Norwich Sewage Division of the Anglian Water Authority serves a population of 200 000 and has a DWF (dry weather flow) of $55\,000\,m^3\,day^{-1}$. The final effluent, discharging to the River Yare, must not contain more than 30 mg litre^{-1} suspended solids and 20 mg litre^{-1} BOD.

The plant includes screens, disintegrators, detritors, percolating filters, activated sludge plant, heated anaerobic sludge digestion tanks and pressure filtration. The various treatment units are substantially automated. Control, data acquisition, monitoring, using quantity and in some cases quality sensors and data processing are performed by minicomputers. Software makes extensive use of a high level process sequencing language; 20 routines were specially developed and are capable of overriding normal control instructions in the event of electrical or mechanical failures of the plant or under storm conditions.

The operational program occupies approximately 14K of core memory and contains some 60 different programs and 174 plain language messages. Further programs control and monitor the inlet screens, flow division, aeration channels, the sequential switching of pumps and valves for recirculation or double filtration techniques and batch feeding of the anaerobic sludge digestion process. The control system is connected to the plant via 436 input and 207 output channels with a total of 32K core memory. Plant operations are monitored and controlled from the central control room where the operator communicates with the system via the operator control panel (OCP) and the logging printer. The OCP has digital displays for presentation of information and push button facilities for entry of data and instructions. The operator can update set-points, retrieve data on demand and initiate various control strategies. In the event of a computer failure, provision has been made for the continuity of control using manual access facilities and a mimic diagram.

The control system which was installed during 1974/75 at a cost of approximately £183 000 (including instrumentation, control system and cabling) represents 3·5% of the total current value of the two treatment plants (1976 costs).

Owing to the major extensions, an assessment of the effects of automatic control is difficult. However, the number of operating staff prior to automation (22) has not changed despite an effective doubling of capacity. A substantial amount of time and effort has been spent in commissioning the control systems and in overcoming operational difficulties with the treatment processes between 1974 and 1976 and a full assessment of the system is currently being undertaken.

4.3. The Carbarns Wastewater Treatment Works of the Strathclyde Regional Council, Lanark Division[27–31]

The treatment works, which serves a population of 42 000 has a DWF of 22 750 m^3 day^{-1}.

Treatment comprises screening, grit removal, settlement, activated sludge and anaerobic sludge digestion. The effluent quality criteria are suspended solids not greater than 30 mg litre^{-1} and BOD not greater than 20 mg litre^{-1}.

The control system at Carbarns also controls two other treatment plants via telemetry links. These are the Clyde Park works having a DWF of 9450 m^3 day^{-1} and the Coursington works with a DWF of 4500 m^3 day^{-1}.

A mini-computer with 12K core memory serves all three works. The system also provides for monitoring and data logging and utilises three tele-typewriters. Very little trouble was experienced with the control and telemetry systems. However, during commissioning, considerable problems were experienced with the measurement of level and flow in sewers and with mechanical and electrical items of plant which are normally reliable. Most of the control systems were installed in 1974, but full closed loop control was deferred until the quality sensing elements were made more reliable.

It has been estimated that a conventional plant would have needed 35 to 40 manual workers and automation has enabled the plant to be operated with only half this number. The cost of the control system (including instruments, cabling, telemetry, etc.) was £108 000 which represents 4·5% of the total current value of the treatment plant (1976 costs).

4.4. In the USA

A USEPA report[32] published in 1976 and summarised by Guarino and Radziul[4] gives the results of a national survey of the instrumentation and automation at 50 wastewater treatment facilities throughout the USA. The technical and economic benefits of current monitoring and control practices were studied to determine cost effective measures for improvements in the performance and reliability of wastewater treatment facilities. It is of interest that only 10 of the plants had computer control systems with only a few process streams under set-point, direct digital, or sequential control and that with most of the computerised systems the operator made the final adjustments based on logged data and calculations.

Also in the summary[4] is evidence of the preponderant need for analysers for wastewater treatment facilities, compared, for example, with the requirements in the petrochemical industry; this is reproduced in Table 1.

Reproduced in Table 2 are instrument performance data[4] from which it can be seen that maintenance problems are relatively severe, probably because of the hostile environment and the diversity of instruments. No mention was made in the report of the maintenance required for computer hardware and software. Limited UK experience indicates that whilst this is

TABLE 1
COMPARISON OF MEASURING INSTRUMENTS USED

Variable	Wastewater treatment plants (%)	Petroleum plants (%)
Flow	30	48
Level	19	22
Density	7	—
Pressure	—	8
Temperature	—	17
Miscellaneous	15	—
Analysers	29	5

TABLE 2
INSTRUMENT PERFORMANCE (AVERAGE)

Variable	Instrument	Maintenance (times per year)
Level	Bubbler	12
Flow	Venturi and magnetic	4, 12
Density	Nuclear	48
Analysers	DO, pH	100, 300
Miscellaneous	Pressure	5

TABLE 3
DISINFECTION BY CHLORINE ADDITION

Control method	Benefits	Advantages
Fixed rate	—	Simple and reliable
Flow proportional	15% labour saving 25% chlorine saving	Reliable and well established
Residual chlorine feedback	15% labour saving 50% chlorine saving	Well established good effluent residual control

TABLE 4
SUMMARY OF AUTOMATED PERFORMANCE[4]

Variable	Improvement
Air/unit BOD removal	21·9
Air/unit volume of effluent	11·6
BOD removed/blower (kWh)	32·1
BOD removal efficiency	13·8
Improvement in sludge volume index	108·6

not insignificant it is far less of a problem than that of maintaining the basic instrumentation. However, the initial cost of software writing is high.

The survey also illustrates that savings in chemicals and power (10–20 %) can be obtained with partial automation and the use of well known control strategies. As an example, the benefits and advantages of chlorination control detailed in the survey have been summarised in tabular form by Guarino and Radziul.[4] This information is reproduced in Table 3.

Additionally, the percentage savings in power costs and improvement in BOD removal from 12 automated activated sludge wastewater treatment plants has been given by the same authors in tabular form; these data are produced in Table 4.

4.5. In Europe, Japan and Elsewhere

Developments in Europe and Japan appear to have fallen somewhere between those in the US, where the greatest expenditure has been in the computer control area and in the development of control strategies aimed at works serving large populations, and developments in the UK, which have been aimed with one or two exceptions at monitoring as an aid to management. Since full details of developments in automation of wastewater treatment are available in the literature[33,34] these will not be discussed further here.

4.6. Current Developments in the UK

Because of the current uncertainties about the real benefit of automation in wastewater treatment apart from the more obvious ones such as improvements in reliability, e.g. centralised logging of equipment status and remote control of simple sequencing operations such as filter backwashing and automatic operation of valves and penstocks, the Water Research Centre at the recommendation of the Working Party on Control Systems for the Water Industry is now involved in a detailed economic appraisal of existing control systems with a view to establishing reliable cost benefit criteria. Additionally in co-operation with the Chiltern Division of Thames Water Authority the Centre is carrying out a detailed experimental programme at Blackbirds Sewage Works. This involves the installation of two mobile monitors for measurement of the concentration of dissolved oxygen, suspended matter, organic matter, oxidised nitrogen and ammonia in the influent and effluent of each unit process taken in turn and, where appropriate, sludge blanket levels, sludge solids concentration and temperature. A Texas 990/10 computer with a 10 megabite disc enhancement is to be installed at the works to log the water quality data and to interface to the remote control system and flow recorders at present in operation. The deterministic model described by Jones[35] will be deployed, as indicated earlier,[17] to develop control strategies and as an aid to the decision taking process. The real-time quality data will be used for model verification and to establish alternative transfer functions for the unit processes.

It is hoped that this detailed experimental work coupled with the economic study will enable the Centre to establish firm guidelines for the cost effective deployment of instruments and control systems in waste water treatment and the River Wear system, described subsequently, will be similarly deployed in the context of water treatment.

5. MONITORING OF SOURCE WATER

Presumably the fundamental reason for monitoring the quality of natural waters is the assessment of their suitability for a specific purpose. The criteria of quality of waters intended to support fish, to serve as a source of public supply, or to serve as an industrial coolant may well be very different and it is clearly impracticable to design an automatic monitoring system in which measurements are made of all the chemical, physical and biological factors involved. It is desirable, however, to devise a system of data collection, storage and dissemination which would accept information resulting from analysis of manual samples as well as from automatic water quality monitoring stations. This requirement was recognised in the US and a data storage and retrieval system (STORET)[36–40] was designed and built under the auspices of the Federal Water Pollution Control Administration (FWPCA) and continues in operation today under the control of the Environmental Protection Agency (EPA).

As early as 1962 Mentink, under the auspices of the FWPCA, produced specifications for an integrated water quality data acquisition system and for a slow speed telemetry system for water pollution surveillance[41,42] and, mainly as a result of experience gained with the Orsanco project which was brought into being by Cleary in 1960,[43] has updated them several times since. The water quality monitoring systems operating in New York harbour, on the River Delaware, on the River Potomac and elsewhere in the US are based almost entirely on Mentink's specifications and the hardware is obtainable from several sources including the Schneider Instrument Company†, Honeywell Controls and the Robert Shaw Controls Company.

† Mention of trade names or company products in this chapter does not constitute endorsement or recommendation for use by the Water Research Centre.

The current Orsanco system has been described by Klein, Dunsmore, and Horton[44] and comprises 14 field stations, eight of which are on the Ohio River and six on tributaries, a central receiving station, and a data processing centre. All field stations are equipped with transmitters for telemetering data to headquarters using exclusively based 0–15 Hz teletype grade lines and can measure some or all of the following variables: pH value, oxidation–reduction potential, conductivity, temperature, solar radiation and the concentrations of dissolved oxygen and chloride ions. The cost of such a system at 1968 prices and converted to pounds sterling would be a capital investment of £68 000, and an annual running cost of £22 000. Assuming a system capability of 650 000 items of processed data, the cost of collection would be about 3p and of processing 1p per item of data. Modern technology, however, will have considerable impact on the costs of data processing and collection and it is of interest in this context that the Philadelphia Water Department conducted an experiment on the transmission of data from the monitoring sites on the River Delaware to a satellite which retransmitted the data to a ground station which subsequently processed the data and rerouted it to user agencies.[45] The success of this experimental project culminated in the Geostationary Operational Environmental Satellite System which collects and distributes river monitor data on a continuous real-time basis. This system provides for advanced warning for floods and for the surveillance of water quality (chemical spills, etc.).

In January 1977 a workshop on Water Quality Monitoring Networks was organised by the World Health Organisation's Regional officer for Europe in collaboration with the Government of the UK. The aim of this workshop was to review the development of water quality monitoring networks in various countries (12) and prepare recommendations for their optimisation. Since progress has been very similar in the US, the UK, Europe and Japan there seems little point in reporting in detail on each country separately, this information being available in the WHO report.[46]

The detailed work discussed subsequently will be based, therefore, to a great extent on developments in the UK with which the author has been personally involved. Certain differences in emphasis and the reasons for these, however, are worthy of comment. In the US and in Europe, since river quality criteria are used as the basis for consents for discharges and because rivers cross state or international boundaries, the emphasis has been on the system or network approach so that data would be immediately available to allow users to be warned of sudden changes in quality and to enable sources of pollution to be quickly detected. In the UK the initial requirement was for data for planning, for research and for following trends in quality, hence the emphasis was on the development of package water quality monitors in which the data were logged on autographic recorders and/or magnetic tape for subsequent off-line processing. Recently, however, a detailed economic appraisal of methods of monitoring water quality has suggested that in the UK also the justification for on-line instrumental methods must be that of a data requirement for day to day management. As a consequence, recent work in the UK has been directed towards a systems approach and to the development of robust, reliable and maintenance-free systems. In contrast to the USA and Europe, because of the relatively small size of river basins, the use of satellites does not yet seem appropriate for river management in the UK.

The data required for river management, including, in particular, those required for protection of intakes and for facilitating feed-forward control of water treatment processes, may be divided into two classes.

1. Variables that need to be monitored continuously or semicontinuously; this may be because they vary rapidly either in the source water itself or in a sample bottle (for example, temperature, BOD, colour and concentrations of dissolved oxygen, ammonia, suspended matter and organic matter) or because they form the basis of an automatic alarm or control system.

2. Concentrations of stable substances, such as soluble inorganic solids, when a knowledge of long-term trends alone is required; these data can be obtained by manual or automatic sampling followed by laboratory analysis.

Variables which are thought to require continuous or semicontinuous recording are listed in Table 5, together with preferred units and limits of accuracy.

Other variables which need to be measured, but not necessarily continuously or at all stations unless required for automatic control purposes, include cyanide, phenol, copper, zinc, nickel, cadmium, chromium, pesticide and herbicide residues, colour, COD, toxicity and substances responsible for taste and odour. Additionally, for waters required for potable supply and irrigation, the bacterial content and concentrations of sodium, boron, heavy metals and suspended solids (for spray irrigation) are also of importance.

For protection of fisheries, and possibly for protection of intakes to water treatment plants, a continuous measurement of toxicity can be made by recording the activity of fish in a tank at a water quality monitoring station.

TABLE 5
PREFERRED UNITS AND LIMITS OF ACCURACY FOR DATA REQUIRED FROM AUTOMATIC WATER QUALITY MONITORS

Data	Unit	Range
Temperature	°C	-10–40 ± 0.5°C (linear scale)
Dissolved oxygen	% of air saturation value	0–100 ± 1% of saturation 0–200 ± 2% of saturation (linear scale)
Ammoniacal nitrogen	mg N litre^{-1}	0–5 ± 5% of reading (log scale) 0–10 0–50
Organic matter	mg C litre^{-1}	0–10 ± 5% of reading (log scale) 0–100
Colour[a]	°Hazen	0–10 ± 5% of reading (log scale) 0–200
Suspended matter	mg litre^{-1} based on formazin standard	5–500 ± 5% of reading (log scale) 50–5000
Conductivity	micromhos cm^{-2}	5–5 000 ± 5% of reading (log scale) 50–50 000
Chloride	mg Cl litre^{-1}	0·5–500 ± 5% of reading (log scale) 25–25 000
Hardness	mg litre^{-1} as CaCO$_3$	10–1 000 ± 5% of reading (log scale)
pH value	pH units	2–11 ± 0.1 (linear)
Sunlight intensity	cal cm^{-2} h^{-1}	0–120 ± 1.2 (linear)
Dissolved carbon dioxide	mg litre^{-1} as CO$_2$	0–100 ± 5% of reading (log scale)

[a] In the context of control of water treatment only.

5.1. Equipment

A number of manufacturers now offer a wide range of discrete instruments and integrated monitors capable of measuring one or more of these parameters. (Examples are shown in Fig. 1.) Those manufactured by Electronic Instruments Ltd, Plessey Radar Ltd and Philips Pollution Monitoring measure temperature, dissolved oxygen, conductivity, turbidity (suspended solids) and pH value; the Philips monitor also measures redox potential (ORP) and chloride ion concentration in the standard instrument. The costs of individual monitors, which range between £5000 and £18 000 (1976 prices), are reflected in the special facilities available with each type; these are listed in Table 6.

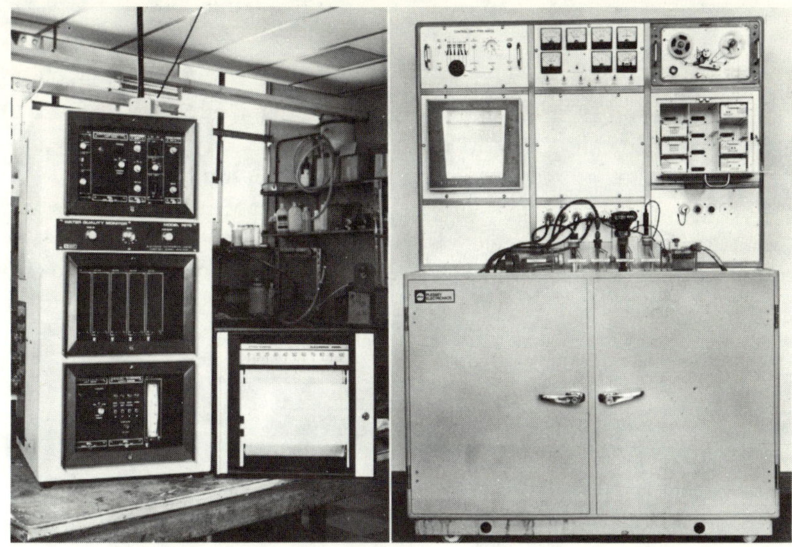

FIG. 1. Examples of commercially available integrated water quality monitors.

TABLE 6

FACILITIES AVAILABLE WITH THREE COMMERCIAL WATER QUALITY MONITORS

Electronic Instruments type 7972	*Plessey Radar type MM5*	*Philips Pollution Monitoring (AWMS)*
Automatic cleansing at 6 or 12 h intervals, lasting 0·5 h. Chemical injection system. Flow failure indication. Sensor outputs fed to meter and autographic chart recorder. Optional magnetic tape data logger and/or line telemetry with additional sensor–interface buffering. Mains-powered, small, portable and wall-mounted. Pumping and external plumbing supplied by user.	Automatic cleaning or calibration at 12 or 24 h intervals lasting 4 min, by chemical substitution technique. Battery powered. External sampling at discrete 0·25, 0·5 or 1·0 h intervals. Sensor contamination thus minimised. Automatic sample taking when alarm conditions are indicated. Sensor outputs fed to meters, autographic chart recorder and magnetic tape data logger. Telemetry optional extra.	Automatic ultrasonic clearing of individual sensors (except turbidity) at 1·0 h intervals. Automatic individual sensor calibration at low and high values of ranges at 12 or 24 h intervals. Monitor supplied in stand-alone steel cabinet. Automatic sample taking and refrigerated storage facility optional extra. Sensor outputs to autographic chart recorders (2 per channel). Variable stage pumping facility provided with monitor. Line or radio telemetry optional extra.

Each of these monitors has been evaluated at the Water Research Centre between 1972 and 1975. Results have indicated that they can be expected to operate automatically for periods varying from a few days to several weeks, depending on the application and the type of monitor.[47-49]

For use in remote areas where mains power is not available and where vandalism may occur, a range of battery powered, portable, submersible equipment has been developed (Fig. 2). Again these monitors vary in cost

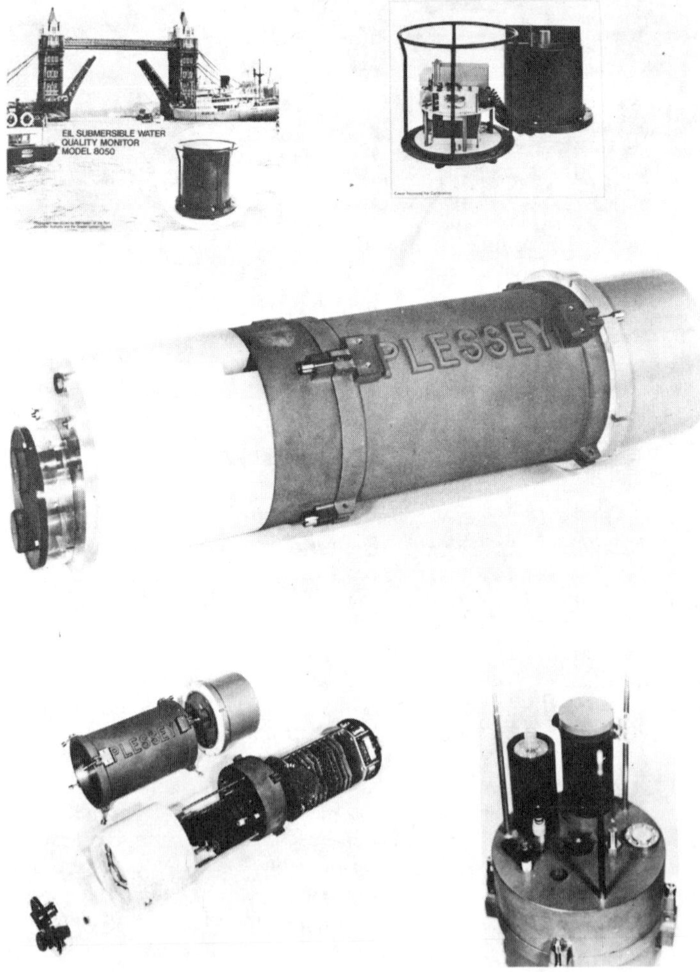

FIG. 2.   Submersible water quality monitors.

and complexity, ranging from a simple temperature and dissolved oxygen recorder marketed by Electronic Instruments Ltd at about £800 (1976 price) to a multi-parameter unit developed in co-operation with Plessey Radar Ltd, which records data originating from temperature, depth (pressure), turbidity (suspended solids), dissolved oxygen, pH, and salinity (conductivity) sensors on an incremental magnetic tape deck and costs about £9000 (1976 price). An evaluation[50] carried out at the Stevenage Laboratory and in the field indicated that in mildly polluted waters satisfactory data were obtained for about 95% of the 4 month period provided the equipment was cleaned every 5 days.

Several of these monitors have been installed in the UK in recent years (Table 7) mainly for evaluation purposes. Few have so far been shown to be cost effective in terms of river management although in applications such as protection of the River Wear intake (described subsequently) the potential economic benefit has been clearly demonstrated.

The deployment of similar monitoring stations on the mainland of Europe is given in Table 8.

5.2. Telemetry

Experience has shown that, even when skilled staff carry out regular preventative maintenance procedures on these monitors, the integrity of the recorded data cannot be guaranteed. Even with automatic cleaning and/or calibration of sensors, the performance of the equipment should be monitored continuously, particularly where the signals are used for provision of early warning of spills or for control purposes. In such situations the use of telemetry networks with a computerised control station has been shown to be extremely valuable and has the additional advantage that the operations of the monitor itself can be remotely controlled.

The Centre, in close co-operation with the Sunderland and South Shields Water Company, has designed and built a water quality monitoring station which is in operation on the River Wear and has the specific objective of protecting a water intake. When the company found it necessary to augment its water supplies, a widespread survey indicated that the lower reaches of the River Wear near Chester-le-Street would provide the most suitable source. Although at the site chosen for abstraction the river is scheduled as a Class 1, clean river, there are in the catchment area a number of sewage, trade, and mine effluent discharges. The provision of bankside storage was found to be impracticable and the company, therefore, decided to install an early warning system—a water quality monitoring station some 2·5 miles upstream of the intake. Commercially available water

TABLE 7
WATER QUALITY MONITOR INSTALLATIONS IN UK IN MARCH 1975

Authority	Site	Type
Anglian WA	Chelmer at Chelmsford	EIL
	Neve at Wansford	Plessey
	Welland at Tinwall	Plessey
	Ouse at Roxton	
	Ouse at Bedford	Protech
	Ouse at Bottisham	
	New site in Welland	
	Nene	Plessey (TBA)
Southern WA	Ouse at Barcombe Mills	Plessey
	Cuckmore at Arlington	Plessey (remote alarm)
	Eastbourne Water Works	EIL and Technicon
	Hardham	Plessey and EIL
Wessex WA	Parrett at Langport	EIL
South-West WA	Experimental site	Special—home made
	Exe at Thorverton Bridge	EIL and Plessey
English China Clays Ltd	Exe at Exeter	Plessey
Welsh National Water DB	Dee at Chester Weir	
	Usk at Newport	
	Usk at Chain Bridge	EIL
	Usk estuary at St Julians	
	Taff at Abercynan	Plessey and EIL
	Tawe at Landore Bridge	EIL
	Teifi at Glantaifi	
North-West WA	Kent at Sedgwick	Plessey (prototype)
	Lune at Caton	EIL
	Ribble at Salmesbury	Plessey
	Irwell at Stubbins	EIL
	Bellam at Dunham Massey	Protech
	Eamont at Penrith	EIL
Northumbrian WA	Tyne at Newcastle	Plessey and Arxon W/L
Portsmouth Polytechnic	Mobile in caravan (sewage effluents)	Plessey
Sheffield Polytechnic	Mobile—steel works effluents	Plessey
Clyde RPB	Clyde at Glasgow	EIL
	S. Calder Water at Bellshill	EIL
Tweed RPB	Tweed at Boleside	QMI
Lothians RPB		Plessey
WRC	On loan to Lea Division of Thames WA	Plessey

TABLE 7—*contd.*

Authority	Site	Type
Severn-Trent WA	Stour at Stourport	Protech–Simac
	Severn at Malvern	Protech
	Trent at Colwick	Plessey prototype
	Trent at Nottingham	Protech and EIL
	Trent at Yoxall	Plessey and EIL
	Derwent at Matlock	Plessey and EIL
	Tame at Lea Marston	Plessey and EIL (dual source)
	Marston-on-Dove	Plessey and EIL
	Derwent at Draycott	Plessey and EIL (Wilne Res.)
	Tame at Elford	Plessey and EIL
Thames WA	Thames at Oxford	Plessey
	Thames at Wallingford	EIL
	Thames at Windsor	Plessey
	Lee at Water Hall	EIL[a]
	Lee at Kings Weir	EIL[a]
	Lee at Springfield	EIL[a]
	Lee at Stanstead Abbotts	EIL (TBA)[a]
	Stort at Roydon	EIL (June 1975)[a]
PLA	Thames at London	QMI

[a] Telemetry network: central stations at WRC Stevenage and Lea Division, Waltham Cross.

TABLE 8

WATER QUALITY MONITOR INSTALLATIONS IN EUROPE—DEPLOYING TYPES OF MONITORS EVALUATED AT WRC (1975)

Authority	Site	Type
Gothenburg Water Board	Gota Alv at Nya Alvsborg	Plessey, multi depth
Riza (Netherlands)	Rhine at Lobith	Plessey
RID (Netherlands)	Effluent at Dordrecht	Philips
RIV (Netherlands)	Lith	EIL
Finland	Helsinki	Plessey (for evaluation)
CNDR—Italy	Rome	Plessey
		EIL 'considerable no.'
	Milan	Philips (14 monitors)
Romania	—	Plessey (2 monitors)
Artois—Picardie	Lysat Armentiers	Plessey (H_2S problem)
France	Valencienne	Philips

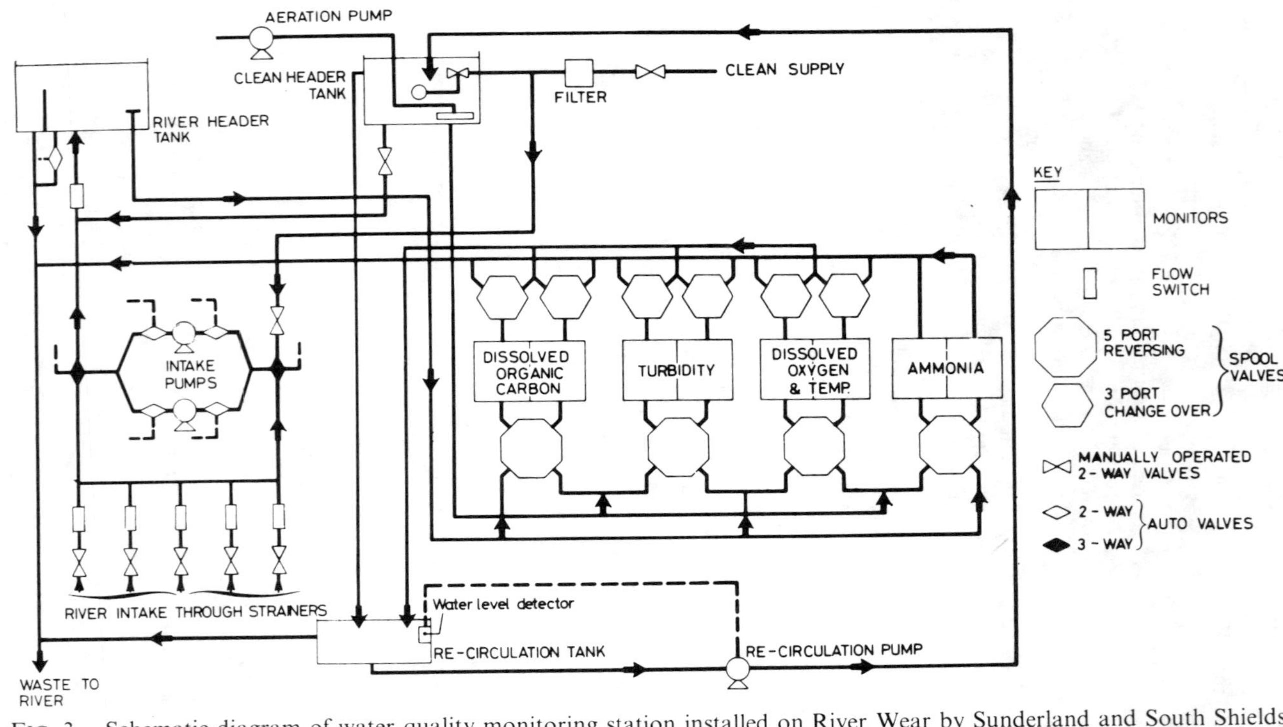

Fig. 3. Schematic diagram of water quality monitoring station installed on River Wear by Sunderland and South Shields Water Company.

quality monitors were ruled out because of lack of flexibility, the limited choice of parameters that could be measured, and the fact that duplicate sensors would be required to give acceptable reliability.

The most appropriate of the commercially available sensors were thought to be those which measured temperature, dissolved oxygen, turbidity, ammonia, organic matter, and water level, although provision was made in the system design to allow additional sensors to be incorporated, and recently pH monitors have been added to provide additional data for treatment process control.

The water quality monitor is shown schematically in Fig. 3 and the control systems for the outstation and central station are shown in Fig. 4.

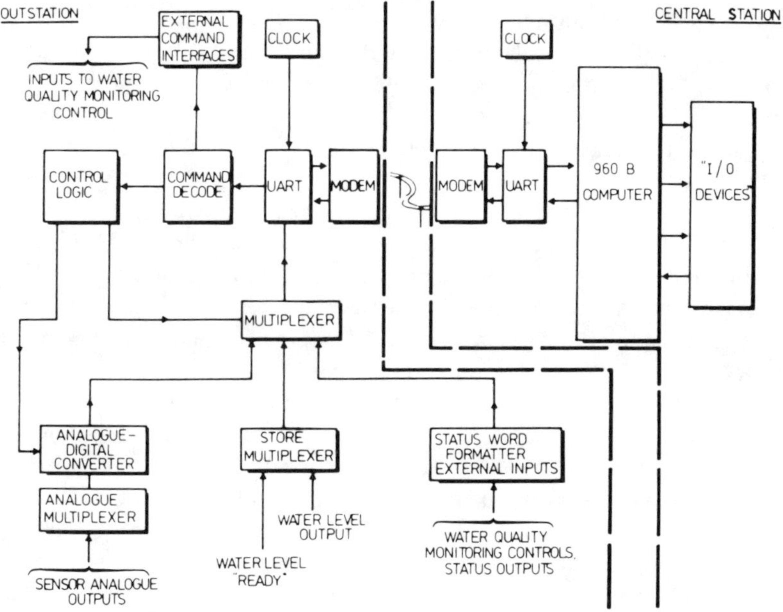

Fig. 4.   Control systems for outstation and central station of the River Wear monitoring scheme.

The system operates as follows. At any given time one sensor is monitoring raw water, the other clean water; if the former indicates a value outside pre-set limits, the sensors are switched over to provide a check. Readings from the outstation will be continuously relayed by telemetric links to the water treatment plant where appropriate action, if necessary, will be taken.

In addition to the Wear being vulnerable to the normal risks of contamination, the intake works are close to a section of a motorway, the A1(M), from which 16 drainage outlets discharge to the river. Accidents involving spillage of toxic or other harmful substances will thus be a continuing threat. A biological monitoring system based on measurement of fish activity has therefore been incorporated into the station.

The system is so designed that it will be possible in the future to use feed-forward control procedures utilising data from the monitoring station to optimise the operation of the treatment works and, at the same time, to log relevant flow data from nearby gauging stations; the system in its original form has now operated reliably for at least 18 months.

The potential economic benefits are therefore considerable, since not only should it allow the cost of the bankside storage to be avoided or reduced, but in addition the cost of the total system is not significantly more than the cost of either a water quality monitoring system based on conventional technology or a conventional telemetry scheme proposed for level and flow recording. There is the added bonus, as stated earlier, of control of the treatment works including a biological pre-treatment stage for ammonia removal.

Much of the experience gained over the past few years in the design, installation and operation of the River Lee Water Quality Monitoring System has been of value in the design of the River Wear scheme.

In the Lee system, developed by the Centre in collaboration with the Lee Conservancy and more recently with the Lea Division of the Thames Water Authority, a number of water quality parameters are measured; these include dissolved oxygen, temperature, conductivity, turbidity, nitrate, ammonia, and pH value. Information from four outstations, at which certain system-performance parameters are also measured, is transmitted over telephone lines as frequency modulated signals. These are decoded at the central station and fed directly to a Texas 960A mini-computer. Automatic dialling and interrogation of the outstations is performed by the computer at regular hourly intervals, via a Post Office automatic dialling unit, and data in SI units (validated and corrected by the computer) are presented on a Texas silent 700 tele-typewriter and on a mimic diagram with appropriate parametric displays. Depending on the operational require-ments, a number of alternative peripherals may be employed; for example, a graph plotter and a magnetic tape for data archiving. Data printouts, including daily or weekly summaries of maxima, minima and mean values of each parameter, may also be presented.

Initially, data were fed to the computerised control centre at the Stevenage Laboratory, but more recently the Lea Division of the Thames

Water Authority have installed their own computerised central station at their headquarters for operational purposes, the station being designed and commissioned by staff of the Stevenage Laboratory.

5.3. Use of Mathematical Models

A deterministic river quality model developed by Knowles and Wakeford[51] has been used by Casapieri[52] of the Thames Water Authority to evaluate the changes in quality which might occur in the Blackwater catchment from future changes in discharge conditions, and it is possible that the model may also be used in the future to protect an intake from the River Lee. It is intended to use the data from the water quality network to validate the model and to update rate coefficients.

Although long-term planning is clearly one of the most important functions of a water quality model, when the model is used within a monitoring system more short-term applications, such as predicting the time of arrival of water of unacceptable quality at an intake, prediction of quality data, and testing out proposed sampling and management schemes, are likely to be of considerable benefit to the water industry. In co-operation with Thames Water Authority the Centre intends to assess whether or not savings may be achieved by predicting the time of arrival of water of sub-standard quality at an abstraction point by a mathematical model and, as a consequence, reducing the number of monitors and manual sampling points needed to protect the supply. Predictions by the model should then provide sufficient information for unmonitored or unsampled stretches.

5.4. Continuous Monitoring of Raw Water Intakes

The protection of raw water intakes is a subject which is currently giving rise to considerable concern. Raw water intakes include some which are subject to sporadic pollution under conditions of heavy rainfall, upland streams which can be 'flashy' and which, as a result, can carry large quantities of suspended matter, lowland rivers which are frequently at risk from various types of pollution (including malfunctioning of industrial and domestic wastewater treatment plants, agricultural run-off and accidental spillages of chemicals, possibly as a result of road accidents), impounding reservoirs, and lakes.

When direct abstraction is practiced, there is a clear case for monitoring on a continuous basis, in all source waters, those variables of greatest significance in the control of treatment processes and for the protection of the consumer. On the other hand, bankside storage can give a degree of protection, so long as the possibility of short circuiting is eliminated,[53] because the nominal 7–10 days retention time usually provided allows effective monitoring by laboratory analysis of intake samples. However, since it is clearly undesirable to contaminate water already in storage, there is still a reasonable case for continuous monitoring of the river water as far upstream as practicable from the raw water intake, even when bankside storage is used.

When abstracting directly from a lowland watercourse it would seem sensible to monitor continuously dissolved oxygen levels, temperature, turbidity, and the concentrations of organic matter, ammonia and nitrate ions, and possibly pH value, since such information would be of great value in the feed-forward control of water treatment processes. In addition, this information could be used either directly or as a result of a decision by staff to close intakes, since major departures from the expected range of variability of these variables would probably be of sufficient concern to necessitate immediate action. The detection of accidental spills of potentially hazardous material is, however, a much more difficult problem, since the equipment being used would have to be capable of monitoring relatively small concentrations of heavy metals, organo-halogens, cyanide, phenols and oils, as well as the variables listed earlier. Even if this approach were technologically feasible, the cost of currently available equipment and its subsequent maintenance in the field would probably be prohibitive in most cases. Attention has, therefore, turned in recent years to the possibility of using biological indicators. It is of interest in this context that the Sunderland and South Shields Water Company has chosen to use a combination of physico-chemical sensors and the monitoring of fish activity to protect a direct abstraction point situated on the River Wear.[54]

The detailed strategy used in any particular situation depends on a number of factors such as type of source, available technology, cost, likely benefit, presence or absence of raw water storage facilities, the ability or otherwise to blend water from a number of sources and, finally, the chance of accidental spills. Detailed control strategies can be analysed by operational staff utilising the Water Intake Simulation model (WISP)[55] developed at WRC and it is possible that, when sufficient confidence in the model has been established, it could form the basis of a closed loop control system.

The water supply system modelled by the program, consists of a river from the point of the pollutant addition to the point of water supply abstraction, a bankside storage reservoir or a pipeline and a water treatment plant. The pollutant concentration/time profile is predicted for the river at the water abstraction point, the reservoir/pipeline outlet and the outlet of the water treatment works as the water enters the distribution system. The model includes representation of:

(1)   dispersion of pollutant in the river,
(2)   pollutant decay,
(3)   dispersion of pollutant in the reservoir including plug flow, complete mixing and short circuit situations, and
(4)   treatability of pollutant in the water treatment works and its rate of removal.

After the pollutant concentration/time profiles have been predicted the following management criteria are applied:

(1)   the maximum pollutant concentration that is permissible for each concentration/time profile, and
(2)   whether or not the pollutant is a cumulative poison.

If the predicted pollutant concentration/time profile exceeds the maximum permissible concentration then the program user is warned of the situation. The time and duration of the predicted excessive pollutant level is given, and if the water abstraction is stopped for that period of time the effect on water supply reserves is calculated and the simulation is stopped at that point. Similarly in the case of all cumulative poisons the simulation is stopped before they are allowed to enter the reservoir and similar warnings are given.

The model can handle a single instantaneous addition of pollutant and an addition made over a period of time. The rate of input need not be constant but the river is modelled assuming plug flow, using the classical dispersion equation.

$$\frac{\partial c}{\partial t} = D\frac{\partial^2 c}{\partial x^2} - \frac{v\,\partial c}{\partial x} \tag{1}$$

where c = pollutant concentration,
D = coefficient of longitudinal dispersion,
v = mean velocity of the river,
x = distance from the point of the addition,
t = time elapsed since the addition.

Two particular solutions of eqn. (1) are used. The first, which does not allow for pollutant decay, is given in eqn. (2) below.

$$c(x, t) = \frac{K}{\sqrt{4\pi Dt}}\exp\left[-\frac{(x - vt)^2}{4Dt}\right] \tag{2}$$

where $K = \dfrac{vM}{Q} = \dfrac{M}{A}$

M = mass of pollutant,
Q = river flow,
A = river average cross sectional area.

The second, allowing for pollutant decay, is given in eqn. (3).

$$c(x, t) = \frac{K}{\sqrt{4\pi Dt}} \exp\left[-\frac{(x - vt)^2}{4Dt}\right] \exp(-\lambda t) \tag{3}$$

where λ = decay coefficient.

The reservoir is simulated for plug flow, complete mixing, or short-circuiting conditions. With the plug flow simulation it is assumed that the reservoir is a wide river and eqns. (1)–(3) are utilised for the simulation. The same equations are used when simulating the short-circuit situation, but both the dispersion coefficient and the apparent volume of the reservoir are reduced as required. The complete mixing situation is represented by the equation:

$$C(t) = [C_R V + (C_I - C_R)Q]/V \tag{4}$$

where C_R = concentration of pollutant in reservoir at time t,
C_I = concentration of pollutant in the river water abstract at time t,
V = volume of reservoir,
Q = rate of abstraction of river water.

If the pollutant decays, the decay factor $\exp(-\lambda t)$ is included.

The water treatment works is simulated by applying the pollutant removal rate to the water input to the works.

6. SENSOR DEVELOPMENTS

In the context of water treatment and supply, probably the most important variables that require to be monitored continuously are flow, turbidity, colour, organic matter, ammonia, nitrate ion and pH value. Considering the water industry as a whole, temperature, dissolved oxygen, sludge level, and sludge-solids concentration are probably the most important additional variables.

Sensors which would clearly be of value also include continuous fluorimeters, since fluorimetry could provide a measure of chlorophyll content and, consequently, of the production and distribution of algae in reservoirs and other source waters. Measurement of toxicity too has important applications in all aspects of the work of the water industry.

Since the viability of any continuous monitoring system depends primarily on the availability of a sufficiently wide range of robust and reliable sensors, even though significantly improved performance can be achieved by careful system design, it seems appropriate to review the current situation in respect of available sensors and to highlight any recent developments of significance.

6.1. Flow

In open channels, conventional techniques based on level measurement are common, but have limitations in unattended operation when applied to liquids containing high concentrations of suspended and/or floating matter. Remote level sensing using pressure or ultra-sonic transducers gives better results for some applications.

Magnetic flow meters are being used increasingly to measure flows of heavily polluted liquids and slurries in pipes. There are instances, however, where large variations occur, and the accuracy of measurement at the lower end of the scale suffers because of zero drift. It has been suggested that magnetic flow meters with smaller internal diameters than the adjoining pipework could be used for the following reasons:

(1) less susceptibility to zero drift;
(2) during periods where the main pipework may not be completely full, adequate measurements could still be made in the reduced section, provided the meter was correctly located; and
(3) since the throughput would necessarily be higher, self-cleaning of the electrodes mounted on the inner wall would be more effective.

However, these advantages must be carefully weighed against the increase in line pressure and the possibility of blockage under high flow conditions.

The turbulence noise technique[56] may be used in both channels and pipes, provided of course that the flow is turbulent. Experiments at the Stevenage Laboratory of the WRC, with mixed liquors of up to 1 % solids concentration, in which the signals from ultrasonic transducers mounted externally on the pipe walls were cross-correlated, have given good results. Measurement of the auto-correlation peak height of the 'noise' output of a transducer, which is proportional to the solids concentration,[57] thus enables mass and volumetric flow rates to be determined simultaneously for sludges at various stages in the process.

Unfortunately, however, sewage and the resultant sludges are rarely in turbulent flow, and two other methods which have been successfully used to measure discharge in rivers and open channels are now being considered.

One is based on the Faraday effect; a moving conductor (flowing sewage or sludge) in a magnetic field (generated by a coil laid beneath the channel) generates an e.m.f. (detected by electrodes immersed in the fluid) which is proportional to the mean flow rate.[58] Experiments have shown that adequate accuracy and reproducibility can be obtained in conditions of weed growth, silting, and obstruction in rivers; hence the method is likely also to be suitable for flow measurement in sewage treatment processes.

The other method employs ultrasonic transducers mounted diagonally on opposite sides of the channel.[59] The difference between transit times of ultrasonic pulses depends on flow rate according to the Doppler effect. Transmission and reception of signals in both directions is used to negate the effects of a number of sources of error, including the effect of temperature on propagation velocity. This technique is ideally suited for channels of well defined cross-section, but in its present form can only measure velocity at one depth. The transducers would ideally be movable under remote control in order to measure the average velocity over the whole section. More sophisticated multi-element transducers are being considered for rivers where large variations in depth occur, but this may prove too expensive for sewage treatment applications.

6.2. Temperature ($-10°$ to $40°C \pm 0.5°C$)

Temperature measurement is seldom a problem. Platinum resistance thermometers give the best results, but in many cases the long-term stability of thermistors is adequate.

6.3. Dissolved Oxygen (0 to 100% $\pm$ 1% or 0 to 200% $\pm$ 2% saturation)

Galvanic (Mackereth)[60,61] or externally polarised (Clark)[62] type dissolved oxygen probes are successfully used to measure dissolved oxygen concentration in flowing samples. However, both rely on the diffusion of gaseous oxygen through a hydrophobic membrane (usually polythene or teflon) and in polluted waters where significant biological activity occurs algal growths or bacterial slimes will readily adhere to the membrane and form a photosynthesising or respiring layer which effectively separates the probe from the sample. In order to achieve the accuracies stated above it is necessary to inhibit these growths from forming, and to calibrate the probe at zero and saturated dissolved oxygen levels on a regular basis and ideally re-establish the corrected calibration curve. In circumstances where anaerobic conditions may occur, the dissolved oxygen probe may become contaminated by gaseous hydrogen sulphide. Special precautions have to be taken, therefore, to minimise the exposure of the probe to the sample. Alternatively a special electrolyte may be utilised which makes the probe tolerant to the presence of hydrogen sulphide. Probes of this type have been found to perform reliably even in settled sewage as has the design of a probe developed at WRC and illustrated in Fig. 5. At constant temperature the steady state current I given by a membrane-covered solid electrode system for oxygen measurement is defined by the equation:

$$I = \frac{nFaP}{b} A_{O_2} \tag{5}$$

where n is the number of electrons involved in the cell reaction:

$$O_2 + 2H_2O + 4e \rightarrow 4OH^- \tag{6}$$

where F = Faraday's constant, a = the area of membranes exposed both to sample and to cathode, P = the membrane permeability coefficient, b = the membrane thickness and A_{O_2} the activity of the oxygen molecule which relates to the concentration of oxygen dissolved in the sample as follows:

$$A_{O_2} = \exp(k_s i_s c) \tag{7}$$

where k_s = the salting out coefficient, i_s = the ionic strength of the sample and c = the concentration of dissolved oxygen.

Temperature dependence is given by:

$$I_T = A \exp(-J/T) \tag{8}$$

where A = a constant and J = 4450K for polythene; this yields a temperature coefficient of about $6\%\ °C^{-1}$ and compensation for this is usually achieved by means of a matching thermistor connected either as the cell load or in the feedback loop of an operational amplifier. The resistance (R_T) of a thermistor at temperature T(K) is given by

$$R_T = B \exp(b/T) \tag{9}$$

where B and b are constants.

     R. BRIGGS

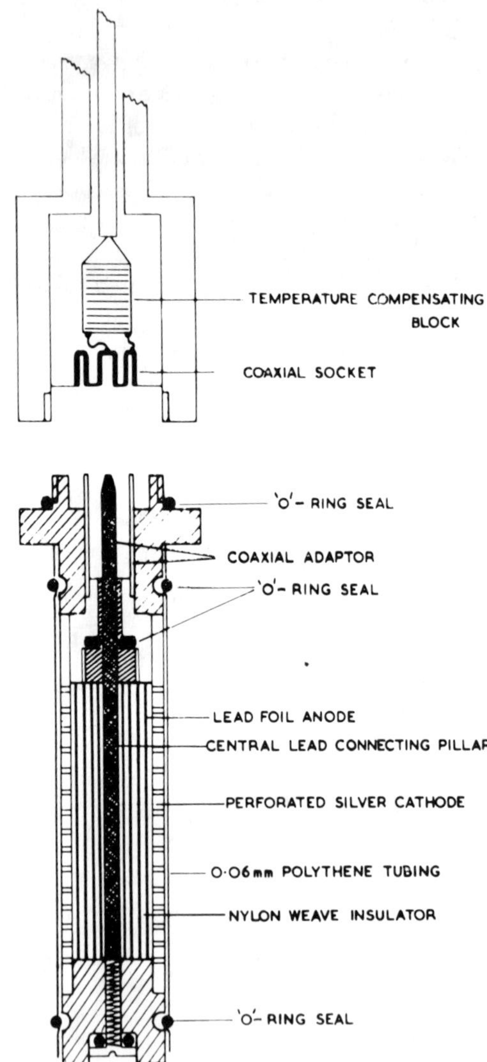

FIG. 5. WPRL galvanic cell oxygen analyser with built in temperature compensation.

It can be seen that if

$$|b| = |J| \tag{10}$$

then perfect temperature compensation can be achieved.

6.4. Oxidised Nitrogen (0 to 50 mg N litre^{-1} $\pm$ 5% of the reading)

Apart from the automatic wet-chemistry analyser approach, which is not generally recommended for unattended monitoring, the only technique known to be in common usage is the deployment of a 'specific ion monitor' fitted with a nitrate ion-selective liquid ion-exchange electrode. The electrode performance is affected by interference from other ions in solution, in particular perchlorate, iodide, permanganate, thiocyanate and zinc.

In addition, the algicide called 'Panacide', which could in other circumstances be used to inhibit algal growth, also has an adverse effect on electrode performance.

However, the specific ion monitor has the facility of mixing the sample with a reagent, in this case a total ionic strength adjustment buffer (TISAB) to stabilise the ionic strength and to reduce the pH value below 4·5 to eliminate carbonate and bicarbonate interference. The means of thermal stabilisation of the sample and electrode assembly, and automatic calibration and standardisation is also built into the monitor and, provided that the sample does not contain a high concentration of suspended solids, the 3 mm bore pipework and peristaltic pumps will operate effectively for up to a week unattended thus providing a measure of nitrate ion concentration in the sample in the range 1·4–140 mg N litre^{-1} with a precision of approximately $\pm 10\%$ of the reading.

The theoretical basis on which these electrodes operate is indicated below and their use in water industry applications has been discussed elsewhere.[63]

Since ion-selective electrodes respond to ion activities, which approach ionic concentration values only at very low total concentrations of all the ions in a test solution, it is necessary either to correct for the total ionic strength in the solution or swamp small natural variations by adding a relatively large concentration of an otherwise non-interfering ion. For many applications within the water industry, calibration in terms of concentration produces a virtually linear relationship over the range of interest.

The ionic strength of a solution is defined by

$$I_\mathrm{C} = 0{\cdot}5 \sum C_\mathrm{i} Z_\mathrm{i}^2 \tag{11}$$

where I_C = the ionic strength,
        C_i = is the molar concentration of an ion,
        Z_i = is the charge of the ion.

Nernst derived the following equation for the potential E of an ideal system:

$$E = E_0 + \frac{2 \cdot 303 RT}{Z_i F} \log_{10} a_i \tag{12}$$

where E_0 = a constant equal to the potential of the system at unit activity,
        a_i = the molar activity of the ion, i, in the sample,
        Z_i = the charge of the ion, i, including its sign,
        R = the universal gas constant, equal to $8 \cdot 314\,33 \, \mathrm{JK^{-1}\,mol^{-1}}$,
        F = the Faraday constant, equal to $96\,487 \, \mathrm{C\,mol^{-1}}$,
        T = the absolute temperature.

It is apparent that the slope factor $2 \cdot 3RT/Z_i F$, which for a monovalent ion (where $Z_i = 1$) has a value of $59 \cdot 16 \, \mathrm{mV}$ at $25\,^{\circ}\mathrm{C}$ for a 10-fold change of activity, varies with temperature, and that the effect of temperature becomes more pronounced as a solution is made more dilute. ('Activity' approaches unity in progressively diluted solutions.) It is worth remembering that there are other effects of temperature such as the variations in potential of the reference electrode—as much as $8 \, \mathrm{mV}$ for a $10\,^{\circ}\mathrm{C}$ change of temperature—and variations in activity coefficients, junction potentials and E_0 itself.

Equation (11) can be simplified, if the activity is held constant, to give the potential change dE corresponding to a concentration change from C_1 to C_2 as

$$dE = \frac{59 \cdot 2}{Z_i} \log \frac{C_1}{C_2} \tag{13}$$

None of the ISEs (ion-selective electrodes) are perfectly specific for one ionic species, although a few approach this ideal, and some are poisoned by certain ions. Therefore it is desirable (but not absolutely necessary) that the constituents in a mixed solution are known, in order to predict the overall effect of interfering ions. Most manufacturers publish tables of selectivity coefficients, which are usually adequate when the total interference is small.

The Nernst equation can be modified to account for the effect of an interfering ion, as shown below.

$$E = E_0 + \frac{2 \cdot 303 RT}{Z_i F} \log_{10} a_i + k_{i,j}(a_j) \frac{Z_i}{Z_j} \tag{14}$$

where, in addition to the symbols given in eqn. (12),

$k_{i,j}$ = the selectivity coefficient,
a_j = the activity of the interfering ion, j,
Z_j = the charge in magnitude and sign, of the ion, j.

Many other interferences are due to complexation of the ion of interest, which results in a lower activity of that ion and a consequent change in electrode potential. In some instances complexation can be employed to remove an interfering ion.

6.5. Ammoniacal Nitrogen (0 to 5, 10 or 50 mg N litre^{-1} ± 5% of the reading)

A specific ion monitor similar to that described for the measurement of nitrate ion concentration may be used for the determination of total ammonia (as NH_3) in the sample. In this case the electrode (Fig. 6) consists of a glass pH electrode situated behind a thin gas-permeable hydrophobic membrane, with a small quantity of ammonium chloride solution in contact with the electrode tip and the membrane. When the probe is immersed in a sample containing free ammonia, the latter diffuses through the membrane until the partial pressure of ammonia is equalised on both sides. The equilibrium between ammonia and ammonium ions in the internal filling is:

$$NH_3 + H^+ \rightleftharpoons NH_4^+ \tag{15}$$

Thus, as the ammonia concentration in the sample changes, the pH electrode detects the change in hydrogen ion concentration and the probe as a whole has a Nernstian response to ammonia. The probe exhibits considerable resistance to contamination by dissolved ions and gases. Carbon dioxide, hydrogen sulphide and sulphur dioxide which might be expected to interfere do not affect the performance at the high pH value at which measurement of free ammonia is made. In practice the reagent added to the sample consists of a mixture of sodium hydroxide solution to increase the pH value to 11–12 and EDTA to minimise the deposition of hardness.

The response time of the probe varies from a few seconds above 1 mg litre^{-1} to several minutes at 0·1 mg litre^{-1}, and when used in the specific ion monitor, will operate unattended in samples containing low concentrations of suspended solids for periods of up to a week. Ammonia concentrations in the range 0·4 to 140 mg N litre^{-1} can be determined with a precision of approximately ±10% of the reading.

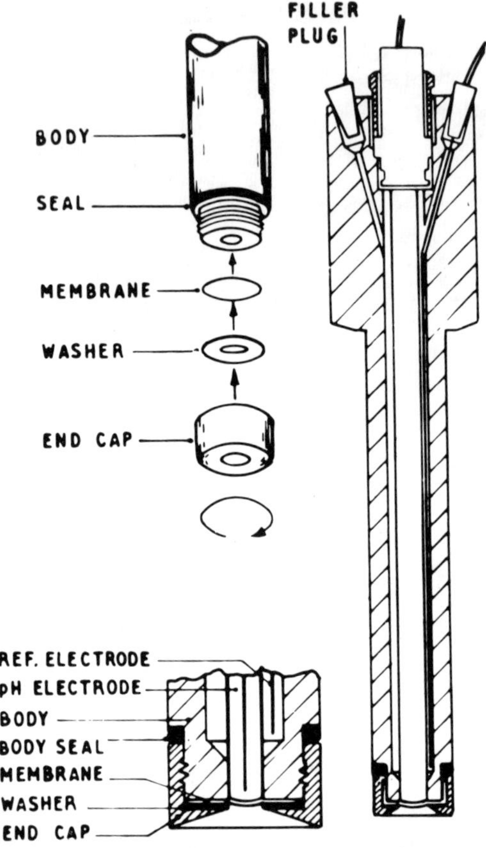

FIG. 6. Ammonia probe assembly.

6.6. Organic Matter (0 to 10 or 100 mg C litre^{-1} $\pm$ 5% of the reading)

The on-line measurement of dissolved organic matter has been the subject of a considerable amount of research and discussion over many years. In an attempt to satisfy the requirement to measure biochemical oxygen demand (BOD) which would be impractical to automate since the test extends over five days various alternatives have been considered. These include the use of wet-chemical techniques to measure the following properties.

(1) Total organic carbon (TOC), by determination of CO_2 liberated from the combustion of a sample at 900 °C.
(2) Total oxygen demand (TOD), by measurement of the amount of oxygen required to oxidise a sample which is combusted at 900 °C.

(3)   Chemical oxygen demand (COD), in which the sample and reagents (sulphuric acid and potassium dichromate) are mixed and heated to between 140° and 180°C. Residual dichromate is detected by mixing with ferrous and ferric ammonium sulphate to change the ratio of ferrous to ferric iron, and the redox potential before and after the reaction is measured, the difference being proportional to the COD. Typical correlations obtained between wet-chemical methods and also ultra-violet light absorption methods are given in Table 9.

(4)   Respiration rate to measure the amount of dissolved oxygen actually consumed by a sample. A variety of manometric techniques have been evaluated[64] and an *in situ* respirometer has been developed at the WRC.[65] In this instrument, a dissolved oxygen electrode which may be used to measure dissolved oxygen in the sample, is periodically used to measure the oxygen consumed by a trapped stirred sample.

(5)   Ultra-violet absorption at 254 nm has been shown to correlate well with TOC for a wide variety of samples ranging from secondary sewage effluent to raw and treated river water,[66] and an instrument has been developed for water quality monitoring applications and for control of water and wastewater treatment processes. When the Organic Pollution Monitor (OPM)[67] first became commercially available, difficulties were encountered because of drifts in the intensities of light emitted in the ultra-violet and visible parts of the spectrum (the latter is used to correct for suspended solids which may be present in the sample). This drawback has now been overcome by the provision of a thermal stabilisation unit around the base of the UV lamp. After initial settling down, which usually takes several hours after initial switch-on, the monitor will operate satisfactorily for at least a week without any attention. The output of the OPM is expressed in absorbance units and *not* in mg C litre^{-1} equivalent TOC or any other carbon related parameter. It is, therefore, necessary to calibrate the monitor empirically against manually analysed samples. This should be carried out when the instrument is first installed and also from time to time, to ensure that the species of organic carbon compounds in the sample has not changed markedly. If an absolute reference is preferred, *p*-hydroxybenzoic acid has been found to exhibit reproducible results, even after several months storage of the standard sample. Several sample cells are available which offer a range of sample

TABLE 9

CORRELATION OF VARIOUS PARAMETERS WHICH MIGHT BE USED TO DETERMINE
DISSOLVED ORGANIC MATTER IN WATER

Source of sample	No. of samples	Correlation coefficient	Mean	Standard deviation	Coefficient of variation (%)
Sewage effluent	39	$\left(\dfrac{\text{BOD}}{\text{COD}}\right) = 0\cdot85$	0·13	0·06	46
		$\left(\dfrac{\text{COD}}{\text{TOC}}\right) = 0\cdot73$	2·39	0·67	28
		$\left(\dfrac{\text{BOD}}{\text{TOC}}\right) = 0\cdot66$	0·32	0·19	59
Sewage effluent	11	$\left(\dfrac{\text{OPM}}{\text{TOC}}\right)^{a} = 0\cdot90$	1·03	0·16	16
Pilot-scale physico-chemical treatment plant	43	$\left(\dfrac{\text{OPM}}{\text{TOC}}\right) = 0\cdot90$	1·00	0·29	29

[a] OPM = organic pollution monitor. OPM readings normalised.

thicknesses to suit the concentration of dissolved organic carbon present, and the instrument offers a viable alternative to the more costly wet-chemical techniques for on-line monitoring of organic matter. (At 1980 prices the OPM costs £1600 whereas the wet-chemical alternatives cost between £5000 and £10 000 and require considerably more frequent and skilled maintenance.)

Typical relationships between UV absorbance, obtained using the Organic Pollution Monitor, and COD and BOD are shown graphically in Figs. 7 and 8, and a block schematic diagram of the instrument is shown in Fig. 9.

In this instrument practical difficulties normally encountered in using optical systems of this kind, including the fouling of optical surfaces and variations in light output, have been largely overcome as stated earlier by recording the ratio of the absorbance in the ultra-violet range to that in the visible range. Compensation is also provided for errors due to the presence of inert suspended matter in the sample, but at the same time the instrument provides a measure of organic particulates.

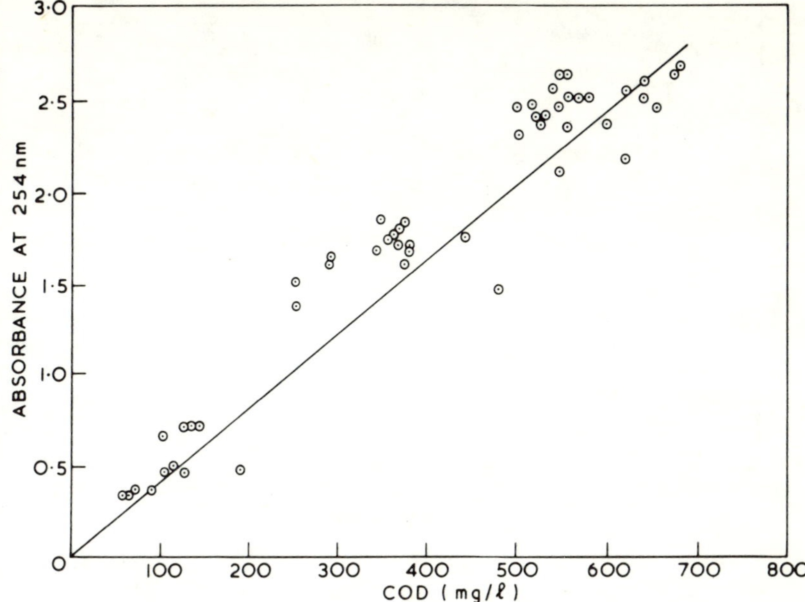

FIG. 7. Relation between UV absorbance and the COD of samples of sewage at various stages of treatment, obtained over four months. COD determination accurate to $\pm 10\%$, absorbance to $\pm 5\%$.

If I_{UV} and I_{vis} represents the UV and the visible output of the lamp, V_{UV} and V_{vis} the output of the UV and the visible light detectors, L the path length through water, and A_C and A_s the light attenuation due to organic matter and suspended solids, respectively, with C and K as constants, then

$$\frac{V_{UV}}{V_{vis}} = C\frac{I_{UV}\exp\left[-L(A_C + A_s)\right]}{I_{vis}\exp\left(-LA_s\right)} = K\exp\left(-LA_C\right) \qquad (16)$$

so that

$$\ln\frac{V_{UV}}{V_{vis}} = \ln K - LA_C \qquad \text{where } K = C\frac{I_{UV}}{I_{vis}} \qquad (17)$$

The term on the left-hand side of eqn. (17) represents the final output of the instrument which, provided K remains constant for all forms of fouling, is dependent only on the path length and concentration of organic matter in the sample.

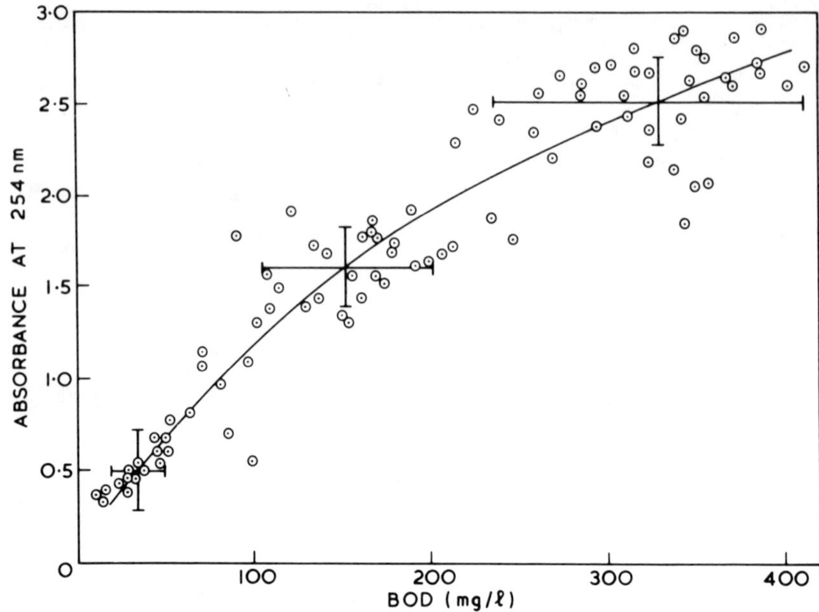

FIG. 8. Relationship between UV absorbance and BOD of samples of sewage at various stages of treatment, obtained over four months. BOD determination accurate to $\pm 10\%$, absorbance to $\pm 5\%$.

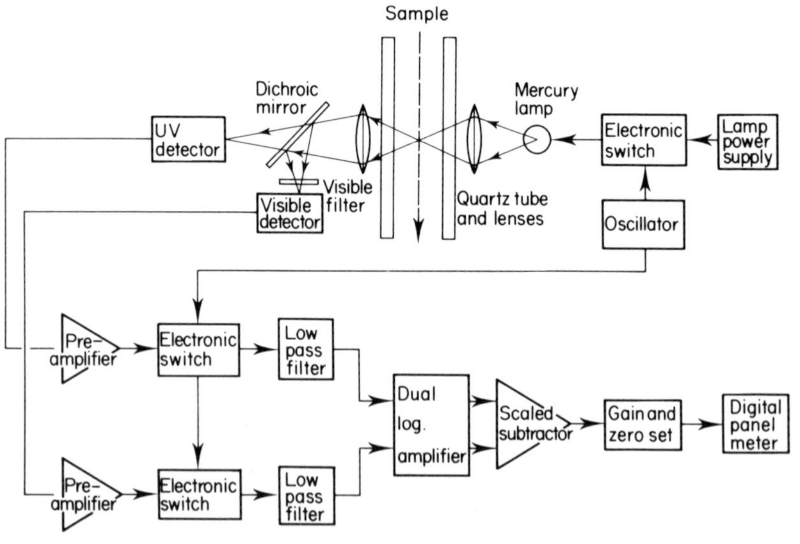

FIG. 9. Block diagram of organic carbon sensor.

6.7. Suspended Solids (5 to 500 and 50 to 5000 mg litre^{-1} ± 5% of the reading)

Strictly speaking, this parameter can only be determined gravimetrically by filtration or centrifugation of a known volume of sample followed by drying and weighing the residue. However, optical techniques have been used for some time to measure turbidity which may be related to the suspended solids concentration provided that variations in the nature of the particulates in suspension, their shape and size distribution are known. Turbidimeters fall into two basic categories, i.e. absorptiometers which measure the absorption of light through a sample, and nephelometers which measure the amount of light scattered at one or more angles to the incident beam. There is now a very wide range of absorptiometers and nephelometers commercially available; these satisfy most operation requirements including the monitoring of ultra-pure waters, river waters, effluents, sludges and slurries whose concentration is measured in % rather than mg litre^{-1}. It should be possible, therefore, by careful selection, to find a turbidimeter suitable for almost any river water quality monitoring application. Some of the better turbidimeters have built-in compensation for fouling of optical surfaces, and/or mechanical means of cleaning those surfaces, and, in some instances, the optical elements are not in contact with the sample at all. The concentration ranges listed earlier should perhaps be revised. A more useful response might be 0 to 50 or 100 mg litre^{-1} at the lower end of the range, and a non-linear response at higher concentrations up to say 1000 mg litre^{-1}. Calibration by means of the Formazin standard is strongly recommended since this has been shown to be reproducible between samples and stable after several months of storage in recommended conditions.

On-line monitoring of turbidity and by implication suspended solids should no longer present a problem but care should be taken in the design of the hydraulic circuit in order to ensure that a representative sample is taken and that sedimentation does not occur. The theoretical bases for these instruments are given in the following sections.

6.7.1. *Turbidimetric Methods*

According to the theory developed by Rose[68] the intensity I_t, of a light beam originally of intensity I_0 after passing through length, L, of a sample is given by:

$$\ln\frac{I_0}{I_t} = LC\frac{\pi}{4}\sum_0^n K_z n d_z^2 \qquad (18)$$

where C is the concentration of the suspended matter in $g\,ml^{-1}$, K_z the ratio of the light absorbed by a particle of diameter d_z to that which would have been absorbed if the laws of geometric optics held, and n the number of particles of diameter d_z per gram of suspended matter. The relation assumes that the particles are opaque, that there is no reflection between the particles or between the particles and the sample cell wall, and that any deviations in the light-obscuring power of a small particle from those given by geometric optics are included in the factor K_z which thus depends on the particle size and the wavelength of the light.

It may also be noted that

$$\text{Optical density} = \log_{10}\frac{I_0}{I_t} = \frac{1}{2\cdot303}\ln\frac{I_0}{I_t} \tag{19}$$

Optical density is proportional to the concentration of suspended matter only if the term $K_z nd_z^2$ in eqn. (18) is constant; with river water and effluent samples the proportion of larger particles and the total concentration both increase with flow, resulting in a non-linear calibration. Nevertheless, in other respects the nature of the solids from a given source is sufficiently constant to permit the use of optical methods to determine their concentration using an experimentally determined calibration curve. Usually the glass-fibre filter paper method[69] is used for such calibrations.

6.7.2. *Nephelometric Methods*
For practical purposes, assuming

$$I_0 = I_t + I_s \tag{20}$$

where I_s is the intensity of the scattered light, eqn. (18) becomes

$$\ln\left(1 + \frac{I_s}{I_t}\right) = LC\frac{\pi}{4}\sum_0^n K_z nd_z^2 \tag{21}$$

showing that turbidity may be measured by the ratio of scattered to transmitted light. By suitable design of the instrument the effects of colour on I_s and I_t can be made equal, and the measurement made independent of colour. Direct measurement of the total intensity of scattered light, I_s, is not feasible and, in practice, the proportion of the light scattered within a finite angle to the incident beam is measured.

For continuous operation and recording automatic compensation must be provided for variations in incident light intensity and other sources of error. These requirements have been partly met by the 'suspended solids monitor' which was developed to record changes in the suspended solids content of effluents from 'extended-aeration plants' and has since found many other applications.[70]

In this instrument light from a central source passes through two different thicknesses of sample of length L_1 and L_2 and falls on two matched photo-conductive cells. These components are encapsulated in a single unit which is immersed in the system being studied. Then, if the intensities of light emerging are I_1 and I_2 respectively, it may be shown that

$$\ln \frac{I_1}{I_2} = \frac{\pi}{4} \sum_0^n K_z n d_z^2 (L_1 - L_2) C \tag{22}$$

which reduces to

$$\ln \frac{I_1}{I_2} = KC(L_1 - L_2) \tag{23}$$

where K is a constant depending on the type of suspended matter. Thus, the ratio of the light intensities reaching the photocells is a function only of the difference in path lengths and the concentration, C.

Since the photocells chosen obey the law

$$\frac{\Delta I}{I} = \frac{\Delta R}{R} \tag{24}$$

where R is the photocell resistance and I is the incident light intensity, it is possible to measure the ratio of the light intensities reaching the photocells by connecting them as adjacent arms in a Wheatstone bridge.

A suspended solids recorder in which two beams of light derived from a single source are deflected by mirrors to enter the sample at right angles has been described.[71] One beam falls directly onto a photocell, giving a signal proportional to the intensity of the transmitted light. Light scattered at a right angle from the other beam falls onto the same photocell, giving a signal proportional to the intensity of the scattered light. The intensity of this scattered light is a measure of the suspended solids content of the sample and by taking the transmitted light as the standard, compensation can be provided for the effects of variations in the intensity of the light source.

Before this comparison can be made the effects of the two light beams must be separated. In the original instrument this was done by interrupting the two beams at different frequencies, so that the mixture of frequencies in the output of the photocell can be separated by electrical filter circuits. A rather different procedure involving the use of electronic gating circuits has been adopted in the commercial version. The ranges of these instruments can be varied from 5 mg litre^{-1} full scale to 2000 mg litre^{-1} full scale. There is an upper limit because, at high concentrations, scattered light is subject to further scattering and absorption before it reaches the detector. Eventually the measured scattered light intensity decreases with a further increase in particle concentration.

This system of two beams and one photocell has other advantages. Since the cell is common to both circuits, changes in the characteristics of the cell are largely compensated for. Also, since the sample path lengths travelled by transmitted and scattered light are approximately equal, there is also automatic compensation for dissolved colour.

A difficulty which occurs with any form of optical instrument continuously immersed in polluted water is that a film of micro-organisms forms on the glass surfaces. Over short periods it is often found that the growth is uniform over all the windows, and under these conditions the effect of the fouling of the windows will be corrected by the compensating property of the instruments. It is necessary, in general, to wipe the windows frequently at intervals which depend on the nature of the water and to remove the residual micro-organisms by treatment with hypochlorite solution. For more rigorous applications other varieties of instruments exist including some which measure the optical density of a free falling sample and some which measure light scattered from a free surface.[72]

Another useful method of minimising all instrumental sources of error including non-uniform fouling of optical surfaces is to utilise two light sources and two matched photocells.[54] The light sources are energised alternately so as to transpose the functions of the two photocells which can be used either to measure the ratio of scattered to transmitted light or the absorbance of two sample paths of different length. The square root of the product of the instrument readings obtained during its two modes of operation is then computed and presented as the output of the device with no component drift or fouling.

$$\text{Output}_1 = \left[\frac{Op_1}{Op_2} \cdot \frac{Op_2}{Op_1}\right]^{1/2} \tag{25}$$

Within the dynamic range of the instrument, therefore, the effects of any source of error such as lamp or photocell drift, uniform or non-uniform fouling of optical surfaces are automatically eliminated since they appear as multiplying constants, say, K_1 and K_2 to the readings Op_1 and Op_2:

$$\text{Output}_2 = \left[\frac{K_1}{K_2} \cdot \frac{Op_1}{Op_2} \cdot \frac{K_2}{K_1} \cdot \frac{Op_2}{Op_1} \right]^{1/2} \tag{26}$$

Although the use of instruments which measure the optical properties of a sample as a means of determining the concentration of suspended matter in a flowing sample has been criticised by some, there is now a substantial body of evidence in the literature which supports this practice. Briggs, Melbourne and Eden,[70] for example, have described wastewater treatment and river monitoring applications in which readings were maintained within $\pm 5\%$ of full-scale for substantial periods of time, the ranges being varied between 0–58 mg litre^{-1} and 0–200 mg litre^{-1} for the different applications. A typical calibration curve is shown in Fig. 10. It was necessary, however, to clean the optical surfaces at frequencies varying between once per day and once per week dependent on the particular application and this was carried out automatically. Fleming[73] has also provided a comparison between the performance of three instruments used to assess sediment transport in rivers and has reached similar conclusions in respect of the degree of correlation obtained between instrument readings and concentration of suspended matter present in the system.

6.8. Sludge Blanket Level and Sludge Solids Concentration

The rewards for minimising the volume of sludge passing forward from settlement tanks are considerable, since sludge disposal accounts for at least 40% of the cost of sewage treatment. Even the manual control of desludging of primary settlement tanks, using a simple battery powered sludge detector developed at the former Water Pollution Research Laboratory, achieved a doubling of the solids content of the sludge withdrawn. This instrument[74] is now being used successfully at an increasing number of sewage treatment works.

For the automatic withdrawal of sludge, with the possibility of improved digester performance from optimisation of the sludge solids concentration, several techniques have been investigated. Ultrasonic sensors have been successfully used by the Greater London Council[75] for the control of sludge withdrawal, and devices based on gamma-ray absorption and backscatter have been used in the USA. Density measurement using a radioactive source and an ionisation chamber on opposite sides of a pipe has been found to be less successful in UK applications and was replaced (by GLC)

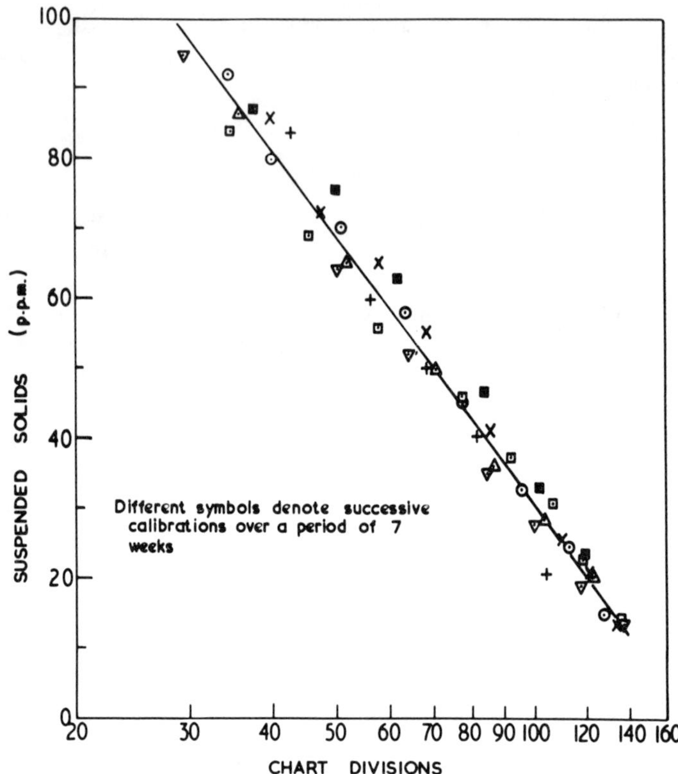

FIG. 10. Typical calibration curve obtained with WPRL suspended solids
recorder.

by remote manual control using closed circuit television, to monitor the
appearance of upward-welling sludge at each draw-off point. While this
necessitates the continuous manning of the TV receiver, results, though
more subjective, have been useful and reliable. It is hoped that the
turbulence 'noise' technique discussed earlier and further developed by
Balachandran,[76] will provide the reliability and immunity to contamination needed to allow progress in this area.

Two other useful possibilities worth further consideration are as follows.

1.   The use of pulsed gallium arsenide lamps which emit infra-red
     radiation at 900 nm. Hultman of the Department of Water Supply
     and Sewage Engineering and Water Chemistry, Royal Institute of
     Technology, Stockholm, has recently developed a simple sludge

solids meter based on this principle which can record in the range 0 to 50 000 mg litre^{-1}.

2. The use of methods based on measurements which are related to viscosity. For example, in the mid-1960s Richards and Kirk[77] developed a system for sludge withdrawal in which the rate of flow of sludge delivered at a constant head was monitored using an electromagnetic flow meter, and more recently an on-line rotating-vane viscometer, reputedly suitable for on-stream application, has been marketed by Eur-Control. Earlier experience at Stevenage, however, has indicated that rotating devices become fouled extremely rapidly in the presence of fibrous material, and the use of a nutating cylinder would probably be more practicable.[78]

6.9. Filtrability of Sludges

An important parameter in the characterisation of a suspension is its specific resistance to filtration. Baskerville and Gale[79] have developed an instrument which, by utilising the capillary suction pressure of a porous medium to achieve filtration, measures a parameter—the capillary suction time—which can be related to specific resistance. A number of versions are now commercially available from Triton Electronics. These have been shown to be of considerable value in the assessment of the dewaterability of sludges originating from sewages and trade wastes, in the control of coagulant addition in the conditioning of sludges, and in the control of the operation of filter presses.

These devices, however, are not suitable for on-line use and a number of other possibilities are, therefore, being investigated. The measurement of turbulence-induced noise referred to earlier is thought to offer some interesting possibilities, since spectral analysis of the noise signal indicates that a shift of the frequency distribution to the high-frequency end occurs with decreasing particle size and decreasing viscosity, each of which leads to poorer dewaterability. Wuhrmann[80] has observed that if a varying shear stress is applied to a sludge, then the change from thixotropic to Newtonian behaviour occurs at a level of shear which increases as the ease of dewaterability of the sludge decreases. By applying a steadily increasing shear, therefore, and using non-contact sensors to detect the onset of turbulence-induced noise, it would be possible to have an on-line measurement of dewaterability—since measurement of the applied shear would provide a measure of viscosity, measurement of noise amplitude at constant shear in the turbulent region would provide an indication of suspended solids concentration, and at the same time, by using two sensors in series and obtaining a cross-correlation peak using a variable time delay circuit, sample flow rates could also be obtained.

6.10. Conductivity (5 to 500 and 50 to 50 000 microsiemens cm^{-1} $\pm$ 5% of the reading)

The usefulness of this measurement has frequently been questioned, but as a gross detector of total dissolved solids, it is probably worth while including, particularly in circumstances where chemical pollution or saline intrusion might occur.

Conductivity probes may have from two to six electrodes, depending upon the precision required and the various methods devised to overcome electrode fouling. Probably the simplest versions would be adequate if some effective cleaning technique could be devised to minimise the build-up of algal growth or bacterial slimes on the electrodes. However, in an effort to overcome errors caused by fouling of the probe and/or the presence of external electrical noise, further electrodes have been added and conductivity meters are now available to cover a wide range of conditions from ultra-pure water to fully saline conditions, including electrodeless versions dependent on inductance principles. Temperature compensation for solubility of dissolved matter should be included; this can vary from approximately 1·8% to 2·2% $°C^{-1}$ depending upon the ionic species present, and the results should be referred to a standard temperature, usually 25°C.

6.11. Chloride (0·5 to 500 and 25 to 25 000 mg Cl litre^{-1} $\pm$ 5% of the reading)

There are basically two types of chloride ion selective electrodes: the solid state membrane and the liquid ion exchange. Each have their merits and also their disadvantages, for example, the liquid ion exchange type is comparatively immune to interference from sulphide, cyanide, ammonia and reducing solutions, but suffers interference from perchlorate, nitrate, sulphate, bromide and iodide. The solid state membrane is more intrinsically stable, but suffers interference from bromide, iodide, sulphide, thiosulphate and cyanide and can be damaged by reducing solutions.

Chloride ion concentration is not normally monitored in rivers, unless pollution by industrial wastes or saline intrusion is suspected, in which case a specific-ion monitor similar to those described for nitrate and ammonia could be used. Buffering is only necessary when one or more of the above interfering ions is present, and it should be possible to monitor chloride ion concentration in the range 0·2 to 350 mg Cl litre^{-1} with a precision of $\pm 10\%$ of reading for up to one week's unattended operation.

6.12. Hardness (10 to 1000 mg litre^{-1} as $CaCO_3 \pm 5\%$ of the reading)

There are several divalent cation selective-ion electrodes commercially available, some of which may be used to monitor temporary and/or permanent hardness, e.g. calcium and magnesium sulphate and chloride. The electrodes are of the liquid ion exchange type and, since they respond to divalent cations, give only half the Nernstian response per decade change in concentration. Interferences are caused by the presence of cupric, zinc, ferrous, nickel, strontium and barium ions and in practice because of the unfavourable selectivity coefficients, care would have to be taken to complex these in order to make an accurate determination of hardness, although strontium may be considered to contribute to hardness. However, the value of this measurement in on-line monitoring applications must be questioned since the hardness of a natural water does not normally vary significantly in a river system, though there may be considerable regional variations. This measurement is more likely to be used in the control of water treatment processes or other industrial applications.

6.13. pH Value (2–11 pH units, $\pm$ 0·1)

Early attempts to measure the pH value of flowing samples taken directly from rivers gave poor results because it was not realised that, with the sample at natural earth potential, and other active sensors such as dissolved oxygen and conductivity probes situated in close proximity to the pH electrode, interference could occur with the measurement and care had to be taken in the screening of the probes. For this to be effective the reference electrode, which ideally should be of the double junction type, should not be electrically grounded or present a low impedance to ground since this would negate its function. In practice it was found necessary to place an earthed 'guard' electrode around the pH probe and connect the glass and reference electrodes to a dual-input balanced-differential amplifier with very high input impedance (10^{13} ohms). This served to overcome the drift problems, and provided that periodic mechanical (brush or ultra-sonic) or chemical (algicide and bactericide) cleaning techniques were also used, it was found possible to monitor pH value in the range 2 to 12 pH units with a precision of $\pm 0·2$ pH units for periods of up to one week's unattended operation. However, the interval between servicing has been extended considerably by feeding low and high calibration solutions to the probe on a daily basis and correcting the instrument calibration curve automatically. Provided these precautions are taken, commercially available glass sensing and reference electrodes may be used with confidence.

6.14. Sunlight Intensity (or Solar Radiation) (0 to 2 langleys min^{-1} $\pm$ 0·02 langleys min^{-1})

For conditions where sunlight intensity may combine with chemical pollutants in the water to cause undesirable effects, e.g. algal blooms, short wave solar radiation may be measured with a solarimeter which usually consists of a thermopile mounted beneath a pair of glass domes (to minimise thermal convection effects). These are very robust, reliable and stable devices, giving a linear relation between instrument readings and incident solar radiation. Instantaneous or integrated solar radiation measurements may be made, but in locations where airborne dust and particulates may contaminate the glass dome, regular (weekly) cleaning should be carried out. This measurement can be made without undue difficulty and produces records of solar radiation within the range and accuracy limits stated above.

6.15. Dissolved Carbon Dioxide (0 to 100 mg litre^{-1} as CO_2 $\pm$ 5% of the reading)

Several probes are commercially available; these are based on similar principles to those of the ammonia sensing probe (i.e. the dissolved CO_2 diffuses through a hydrophobic membrane into a filling solution and causes a change in pH value which is detected by a conventional pH electrode situated within the membrane). The sample must be buffered to below pH 4, and interference from volatile acids is severe, particularly sulphur dioxide, nitric oxide, nitrogen dioxide and, to a lesser extent, acetic acid. However, the value of this determinand is questionable in other than specialised applications such as the study of the intrinsic toxicity of CO_2 to fish and the additional toxicity of ammonia in the presence of CO_2 and perhaps the monitoring of $CaCO_3$ deposition or solution properties of water entering a distribution system.

6.16. Heavy Metals

In most monitoring applications the need for continuously determining heavy metal concentrations seems doubtful since these are conservative substances and trends in their concentrations can usually be established by periodic sampling and off-line analysis. In the context of protection of raw water intakes, however, the ability to detect accidental spills of liquors containing heavy metals is of considerable importance. Recent developments in ion-selective electrode technology,[81,82] particularly that carried out at the Canada Centre for Inland Waters and that resulting from contract work carried out for WRC by the University of Edinburgh Micro-Electronics Liaison Unit and, more recently, by STL Harlow, may make continuous monitoring of heavy metals practicable in the not too distant future. In this context the recent availability from STL of phosphate and borate glass from which metals may be leached at a controlled rate may well add impetus to these developments as well as providing a useful means of supplying biocides to monitoring equipment at a controllable rate.

Given that the purpose of the monitor is firstly to detect the presence of significant contamination of the raw water, secondly to provide an indication of when the polluted water has passed the intake and thirdly to control a sampling programme rather than to provide a continuous and accurate record of metals at concentrations approaching drinking water standards, then other possibilities may well be practicable, for example, polarographic techniques such as those recently developed at the University of Strathclyde, or simplified colorimetric or flameless atomic absorption techniques. These possibilities are under active consideration at WRC at the present time.

6.17. Trace Organics

In general, the wide range of compounds encountered, the fact that they are usually present in microgram quantities, and the uncertainty in respect of their potentially hazardous nature implies a need for sampling followed by sophisticated analytical techniques. Gas chromatography/mass spectrometry, for example, is often required to obtain qualitative and quantitative data of a sufficiently reliable nature to establish trends. However, again for the specific purpose of protecting intakes and indeed in the context of assessing the efficacy of a particular treatment process the ability to monitor trace organics continuously is clearly desirable.

A number of possibilities are being considered at present. The first of these is the development of a robust GC/MS system for on-line use such as that currently deployed in aircraft in air pollution studies;[83] a major difficulty, however, would be removal of water from the sample. The second possibility is the development of electrodes based on special glasses, lipid membranes or indeed on specific enzymic reactions. Limited work in this area has shown promise.[84] Alternatively, it might be possible to strip volatiles, absorb them onto and then desorb them from a continuous filament of activated carbon fibre or to measure in the head space using gas-sensitive semiconductors. Recent work at EMI along these lines appears to be promising.

6.18. Oil

A number of devices are currently available for monitoring oil. Surface films are reasonably easily detected by utilising the change in refractive index,[85] measurement of UV fluorescence[86] or by a novel device described by Malz.[87] It comprises a polythene disc on which is mounted a number of conducting sectors. The disc is slowly rotated in the vertical plane partially submerged in the water. The conductivity between sectors is measured and the disc is wiped clean between measurements. Since oil has a far greater affinity for polythene than has water, a significant change in conductivity results if the disc passes through an oil film.

Dispersed oil is of far greater significance, however, since it can readily enter intakes and seriously contaminate treatment works and reservoirs even though the intake is located below the surface. Probably the more reliable methods of detection of significant amounts of oil would be either to use the Malz development within the monitoring station or, alternatively, a recently available instrument from Fisher Controls, based on solvent extraction followed by infra-red analysis.

6.19. Toxicity

At the present time (and indeed in the foreseeable future) there are limits to the scope and range of information that can be obtained at reasonable cost from monitors based on physical and chemical sensors. Therefore, attention has been directed to the use of biological monitoring techniques. Holland, Green, Stroud and Jones[88,89] for example have developed a monitor based on the response of *Nitrosomonas* supplied with the water under test, augmented with a controlled addition of an ammonium salt. The efficiency of culture is indicated by the level of removal of ammonia on a continuous basis by means of a proprietary electrode which responds to ammonia (as NH_3).

According to Holland[90] the system located on the River Severn operated effectively for about 95 % of the time and when deployed on a site on the River Derwent the effective operational time was about 86 %. He also reported that the monitors responded particularly well to levels of cyanide of less than 0.1 mg litre^{-1}, but that in the case of heavy metals significantly higher levels had to be present for a response to be obtained.

At the WRC the major effort in recent years has been directed towards the development of water quality monitors based on measurement of the

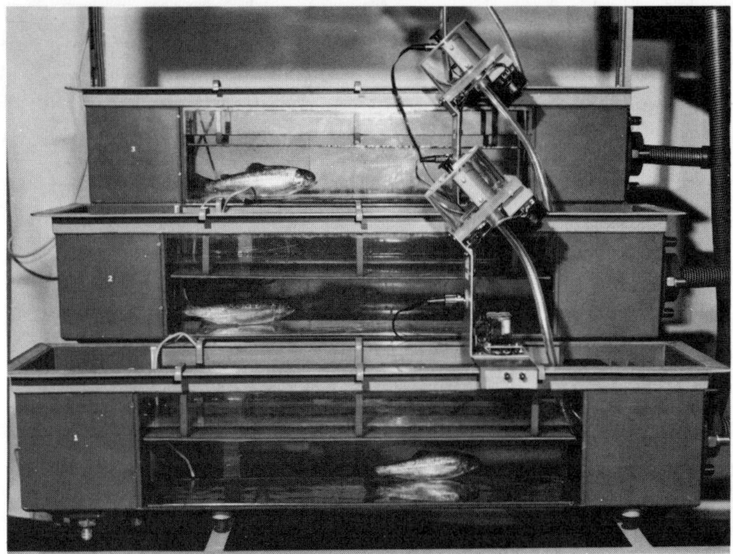

FIG. 11.   WRC fish activity monitor.

activity of captive fish (Fig. 11). The WRC system, which has been described in detail by Miller,[91] is based on the technique developed initially by Spoor et al.[92] The test fish, in this case rainbow trout (*Salmo gairdneri*), are kept in a series of tanks through which the test water is pumped at a controlled rate. Electrodes placed in the tanks above and below each fish pick up electrical signals generated as a result of their various physiological activities. These signals, which are at the few microvolt level, are fed to a pre-amplifier with a high noise rejection capability and then processed to determine the health and behaviour of the fish. Signal components from the following sources have been identified:

(1)   muscle movements,
(2)   gill (opercular) movements,
(3)   heart beat, and
(4)   coughing reflexes.

The total power content of the composite activity signal averaged over an appropriate time interval (Fig. 12(a)) is passed to a series of electronic comparators which provide digital outputs corresponding to four levels of activity. The lowest corresponds to death, the second and third to normal activity, and the highest level to distress or avoidance. In addition, by use of low and high pass filters, opercular signals including those produced by coughing (Fig. 12(b)), and heart-beat signals (Fig. 12(c)) can be separated out. It is hoped that this additional information might be of use in the characterisation of the toxicant. Considerable further research is, however, still required and a detailed test programme has commenced.

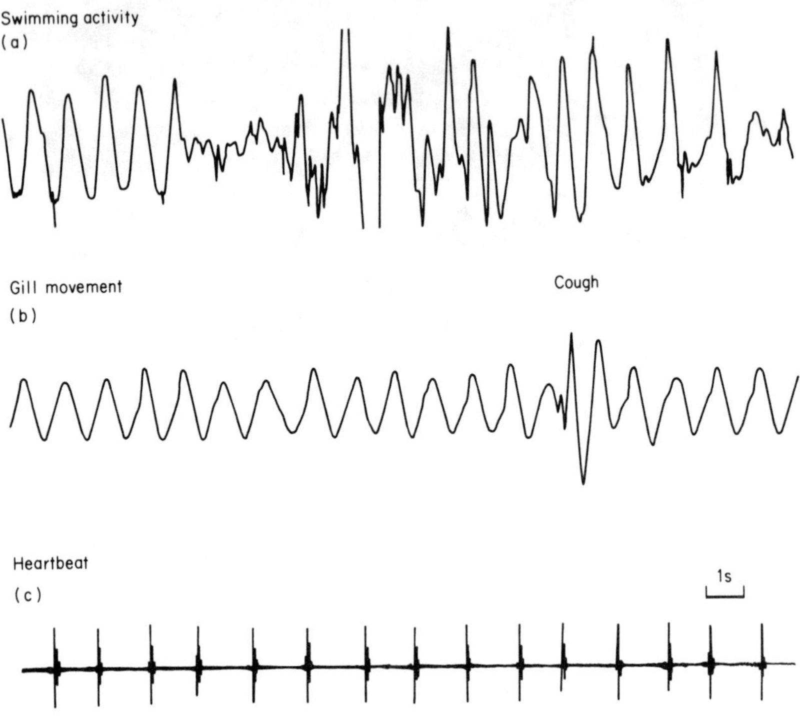

FIG. 12.   Typical signals obtained from the WRC fish activity monitor.

It is of interest in this context that Morgan,[93] using rather similar equipment and three species of fish, found that the response limit for a wide range of toxicants lay between 5 and 10 % of the 48 h lethal limit. He also commented that, although his system did not identify the toxicant, the severity of its effect could be judged by a consideration of the percentage of fish which elicit a response as well as the lag time between initial and final fish sensor responses. More recently Sloof[94] has published even more encouraging data obtained using equipment based on that of Spoor et al.[92] His data are reproduced in Table 10 below.

TABLE 10

THE RELATIVE SENSITIVITY OF A BIOLOGICAL MONITORING SYSTEM WITH DUAL EXTERNAL ELECTRODES, BASED ON CHANGES IN RESPIRATION FREQUENCY OF FISH TO SEVERAL ORGANIC AND INORGANIC COMPOUNDS

Substances tested	Toxicity to fish (model experiments)		Toxicity to mammals (based on literature data)	
	Detection limit of the biological monitoring system $(mg\,litre^{-1})^a$	48 h LC_{50} for zebra fish $(mg\,litre^{-1})$	LD_{50} for rat, oral $(mg\,kg^{-1}$ b.w.$)$	Threshold concentration for man $(mg\,litre^{-1})^b$
Acrylonitrile	5	15	81	2·3
Cadmium (chloride)	0·025	2·5	150	4·2
Chloroform	20	100	2 000	56
Copper (sulphate)	0·06	0·06	120	3·4
Cyanide (potassium)	0·13	0·44	10	0·3
o/m-Dichlorobenzene	0·5	10	500	14
γ-Hexachlorocyclohexane	0·04	0·12	76	2·1
Hexachlorobutadiene	0·05	1	200	5·6
Pentachlorophenol	0·07	0·4	180	5·1
Phenol	4	60	530	14·8
Toluene	2·5	25	5 850	163·8
Trichloroethylene	5	60	4 920	137·8
Xylene	2	20	4 000	112

[a] Rainbow trout were used. Defined as the concentration at which an alarm is caused within 24 h.
[b] Defined as LD_{50} (rat) in $mg\,kg^{-1}$ b.w. $\times$ 70 kg/(2·5 litres $\times$ 1/1000).

7.   IMPROVED WATER QUALITY MONITORS

Considering the total process of transferring information about water quality from the sensor to the final user, the least reliable element is usually the first in line—the sensor. Improvements in the reliability of information received from the sensor should, therefore, be the first concern of those building water quality monitoring networks. Two approaches are possible —these may be termed intrinsic methods and extrinsic methods.

Intrinsic methods involve the development of new sensor mechanisms and the refinement of existing ones. Extrinsic methods may involve the use of computers to detect and correct sensor failures or faults as they occur. These methods usually employ more than one sensor for each determinand,

and a source of calibration water with known properties. One method would be to use three sensors for each determinand and take, as the value of the measured quantity, the average of the two sensors which agreed most closely. Although superficially attractive because of its simplicity, this method, or an extension using more than three sensors would be costly if the actual sensors are costly, and, more seriously, would only detect catastrophic failures, not gradual degradation affecting all three sensors equally.

The patented method[95] used in the River Wear monitoring scheme which has been described earlier is thought to be more promising. Two similar sensors are arranged so that one is connected to the source water to be measured and the other to a source of clean water with known properties. An arrangement of electro-pneumatically operated spool valves may be used to interchange the sources of the water passing through the sensors. These values are under the control of a mini-computer, to which the sensor outputs are transmitted. The sensors are interrogated by the computer every few minutes and the values obtained are compared, as applicable, with high or low limits and with previous values, held in the computer memory. If the measured values of the determinands do not exceed the limits, and do not show sudden changes from previous values, they are recorded as true data and the only action needed is to exchange the sensors about once a day to equalise fouling and wear. If the above conditions are not met, the computer programs are designed to interchange the flows through the sensors and thus obtain new readings.

The four sensor readings now available are:

(1)   RA River measured by Sensor A,
(2)   RB River measured by Sensor B,
(3)   CA Calibration water measured by Sensor A, and
(4)   CB Calibration water measured by Sensor B.

These are used to determine whether the alarm state is genuine or whether it resulted from failure of either sensor or calibration water. For example, if Sensor A had failed in such a way that its output was always at zero, then readings RA and CA would be both low and similar, and the failure could be detected. By comparing RA, RB, CA, CB in pairs it is possible to detect any of the four possible types of failure, providing that only one occurs at a time.

In the case of sensor failure the good sensor is switched to monitor the river until the other has been repaired. Central to the success of such a scheme is the ratio of the mean time between failures for a sensor to the mean time to repair it. There must be a low probability of both the sensors in a pair being out of action at the same time. This implies that management must ensure that an efficient communication channel exists at all times between the person who reads the computer log and the one who repairs the sensors.

Efficient mechanisms should also exist for the repair of non-redundant parts of the system such as the computer and telephone line.

8. DESIGN OF SAMPLING PROGRAMMES

Much of the previous discussion has been concerned with problems associated with on-line monitoring, since continuous records form an ideal basis for the assessment of those qualities which vary continuously with time. However, as stated earlier, a comprehensive network which would include the continuous monitoring of all major effluents would be impractical for both financial and technical reasons.

Subsequent discussion, therefore, will be concerned with sampling both for on-line and off-line analysis since at present most pollution control relies on data acquired by the latter method.

Montgomery and Hart[96] have published a detailed account of the considerations involved in the design of sampling programmes for river waters and effluents. This information, together with particular details which affect sampling for on-line analysis, is summarised below.

Because it is necessary for pollution control purposes to rely largely on data obtained by intermittent sampling and subsequent analysis, a compromise must be made in which the amount of information gathered is balanced against the frequency of sampling and the attendant labour and costs. The most effective compromise can usually be judged only from a consideration of the individual circumstances, and it is not possible to provide a 'blue print' which will cover all cases. These circumstances include vagaries of weather and a wide range of human activities, of which some are continuously variable, some intermittent, and some unique. Before undertaking any sampling programme, therefore, it is essential to determine the exact nature of the information required from the sample or samples. In many cases, discrete values of concentration or load (mass per unit time) as measured by sampling and analysis are distributed according to statistical patterns with well established properties, such as the normal and log-normal curves of error, and in these circumstances it is often possible for plant or river management purposes to draw inferences, for example about the number of samples needed to establish a conclusion with given precision using the known properties of such distributions. These can be found in any of the standard text books on statistics. This approach involves making use of existing data to estimate statistically the frequency of sampling which would be needed to establish the required quality characteristic with stated precision at a stated level of confidence; the quality characteristic might be either a mean or percentile value in the frequency distribution of concentration or less.

Mean or percentile values do not yield some of the information desirable for management purposes, such as the probability of dangerous concentrations persisting for critically long periods. For example, if the 10 percentile concentration of dissolved oxygen was $3.6\,\mathrm{mg\,litre}^{-1}$, a fish population would be more likely to survive if the low concentrations, though totalling 36·5 days (10 % of the year) in duration, occurred for short periods evenly distributed throughout the year, than if the concentration remained continuously below $3.6\,\mathrm{mg\,litre}^{-1}$ for 36·5 days. However, the raw data from which the frequency distributions are derived might well provide valuable indications of such contingencies. The best way of obtaining the duration and/or frequency of occurrence of concentrations above or below a stated value is by continuous monitoring. If this is not possible, attempts should be made to define the conditions of flow, temperature, and pollution under which critical concentrations are most likely to occur, then arrange for no less than six samples to be taken during each period when the defined conditions are expected to be present.

8.1. Frequency of Sampling

More generally, in most rivers in the UK and elsewhere, the rate of change of water quality is such that data collection at an automatic monitoring station need not be more frequent than at hourly intervals. In certain circumstances, however, for example when monitoring relatively small streams receiving sporadic discharges of polluting material, it may be necessary to increase the sampling frequency to once every 15 min. This is illustrated by an analysis of six months oxygen records for a polluted stream carried out by Gameson and Griffith.[97] Recording of an integrated hourly reading, particularly in the case of rapidly fluctuating parameters, would in many cases be desirable. With respect to remote sampling for laboratory analysis it is impossible to generalise. When sampling chemically stable and non-biodegradable substances, an ideal solution would be a 24 h composite sample, bulked according to flow and taken at intervals of eight days so that, over a comparatively short period of time, samples are taken on all days of the week. When variables are being measured for alarm purposes then the relationship of the sampling point to the intake being protected largely dictates the sampling frequency; for example, if with normal flows the retention time between the sampling point and the intake is two days, daily sampling is probably adequate unless sporadic discharges of short duration occur, in which case a 24 h composite sample is necessary.

With respect to intermittent sampling and subsequent analysis, if past records are available for periods similar to that for which the sampling programme is intended (this would often be one year) these will afford the most useful guide; records for say one month are not much use if a year's sampling is being planned, but they might have to be used if nothing better exists. The results are plotted on probability paper[98] and the distribution is judged as closer to normal or log-normal.

When there are few or no suitable data in existence, a hypothetical probability plot of results should be set up based on analogy with other parameters in the same river or effluent or with the same parameter in other similar rivers or effluents. Alternatively the results from three or more intensive surveys, if made under widely differing conditions of flow or composition, might be used.

An estimate, $\bar{\sigma}$, of the standard deviation, σ, is then made from a straight line fitted by eye to the plotted points, those nearest the middle of the probability graph being regarded as the most important for the purpose of fitting the line. In the normal case $\bar{\sigma}$ is taken as $\frac{1}{2}$(84 percentile value − 16 percentile value) and in the log-normal case $\bar{\sigma}$ is found in logarithmic units as $\frac{1}{2}$[log (84 percentile value) − log (16 percentile value)], the 16 and 84 percentile values being taken from the line.

The confidence level, C, and the precision, p, with which the result must be known are chosen, and the corresponding value of k obtained from Table 11 below; k is a constant in the expression $N = (k/p)^2$, where the value of k is dependent on the confidence level chosen and N is the number of samples required.

For many purposes it will probably be satisfactory to take C as 95 %, but where toxic substances are concerned, or where legal action might be

TABLE 11
RELATION BETWEEN k VALUES AND CONFIDENCE LEVELS

Confidence level (%)	99	98	95	90	80	68	50
k	2·58	2·33	1·96	1·64	1·28	1·00	0·67

involved, C might perhaps need to be set higher. The value of p should be chosen with great care since N, the number of samples required, is a function of p^2.

8.2. Compositing

Analytical effort can be saved by combining samples into composites, but only when an average is required. Compositing is not permissible in the case of determination of dissolved oxygen, free carbon dioxide, temperature, pH value, free cyanide, and dissolved (as opposed to total) heavy metals, or of other constituents whose concentrations may be affected by the compositing process or otherwise changed before analysis. The volumes used in compositing should be equal to obtain a time-based average, or in proportion to flow for a flow-weighted average.

8.3. Location of Sampling Points

Samples are taken only where the composition is demonstrably homogeneous over the cross-section (unless it is desired to study stratification or mixing). One sampling point will usually be sufficient for the study of an effluent, but in the case of a river system samples should preferably be taken of important effluents and tributaries just before they reach the main river; in the main river they should be taken from suitable positions just above and below confluences with important tributaries and effluents, below weirs and also above them if reaeration is being measured, and, if necessary, at intermediate points. Sampling points should be well away from any possible disturbing influences, such as pools, stagnant zones, heavy growths of weed or sewage fungus, or points where groundwater enters (unless it is desired to study specifically their effects on water quality).

9. CONCLUSIONS

Although it has not been possible in a chapter of this length to deal with all aspects of the monitoring of natural waters and effluents or indeed to deal with any aspect in depth it is nevertheless hoped that some useful guidelines have been provided which will enable the reader to take a pragmatic approach to the setting up of a cost effective monitoring programme.

In planning such a programme, objectives must be clearly defined, variables must be carefully chosen taking into account their real significance in the satisfactory achievement of the chosen objectives. The required precision in respect of each determination must be established and so too must the frequency of sampling; frequency will relate both to the precision required and to the lead time available before control action must be taken.

It is preferable in this context to define effluent standards and other critical concentrations in terms of probability of occurrence; confidence limits at a stated percentage level should also be stated when average or percentile values of concentration are to be determined.

Cost effective monitoring networks will inevitably be based on the sensible deployment of a suitable selection of the currently available technologies; these will include on-line instrumentation when the required sensors exist in a robust and reliable form and when data are required immediately for alarm or control purposes. A choice exists between the deployment of portable instrumentation from banks of rivers or effluent channels, or from boats in larger bodies of water, and on-line instrumentation when the constituent varies rapidly with time in the source water or is not stable in the sample bottle. In this situation manpower costs will probably be the over-riding factor.

When data are required for planning purposes and when the constituents of major importance are stable, sampling followed by analysis off-line is probably the most appropriate approach, and indeed in many cases is the only approach since the required sensors may not exist in a sufficiently reliable and robust form.

However, some of the developments in systems and sensor technology discussed in this chapter may well result in an increased use of on-line instrumental methods in the future.

REFERENCES

1. Department of the Environment and National Water Council. *Working party on control systems for the water industry, first interim report*, Standing Technical Committee Report No. 9, National Water Council, London, 1978.
2. PEPPER, R. A. and BANKS, W. The telemetry installation for the central control of the Sunderland and South Shields water system, *J. Inst. Wat. Engnrs*, 1969, **23**, 299–349.
3. BURCH, R. H., MARLOW, K. C., GIBBS, G. S. and JENNISONS, M. S. A computer based telecontrol and communications system for a water supply network: Part 1, The project; Part 2, Data transmission and communications; Part 3, Telemetry, *Wat. and Wat. Eng.*, 1973, **77**, 335–9, 397–402 and 453–8.
4. GUARINO, C. F. and RADZIUL, J. V. Water—wastewater, I & A, U.S.A. *Prog. Wat. Technol.*, 1978, **9**(5/6), 35–9.

5. McClelland, N. I. and Mancey, K. H. *Water quality monitoring in distribution systems*, US Environmental Protection Agency, Contract No. 60-03-0043, Dec. 1974.

6. Hultman, B. Trends in instrumentation and automation in North Europe, *Prog. Wat. Technol.*, 1978, **9**(5/6), 25–9.

7. Hiraoka, M. and Nogita, S. The role of computers and automation in effecting economics and improvements in water supply and treatment, and wastewater collection and disposal, *Prog. Wat. Technol.*, 1978, **9**(5/6), 9.

8. Griffiths, J. H. T. Water treatment plant automation in the United Kingdom, *J. Amer. Wat. Works Assoc.*, 1970, **62**, 473–82.

9. Lewis, W. M. An exercise towards waterworks automatic coagulation control, *J. Inst. Wat. Engnrs*, 1968, **22**, 137–49.

10. Melbourne, J. D. and Butcher, R. A. F. Control and instrumentation used in the operation of water treatment plant, in *Proceedings of the Water Research Centre Conference on Instruments and Control Systems for the Water Industry*, Reading, UK, 15–17 Sept. 1975.

11. Hetherington, R. le G. and Roseveare, J. C. A. The River Severn scheme for the water supply of Coventry, in *Proc. Inst. Civ. Engnrs, Part III*, 1954, **3**, 652–94.

12. Anon. The River Severn scheme of the City of Coventry water undertaking, *Wat. and Wat. Eng.*, 1953, **57**, 223–30.

13. Jeffrey, J. Development in treatment of River Thames water at Staines, *Wat. Treatment and Exam.*, 1971, **20**, 52–69.

14. Finan, J. Three Valleys Water Committee—Iver Works, Thames Water Authority. Private communication.

15. Kron, C. Water plant goes automatic, *Wat. and Wastes Eng.*, 1975, **12**(5), 59–61.

16. Radziul, J. V. and Suffet, I. H. *Automation of water analysis and its use to control the water purification process*, International Water Supply Association, New York Congress, 1972.

17. Briggs, R. and Jones, G. L. Aspects of automation of the activated-sludge process, *Wat. Pollut. Contr.*, 1978, **77**, 439–51.

18. Cotton, P. City of Norwich sewage works, *Wat. Pollut. Contr.*, 1978, **67**, 454–7.

19. Cotton, P. Survey of some sewage treatment and allied problems at Norwich 1963–68, *Wat. Pollut. Contr.*, 1969, **68**, 627–34.

20. McVie, A. and Cotton, P. Design of a computer system for the control and operation of a water pollution control plant, *Wat. Pollut. Contr.*, 1972, **71**, 606–17.

21. McVie, A., Cotton, P. and Yallop, A. Automation of Whitlingham Works, Norwich, in *Instrumentation Control and Automation for Waste-Water Treatment Systems*, Andrews, J. F., Briggs, R. and Jenkins, S. H. (Eds.), Progress in Water Technology, Vol. 6, Pergamon Press, Oxford, 1974, 372–6.

22. Cotton, P. and McVie, A. Interfacing the computer and the plant to the operator, in *Instrumentation Control and Automation for Waste-Water Treatment Systems*, Andrews, J. F., Briggs, R. and Jenkins, S. H. (Eds.), Progress in Water Technology, Vol. 6, Pergamon Press, Oxford, 1974, 452–6.

23. COTTON, P. Automation of the control and operation of water pollution control works, *Wat. Pollut. Contr.*, 1973, **72**, 653–7.
24. McVIE, A. The extension and automation of Whitlingham purification works, Norwich, *Paper presented at an Inst. Municip. Engnrs Dist. meeting, Norwich,* 17 July 1973.
25. JONES, C. E. and COTTON, P. Computer control of sewage works, progress at Norwich, *Pub. Health Engnr*, 1975, 46–51.
26. COTTON, P. The Whitlingham sewage treatment works of the Anglian Water Authority, Norwich Sewage Division, First progress report. Private communication.
27. DUNBAR, J. M., STEVEN, W. and WHITTLE, G. M. Burgh of Motherwell and Wishaw: improvements to Carbarns Sewage Treatment Works, *Wat. Pollut. Contr.*, 1973, **72**, 349–59.
28. DUNBAR, J. M. and STEVEN, W. Computer control of sewage works: progress at Motherwell and Wishaw, *Pub. Health Engnr*, 1975, 41–5.
29. STEVEN, W. Process control as an aid to pollution control, *Wat. Pollut. Contr.*, 1975, **74**, 516–23.
30. STEVEN, W. First progress report: Carbarns Sewage Treatment Works (Strathclyde Regional Council, Lanark Division). Private communication.
31. STEVEN, W. Second progress report: Carbarns Sewage Treatment Works (Strathclyde Regional Council, Lanark Division). Private communication.
32. US Environmental Protection Agency. *Instrumentation and automation experience in wastewater-treatment facilities*, EPA 600/2-76-198, Oct. 1976.
33. ANDREWS, J. F., BRIGGS, R. and JENKINS, S. H. (Eds.). *Instrumentation Control and Automation for Waste-Water Treatment Systems*, Progress in Water Technology, Vol. 6, Pergamon Press, Oxford, 1974, 570 pp.
34. ANON. Instrumentation and control for water and wastewater treatment and transport systems, in *Proc. Internat. Workshop*, London and Stockholm, May 1977, *Prog. Wat. Technol.*, 1978, **9**, (5/6).
35. JONES, G. L. A consolidated approach to activated sludge process design: a microbiological view, *Prog. Wat. Technol.*, 1975, 7(1), 199–207.
36. GREEN, R. S. *The storage and retrieval of data for water quality control*, US Dept. of the Interior, Fed. Wat. Pollut. Contr. Admin., Washington, DC, 1964.
37. DUBOIS, D. P. *Storage and retrieval of data for open water and land areas*, US Dept. of the Interior, Fed. Wat. Pollut. Contr. Admin., Washington, DC, 1966.
38. FWPCA. *STORET system development report—decimal input program*, US Dept. of the Interior, Fed. Wat. Pollut. Contr. Admin., Washington, DC, Feb. 1966.
39. FWPCA. *Parameter code list for the STORET system*, US Dept. of the Interior, Fed. Wat. Pollut. Contr. Admin., Washington, DC, 1966.
40. FWPCA. *STORET system development report—statistical analysis*, US Dept. of the Interior, Fed. Wat. Pollut. Contr. Admin., Washington, DC, Mar. 1967.
41. MENTINK, A. F. *Specification for an integrated water quality data acquisition system*, 8th edn, US Dept. of the Interior, Fed. Wat. Pollut. Contr. Admin., Divn Pollut. and Surveill., Jan. 1968.
42. MENTINK, A. F. *Specifications for a slow speed telemetry system for water*

pollution surveillance, 1st edn, US Dept. of Health Education and Welfare, Fed. Wat. Pollut. Contr. Admin., Basic Data Program, Water Quality Activities: Engineering and Field Operations, Apr. 1966.

43. CLEARY, E. J. An electronic monitor system for river quality surveillance and research, in *Advances in Water Pollution Research*, Vol. 1, Southgate, B. A. (Ed.), Pergamon Press, Oxford, 1962, 63–73.

44. KLEIN, W. L., DUNSMORE, D. A. and HORTON, R. K. An integrated system for water quality management in the Ohio Valley, *Paper presented at the Natl. Meet. Amer. Chem. Soc. Symp. Instrumental and Automated Methods of Chem. Anal. Wat. Pollut. Contr.*, San Francisco, California, 3 Apr., 1968. Ohio Valley Sanitation Commission, Cincinnati, Ohio, 45202.

45. PAULSON, R. W. The use of ERTS-1 for relaying hydrologic data in the Delaware river basin, *J. Amer. Wat. Works Assoc.*, 1974, **66**, 301–5.

46. World Health Organisation. *The optimisation of water quality monitoring networks*, Report on a Workshop, Reading, 4–14 Jan. 1977. WHO, Regional Office for Europe, Copenhagen.

47. Water Pollution Research Laboratory. *Evaluation of water quality monitors: 1, The Plessey MM5*, WPR Report No. 382R, Stevenage, UK, May 1972.

48. Water Research Centre. *Evaluation of water quality monitors: 3. The Electronic Instruments Ltd Series 72 Monitor*, WRCS Report No. 454R, Stevenage, UK, Aug. 1974.

49. Water Research Centre. *Evaluation of water quality monitors: 4. The Philips Automatic Water Monitoring Station*, WRCS Report No. 478R, Stevenage, UK, Jan. 1975.

50. Water Pollution Research Laboratory. *Evaluation of water quality monitors: 2. The Plessey Submersible Water Quality Station Type MM4*, WPR Report No. 439R, Stevenage, UK, Nov. 1973.

51. KNOWLES, G. and WAKEFORD, A. C. A validated river-quality model, *Effluent and Wat. Treatment J.*, (in prep.).

52. CASAPIERI, P. The use of a steady-state deterministic model in evaluating water-quality for management of the Blackwater catchment, *Effluent and Wat. Treatment J.*, (in prep.).

53. WHITE, K. E. and DAVIS, J. M. WRC Technical Report, (in prep.).

54. WALLWORK, J. F., HESLOP, R. T. and REDSHAW, N. L. A river monitoring station for protection and control of water treatment, *Prog. Wat. Technol.*, 1978, **9**, (5/6), 215–20.

55. WAKEFORD, A. C. WRC Technical Report, (in prep.).

56. ONG, K. H. and BECK, M. S. Slurry flow velocity, concentration and particle size measurement using flow noise and correlation techniques, *Proc. Inst. for Measurement and Control Symp.*, Kent, Oct. 1974.

57. WORMALD, C. N., BECK, M. S., BRIGGS, R. and CORNISH, A. 'Sludge solids concentration and velocity-flow measurement using electrical noise-techniques, *Instrumentation Control and Automation for Waste-Water Treatment Systems*, Andrews, J. F., Briggs, R. and Jenkins, S. H. (Eds.), Progress in Water Technology, Vol. 6, Pergamon Press, Oxford, 1974, 114–23.

58. HERSCHEY, R. M. and NEWMAN, J. D. Electromagnetic river gauging, *Proc. Wat. Res. Centre Symp. on River Gauging by Ultrasonic and Electromagnetic Methods*, Reading, UK, Dec. 1974.

59. HERSCHEY, R. M. and LOOSEMORE, W. R. The ultrasonic method of river flow measurement, *Proc. Wat. Res. Centre Symp. on River Gauging by Ultrasonic and Electromagnetic Methods*, Reading, UK, Dec. 1974.
60. MACKERETH, F. J. H. An improved galvanic cell for determination of oxygen concentration in fluids, *J. Sci. Instruments*, 1964, **41**, 38–41.
61. BRIGGS, R. and VINEY, M. The design and performance of temperature compensated electrodes for oxygen measurements, *J. Sci. Instruments*, 1964, **41**, 78–83.
62. CLARK, L. C., WOLD, R., GRANGER, D. and TAYLOR, Z. Continuous recording of blood oxygen tensions by polarography, *J. Appl. Physiol.*, 1953, **6**, 189.
63. BRIGGS, R. and MELBOURNE, K. V. Ion-selective electrodes in water quality monitoring, *Proc. Conf. on Measurement Techniques in Air and Wat. Pollut.*, Institution of Mechanical Engineers, London, 12 January 1972, 37–64.
64. MONTGOMERY, H. A. C. The determination of biochemical oxygen demand, *Wat. Res.*, 1967, **1**, 631–62.
65. BRIGGS, R. Instrumentation for monitoring water quality, *Wat. Treatment and Exam.*, 1975, **24**, 23–45.
66. BRIGGS, R., SCHOFIELD, J. W. and GORTON, P. A. Instrumental methods of monitoring organic pollution, *Wat. Pollut. Contr.*, 1976, **75**, 47–57.
67. BRIGGS, R. *Improvements in or relating to optical density measurement*, UK Pat. App. 6568/73, 1973.
68. ROSE, H. E. The analysis of water by assessment of turbidity, *J. Inst. Wat. Engnrs*, 1951, **5**, 521–45.
69. MELBOURNE, K. V. Determination of suspended solids in sewage and related suspensions, *J. and Proc. Inst. Sewage Purification*, 1964, 392.
70. BRIGGS, R., MELBOURNE, K. V. and EDEN, G. E. The monitoring of water quality, in *River Management*, Isaac, P. C. G. (Ed.), Applied Science Publishers, London, 1967, 38–55.
71. BRIGGS, R. Continuous recording of suspended solids in effluents, *J. Sci. Instruments*, 1962, **39**, 2.
72. PAGE, H. R. S. Alternative methods of measurement of suspended solids, *Paper presented at PIRA Seminar*, 7 Dec. 1977.
73. FLEMING, G. Suspended solids monitoring: a comparison between three instruments, *Wat. and Wat. Eng.*, 1969, **73**, 377–82.
74. WILLIAMS, G. and OWNSWORTH, R. A. A simple photoelectric sludge-level detector, *Wat. Pollut. Contr.*, 1967, **66**, 282–5.
75. BARNES, N. The development of a system for the automatic withdrawal of raw sludge from a primary sedimentation tank, in *Instrumentation Control and Automation for Waste-Water Treatment Systems*, Andrews, J. F., Briggs, R. and Jenkins, S. H. (Eds.), Progress in Water Technology, Vol. 6, Pergamon Press, Oxford, 1974, 137–9.
76. BALACHANDRAN, W. *Measurement of suspended-solids concentration and volumetric flow of slurries and sludges*, Ph.D. Thesis, University of Bradford, 1979, 134 pp.
77. RICHARDS, G. M. and KIRK, W. T. The design of the Bristol primary treatment plant, *J. and Proc. Inst. Sewage Purification*, 1965, 55–73.
78. Department of Scientific and Industrial Research. Determination of solids content of sludges, *Wat. Pollut. Res.*, 1962. HMSO, London, 1963, 112–13.

79. BASKERVILLE, R. C. and GALE, R. S. A simple automatic instrument for determining the filtrability of sewage sludges, *Wat. Pollut. Contr.*, 1968, **67**, 233–41.

80. WUHRMANN, K. A. *Information presented at Workshop at 3rd Internat. Wat. Conserv. Exhibit. and Conf.*, Jönköping, Sweden, 1–5 Sept. 1975.

81. SEKERKA, I. and LECHNER, J. F. Preparation and evaluation of halide ion-selective electrodes based on mercury (II) sulfide matrices, *J. Electroanalytical Chem. (and Interfacial Electrochem.)* 1979, **69**, 339.

82. KELLY, R. G. Micro-electronic approaches to solid state ion selective electrodes, *Electrochimica Acta*, 1977, **22**, 1.

83. EVANS, J. E. and ARNOLD, J. T. Monitoring organic vapors, *Environ. Sci. Technol.*, 1975, **9**, 1134–8.

84. PHILIP, M. A. and DRAKE, C. F. Standard Telecommunications Ltd. Private communication.

85. BRIGGS, R. and MIDDLEMASS, J. N. *Detection of Surface Films*, UK Pat. App. 39961/62, 1962.

86. RICCI, R. J. and SOMERVILLE, N. Instrumentation reliability for oily waste discharge surveillance, *Instrument Soc. Amer. Ann. Conf.*, 1977, **32**(2), 137–44.

87. MALZ, F. Emschergenossenschaft und Lippeverband. Private communication.

88. HOLLAND, G. J. and GREEN, A. Development of a gross pollution detector: laboratory studies, *Wat. Treatment and Exam.*, 1975, **24**, 81–99.

89. STROUD, K. C. G. and JONES, D. B. Development of a gross pollution detector: field trials, *Wat. Treatment and Exam.*, 1975, **24**, 100–19.

90. HOLLAND, G. J. Water quality monitoring in the Severn-Trent area, *Proc. WRC Seminar on Practical Aspects of Wat. Qual. Monitoring Systems*, Stevenage, UK, 7 Dec. 1977.

91. MILLER, W. F. Development of the WRC water quality monitor using fish, *Proc. WRC Seminar on Practical Aspects of Wat. Qual. Monitoring Systems*, Stevenage, UK, 7 Dec. 1977.

92. SPOOR, W. A., NEIHEISEL, T. W. and DRUMMOND, R. A. An electrode chamber for recording respiratory and other movements of free-swimming animals, *Trans. Amer. Fisheries Soc.*, 1971, **100**, 22–8.

93. MORGAN, W. S. G. Biomonitoring with fish: an aid to industrial effluent and surface water quality control, *Prog. in Wat. Technol.*, 1977, **9**(3), 703–11.

94. SLOOF, W. Detection limits of a biological monitoring system based on fish respiration, *Bull. Environ. Contam. Toxicol.*, 1979, **23**, 517.

95. PAGE, H. R. S., SCHOFIELD, J. W. and WALLWORK, J. *Fluid Monitoring*, UK Pat. App. 31057/77, 1977.

96. MONTGOMERY, H. A. C. and HART, I. C. The design of sampling programmes for rivers and effluents, *Wat. Pollut. Contr.*, 1974, **73**, 77–107.

97. GAMESON, A. L. H. and GRIFFITH, D. Six months oxygen records for a polluted stream, *Wat. and Waste Treatment J.*, 1959, **7**, 198–201.

98. HAHN, G. J. and SHAPIRO, S. S. *Statistical Models in Engineering*. Wiley, New York and London, 1967, p. 260.

Chapter 7

WATER SUPPLY

G. F. G. Clough, B.Sc.(Eng.), C.Eng., M.I.Mech.E., M.I.E.E.,
F.I.P.H.E., F.I.W.P.C.

Consultant Engineer, Macclesfield, Cheshire, UK

SUMMARY

A reliable supply of wholesome water is one of the more essential requirements for a civilised existence. In the UK piped supplies have been almost universally available for many years. In many western countries the situation is similar, but not necessarily so in, for example, the developing countries.

Water supply installations are expensive and long-lasting and the demand for water changes only slowly; the rate of introduction of new technical developments can, therefore, only be slow. Nevertheless steady technical progress is being made and a number of such developments are described under the headings of water resources, water treatment and water distribution.

Administrative changes can be introduced more quickly and the gathering together of the control of all aspects of water use and disposal under the Regional Water Authorities in 1974 represents probably the major development of the last decade. The advantages, but not necessarily the economies, of scale have been felt throughout the water services. This chapter ends with a brief discussion of possible future developments.

1. INTRODUCTION

'Water, water everywhere nor any drop to drink.' The writer was at sea and seawater is not of a quality suitable for drinking. In the absence of a water supply and distribution system the same might easily apply, at times, on land for, whilst this natural resource is often readily available, only occasionally is it of the right quality, in the right place at the right time. These three needs are met by the water treatment and distribution system. Whilst the main demand is for water for human consumption, it is also used for a wide variety of other uses. Table 1[1] indicates the relative importance of some of the parameters reflecting the quality of water for different uses.

Whilst it is possible to produce any given quality of water starting from

TABLE 1

CHARACTERISTICS OF WATER FOR VARIOUS USES

	Total solids	Suspended solids	BOD	Toxicity[a]	Bacteria
Floating ships	NC	NC	NC	NC	NC
Water power	NC	NC	NC	NC	NC
Transport—ash, sugar beet, potatoes	NC	NC	NC	NC	NC
Flushing WCs	NC	low	NC	low	NC
Recreational					
contact sports	NC	low	low	v. low	v. low
non contact	NC	NC	NC	NC	NC
coarse fishing	NC	low	low	low	NC
game fishing	low	v. low	v. low	v. low	NC
Irrigation	low	low	low	v. low	NC
Washing	NC	v. low	v. low	v. low	low
Paper making	NC	low	low	NC	NC
Textile processing	low	v. low	v. low	NC	NC
General cooling	NC	low	NC	NC	NC
Low pressure boiler feed water	$\lfloor 3\,000$ mg litre^{-1}	low	NC	NC	NC
Cooling canned foods	NC	low	v. low	low	nil
Drinking and food preparation	$\lfloor 1\,000$ mg litre^{-1}	v. low	v. low	nil	nil
High pressure boiler feed water	v. low	v. low	NC	NC	NC
General laboratory use	v. low	—[b]	—[b]	—[b]	—[b]
Electronics manufacturing	—[b]	—[b]	—[b]	—[b]	—[b]
Injections for medical use	nil	nil	nil	nil	nil

[a] Although for some uses toxic substances are not unacceptable, they may prove embarrassing when the water has to be disposed of.
[b] Negligible.
NC = not critical.
Taken from reference 1.

low quality water, economic considerations usually limit the practical options. In particular the removal of dissolved solids may require relatively large amounts of energy in the form of heat, to effect a phase change, in the form of pressure if reverse osmosis is used or as chemicals to regenerate ion exchange resins. In practice, therefore, where water of high purity is needed a high quality source is used.

TABLE 2

WORLD HEALTH ORGANISATION INTERNATIONAL STANDARDS FOR DRINKING WATER[2]

Parameter	Highest desirable level	Maximum permissible level
Discoloration	5 Hazen units	50 Hazen units
Odour	Unobjectionable	Unobjectionable
Taste	Unobjectionable	Unobjectionable
Suspended matter	5 FTU	25 FTU
Total solids	500 mg litre^{-1}	1 500 mg litre^{-1}
pH range	7·0–8·5	6·5–9·2
Anionic detergents	0·2 mg litre^{-1}	1·0 mg litre^{-1}
Phenolic compounds	0·001 mg litre^{-1}	0·002 mg litre^{-1}
Total hardness	100 mg litre^{-1} $CaCO_3$	500 mg litre^{-1} $CaCO_3$
Chloride	200 mg litre^{-1}	600 mg litre^{-1}
Copper as Cu	0·05 mg litre^{-1} as Cu	1·5 mg litre^{-1} as Cu
Calcium as Ca	75 mg litre^{-1}	200 mg litre^{-1}
Iron, total as Fe	0·1 mg litre^{-1}	1·0 mg litre^{-1}
Magnesium as Mg	Not more than 30 mg litre^{-1} if there are 250 mg litre^{-1} of sulphate; if there is less sulphate up to 150 mg litre^{-1} may be allowed	150 mg litre^{-1}
Manganese as Mn	0·05 mg litre^{-1}	1·5 mg litre^{-1}
Sulphate as SO_4	200 mg litre^{-1}	400 mg litre^{-1}
Zinc as Zn	5·0 mg litre^{-1}	15 mg litre^{-1}
Escherichia coli/100 ml	nil	nil
Coliforms/100 ml	nil	3

Tentative limits for toxic substances
(subject to periodic review)

Arsenic as As	0·05 mg litre^{-1}	
Cadmium as Cd	0·01 mg litre^{-1}	
Cyanide as Cn	0·05 mg litre^{-1}	
Lead as Pb	0·1 mg litre^{-1}	
Mercury, total as Hg	0·001 mg litre^{-1}	
Selenium as Se	0·01 mg litre^{-1}	
Radioactivity, gross α	3 pCi litre^{-1}	
Radioactivity, gross β	30 pCi litre^{-1}	

The demand for high quality water has increased during recent years and, although the current recession has reduced the rate of increase to negligible proportions at the moment, it is likely to quicken in the future. High quality sources are limited and hence, in order to make the best use of them, there has been a substantial development in the overall control of water resources in recent years. Drinking water need not be pure in the chemical sense; it would be flat and tasteless if it were. It must be wholesome and this requires that the dissolved solids should not be too high, a virtual absence of suspended solids, clarity, little colour or smell and an absence of harmful bacteria and chemical substances. Table 2[2] indicates the World Health Organisation Standards for Drinking Water. The standards should apply at the point of delivery to the consumer and hence both the treatment plant and the distribution system have to be well designed and operated efficiently if this is to be achieved.

Water from the public supply system is often used as the starting point for water to be treated to higher quality. Much of the water from the same system is also used for purposes for which the quality is needlessly high, for example the flushing of WCs. There would be no difficulty in providing a second distribution system for water of lower quality but at the present time in the UK the saving in treatment costs would not be sufficient to pay for it. Where treatment costs are high, for example where desalination has to be used to provide drinking water, dual systems are used. The objection sometimes raised, the risks arising from inadvertent cross connection, can be minimised by operating the drinking water system at a significantly higher pressure and by adding colour to the low grade circuit.

Where high quality water resources are limited, a separate lower quality supply for some users may be attractive as an alternative to seeking additional resources. One possibility is to take used water, for example the effluent from a sewage treatment works and treat it to a standard suitable for industrial use. Large pilot scale studies have been carried out by the North West Water Authority,[3] at the wastewater treatment plant serving Manchester where a substantial amount of the town's water is used in the adjacent industrial estate.

2.   WATER RESOURCES

Relatively little water is needed to sustain human life—a few litres a day. Rather more is needed if a reasonable level of cleanliness is to be achieved and more again if this is to be maintained in comfort. The consumption per head in the developed countries is of the order of 200 litres day^{-1}, that in the developing countries much lower. In many cases there is no piped supply, hence the current WHO programme to try and ensure that an adequate water supply will be available to all by the end of the decade.

The higher consumption in the developed countries arises mainly from the use of water for sewage disposal and the relevance of a water borne sewage system in areas where water is in short supply is now being questioned. High water consumptions can also arise from the use of baths rather than showers, the latter using only about a tenth as much as the former. The cost of fuel needed to heat the water is similarly reduced and it is significant that with the rise in the cost of fuel, the amount of water used for domestic purposes in the UK appears not to be increasing at the present time.

Economy in the use of water also becomes important from time to time in developed countries. Rain does not fall uniformly during the year, nor even from year to year. If storage facilities are provided to maintain normal supplies at times of drought, occurring only infrequently, part of the capital investment will lie idle most of the time. In effect many millions of pounds may be spent to allow consumers to continue taking baths rather than showers for a period of a few weeks on two or three occasions during their lives. The continuing rise in the cost of water is leading to a critical examination of this point and the more general one of exploiting different types of resources in the most economical way, by conjunctive use schemes.

2.1. Conjunctive Use Schemes

Rain which falls on upland catchments may be collected in reservoirs and distributed by gravity, often with only limited treatment and at low operating cost, although the capital cost of the reservoir and trunk main may be high. Water abstracted from a river will require pumping and more treatment and, therefore, higher operating costs, but the capital costs will be lower. Borehole water may or may not need treatment but the pumping costs may be substantial. The aquifer from which the water is drawn by the borehole also serves as a reservoir, whilst the quantity of water that may be drawn from a river may be limited at times of low flow. There may also be a suspended solids problem at times of flood. The cost of water from each source can be estimated for a given set of conditions and a strategy developed which will give the lowest total cost in a given set of circumstances to take into account different anticipated rainfall patterns. The problem is complicated by the large number of alternatives likely to be

available and the fact that changes in the discount rate on which the
calculations are based will affect the cost of water from each source
differently. The combined use of resources in this way is termed conjunctive
use, a good example of which is the Lancashire Conjunctive Use Scheme,
serving an area of East Lancashire.

The scheme, illustrated in Fig. 1, combines the use of water from upland
catchments (Stocks and Barnacre reservoirs), lowland rivers (Lune and
Wyre) and boreholes into the Bunter sandstone aquifer. Water is pumped

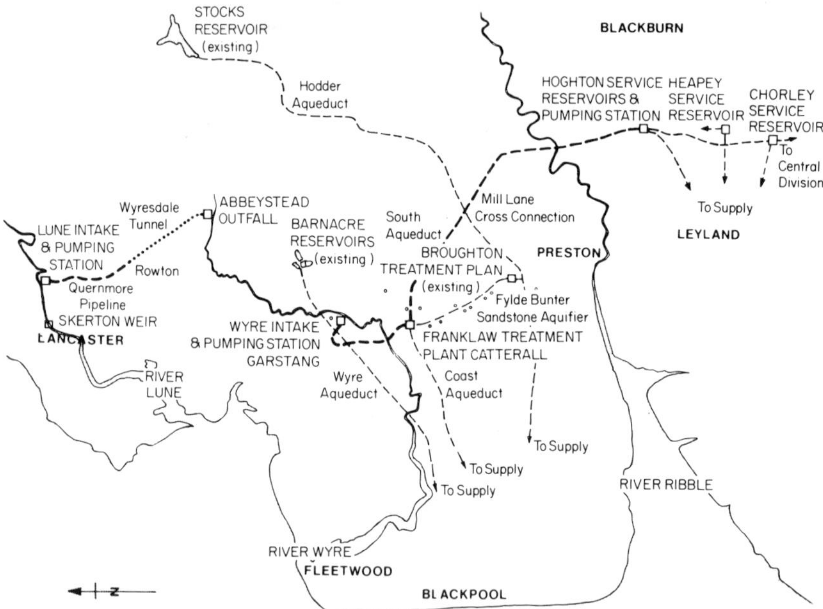

FIG. 1.   Schematic plan of Lancashire Conjunctive Use Scheme. (By courtesy of
the North West Water Authority.)

from the Lune through a tunnel to Abbeystead on the River Wyre, which is
used to carry the water onwards to Garstang. Here it is pumped to
Franklaw Treatment Plant at Catterall and thence to service reservoirs and
the distribution system. Besides improving supplies locally the scheme
reduces the demand on the aqueduct taking water from the Lake District to
Manchester, making more water available for that area.

The principle can be extended by the transfer of water from one supply area to another, either because of differences in rainfall or in population density and, hence, demand. Capital and pumping costs may be minimised by using existing rivers where possible and pumping at times when off-peak electricity is available. Such a scheme is in operation in the South-East of England, where water is transferred from the Ely Ouse river system to more heavily populated areas in Essex.

If rivers are used care must be taken to ensure that a deterioration in water quality does not take place as a result of pollution. The quality of water will also vary from source to source and appropriate treatment has to be provided if consumers are to be spared embarrassing changes in quality.

In some industries water quality is critical and water taken from the public supply is often treated further. For example, water for a brewery may be treated by ion-exchange, to reduce the concentrations of some inorganic salts, followed by the controlled addition of others, to produce beers formerly characteristic of particular locations, elsewhere.

3.   WATER TREATMENT

Water is treated to ensure that it will reach the consumer in a condition fit to drink. It is not sufficient for it only to enter the distribution system in this state; account must be taken of the changes that may take place within the distribution system. It must not attack the system, nor must scale be deposited to such an extent that pipes and fittings become obstructed. Pathogenic bacteria must not be permitted to grow within the distribution system and solids present, whether suspended or dissolved, must not be such that the water is harmful to health or even cause physiological upsets. Preferably it should be suitable also for use by industry in the area, although additional treatment by industrial users is common.

3.1. Standards for Treated Water

The traditional requirement for water for public supply in the UK is that it should be wholesome, not defined in analytical terms but water deemed to be so would certainly be within World Health Organisation standards for drinking water (Table 2). A very much more detailed set of analytical requirements has been put forward by the European Economic Community. These are controversial at the present time, mainly on account of the very low limits placed on some substances. Whilst there are many substances that are undesirable in drinking water there will always be a concentration below which they are very unlikely to have any significant effect. The difficulty lies in deciding on the appropriate concentration.

Part of the difficulty, probably most of it, has arisen from the improvements that have taken place in methods of analysis, which allow concentrations of $10^{-6}\,\mathrm{g\,litre^{-1}}$ of many substances to be measured accurately. Unfortunately, knowledge of the effects of concentrations of this order on the human body are generally not known. Obtaining this information will take a long time and require the expenditure of a great deal of effort. In the meantime the temptation is to specify low levels on the grounds of safety, although this must be based on intuition rather than fact. For example, a person consuming 2 litres of water per day containing $1 \times 10^{-6}\,\mathrm{g\,litre^{-1}}$ of chloroform would ingest, during the course of a year, rather less than is contained in one dose of some cough mixtures. It is extremely difficult to obtain sound evidence of the levels at which known contaminants become harmful to the most susceptible part of the population when ingested over a long period. It is not something which can be determined by experiment. The only reasonable method is to take advantage of local circumstances where populations happen to have been subject to water supplies containing the substances in question.

There are of course severe limitations. A reliable history of the concentrations of particular compounds in the water supply for a period of many years is required. Even if this exists the accuracy of past determinations may be in doubt; analytical techniques have improved considerably during the last few years. In any case some substances in question have only come into widespread use relatively recently. There are likely to be other factors complicating the interpretation of the results; consumption of water is only one of the ways in which man can ingest harmful substances. The controversy over allowable lead concentrations and the origin of lead found in the human body provides a good example of the difficulties likely to be encountered.

Whilst the risk of harm can be reduced by specifying very low levels of contaminants, this is likely to increase the use of resources for water supply and so reduce those available for other activities of benefit to health. For example, the extra resources might be more effectively employed in seeking to reduce the damage to health caused by smoking rather than drinking water. It is an area where controversy is inevitable, if only because of the lack of factual evidence, and it is essential to keep a sense of perspective.

One of the outstanding developments in the analytical field has been the establishment of analytical quality control. This is a means of ensuring that different laboratories will produce similar results when presented with identical samples. The methodology, which has been developed by the Water Research Centre,[4] covers precautions needed in sample preparation, analytical methods used, control procedures and monitoring of the results. Figure 2 shows the improvement in reliability resulting from the adoption of AQC (analytical quality control). The figures are based on results obtained during a survey of lead in drinking water for the UK Department of the Environment and referred to in reference 4.

Where low levels laid down for specific contaminants are exceeded in the raw water supply, the problem of removal arises, an area where, in many cases, detailed information still also has to be obtained. The problem is

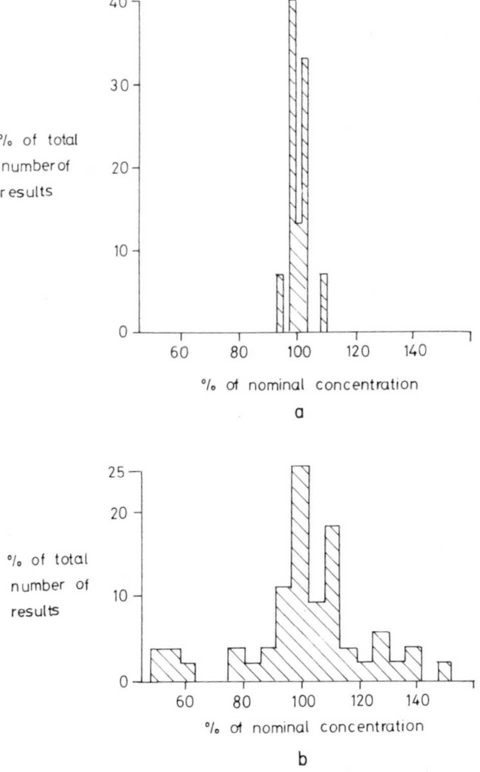

FIG. 2. Results from different laboratories determining lead in portions of standard solutions by laboratories (a) applying analytical quality control, (b) another group of laboratories. (Data is taken from reference 4. Group (a) includes 55 results, the nominal concentration being 180 μg litre^{-1}; group (b) 15 results, the nominal concentration being 46 μg litre^{-1}.)

made more difficult in that any treatment chemicals used must also be to a very high degree of purity. The most likely result of enforcement of standards requiring very low concentrations would be to limit the sources available for drinking supplies. Lowland rivers, some of which have been used for many years without noticeable ill effects, are particularly at risk. An alternative approach would be to limit the manufacture and use of sensitive compounds.

A specific case of an undesirable ion now found in many raw water supplies is that of nitrate. The maximum permissible level, laid down by the WHO is 45 mg litre^{-1}, expressed as NO_3. The explanation usually given is that water containing more than this may cause illness (methaemoglo-binaemia) in very young babies. The disease is very rare in the UK; as far as the author is aware there has been only one case in the last twenty years and that was in rather unusual circumstances, involving a well supplying a single farm. It would be difficult to justify treatment on these grounds alone in the UK, since the problem can be avoided by supplying bottled low-nitrate water to those at risk for the short period necessary. Recently, however, there has been suspicion that under some circumstances nitrate may be involved in the formation of potentially carcinogenic substances, although specific information is not yet available. Fortunately nitrate can now be removed from raw water supplies without undue difficulty.

3.1.1. *Fluoridation*

Occasionally elements may be added to water. Fluoride is a specific example over which there has been much controversy. Children growing up in areas in which there is less than about 1 mg litre^{-1} of fluoride in the drinking water have been found to develop teeth less resistant to decay than those in areas where this level of fluoride is present. The obvious step of introducing fluoride into supplies lacking a natural source has been recommended by almost all UK Area Health Authorities but has not yet been generally adopted. The main objection has been that it is compulsory medication, although the argument seems difficult to justify when fluoride occurs naturally in other supplies. It is fortunate that similar objections have not been raised in the case of chlorine, needed to discourage the growth of pathogenic bacteria in the supply system.

Statistical studies have shown that there appears to be a correlation between soft water and cardiovascular diseases, and the EEC proposed directive gives minimum recommended concentrations of calcium and magnesium. Excessively soft waters are also undesirable in that they may attack plumbing systems.

3.2. The Treatment of Water for Public Supply

The requirements for treatment depend mainly on the characteristics of the raw water. Borehole or deep spring water may require only chlorination, although some may have to be treated to reduce iron and manganese. Surface waters will generally require solids removal and may also require the removal of organics, ammonia and nitrate. The hardness and pH of the water may need adjustment and the water is disinfected before being distributed.

3.2.1. *Solids Removal*

Slow sand filtration is probably the oldest and is still one of the best methods of removing suspended solids. Unfortunately it requires much more space and costs more to build than other methods producing adequate results. The labour needed to clean the surface of the bed has been reduced by the use of mechanical devices but the area of land needed cannot be reduced without departing from the principles of the system.

However, the process is rather more than solids removal alone, the biologically active layer which grows at the surface of the sand will remove bacteria and some organics, reducing the chlorine demand in the later stages of treatment. This aspect is likely to become more important as allowable concentrations of organics are reduced.

The most commonly used method for removing suspended solids is coagulation and flocculation, followed by settlement or clarification and filtration at rates up to fifty times as fast as those used for slow sand filtration.

Coagulation requires the addition of chemicals, traditionally iron or aluminium salts, although polyelectrolytes may also now be used, providing they meet the requirements laid down by the Department of the Environment. This is followed by controlled agitation during which the solid particles in the water are brought into contact with and trapped by the flocs formed. These are then removed by settlement in a clarifier usually of a sludge blanket type. The water then passes through a high rate filter. The water is passed, usually downwards, through media, a bed of coarse granular material, originally a carefully graded sand. The flow of water may be by gravity or, in closed vessels, under pressure. Solids collected in the bed lead to an increase in differential pressure, or a reduction in flow, depending on the method of operation in use. The solids are removed by backwashing, i.e. an upward flow of clean water, usually after scouring with an air flow to loosen dirt from the media. The performance of the filter and the frequency of backwashing depends on the solids load and is, therefore, dependent on the efficiency of the preceding stage. The main feature of development in this area has been the introduction of media using more than one material, termed dual media if two are used or multi-media if more than two.

Ideally a filter bed would be graded from coarse to fine in the direction of flow, so that the fine media are protected from a heavy solids load by the preceding media which will remove the larger particles. Unfortunately if media of varying size but the same density are used the larger particles will tend to accumulate at the bottom of the bed after backwashing, which is the opposite of the requirement.

The effect can be avoided by using media of different densities, for example, fine garnet at the bottom, sand in the middle and coarse anthracite at the top. The advantage of multi-media filtration is that a given unit will handle a greater flow than when single media are used.

Another development is the use of a continuously moving bed of sand. In this case, illustrated in Fig. 3 sand is introduced at the top of the vessel, the water being filtered flows across it and the sand and the solids removed are taken continuously from the bottom. The sand is cleaned and returned to the top of the vessel, the solids also being discharged continuously.

The main developments in this area have been directed towards increasing the rate of flow through a given size of plant. The most effective of these has been the pulsed flow principle introduced by Degremont. In this arrangement, illustrated in Fig. 4 there is a vacuum chamber in the inlet pipe, the vacuum being alternately made and broken. Whilst the pressure in the chamber is falling the water rises in it, so that there is a negligible flow into the settling compartment. Air is then suddenly admitted to the chamber, the water level falls and water enters the clarifier at a relatively high rate for a short period. The cycle is then repeated three times or so per minute.

The advantages of this method of operation are that uniform distribution of water at the base of the clarifier is very much more easily achieved at high flow rates than at low ones and the sludge blanket is more stable. The sludge blanket lifts when the water is admitted and then subsides, the incoming water passing through the bed, clarified water overflowing during each pulse. The period of rest between upward flows allows lateral movement of the sludge to close up any thin places which might form and be kept open if the flow were continuous. Excess sludge flows over a weir into a sludge concentrator in a manner similar to that used for a traditional sludge blanket clarifier. The adoption of the system has been greatly helped by the fact that an existing clarifier can be converted and its capacity increased.

An alternative approach has been adopted in a Hungarian process in the

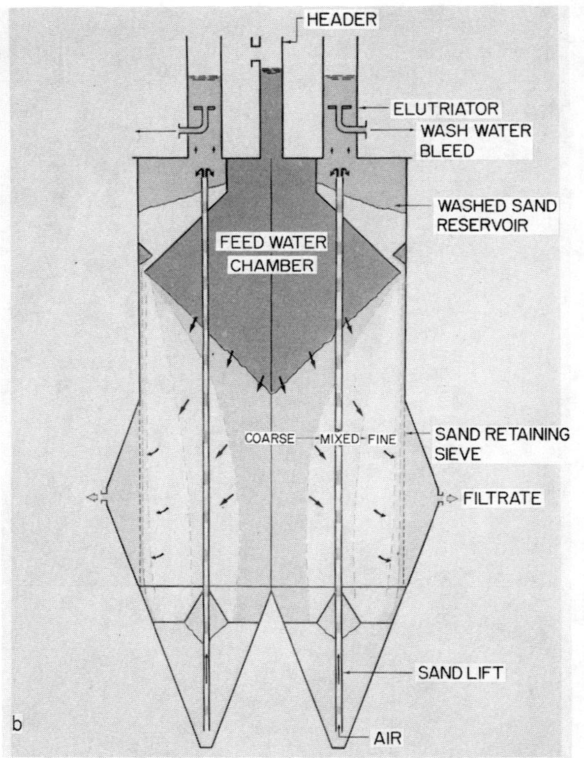
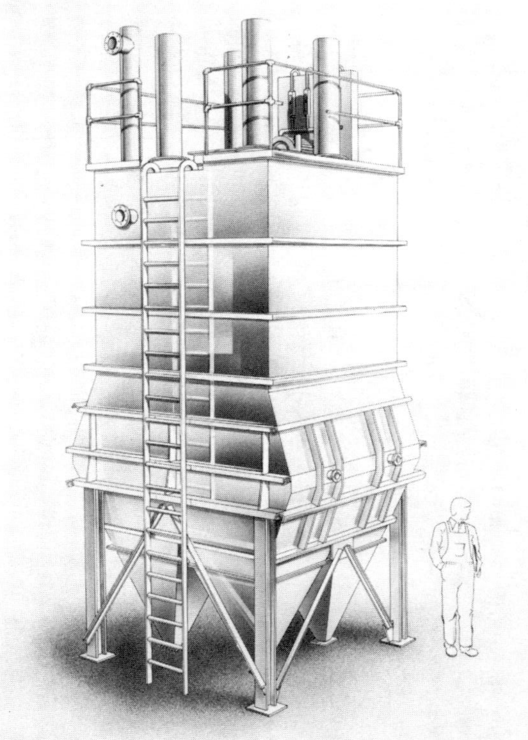

FIG. 3. 'TENTEN' continuous sand filter, (a) exterior (b) cross section. (By courtesy of Simon-Hartley Ltd.)

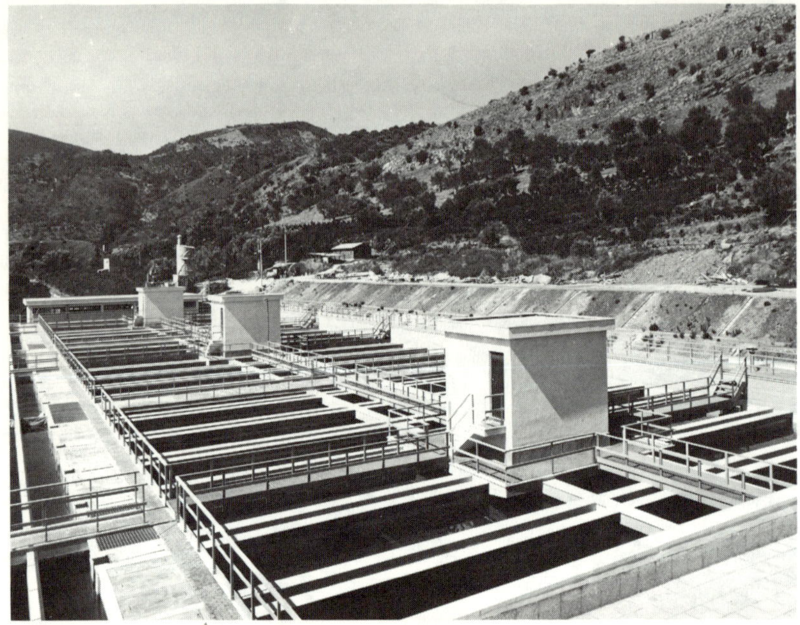

FIG. 4.   Pulsator clarifier.

use of fine sand to weight the floc. The incoming water is treated with a polyelectrolyte and sand, the resulting heavy flocs are settled and subsequently removed. The sand is then cleaned and re-used.

Flocs may also be removed by flotation. Although compact plants at lower capital cost than for sedimentation are possible, more energy is required and the total cost is similar at the present time. The process is, therefore, likely to be adversely affected by a continuing rise in energy costs. It is also more susceptible to variations in the quality of the raw water.

Clarification is normally followed by filtration, to remove stray flocs and solids which may have escaped the earlier process and to serve as a safety device in the case of gross carry-over.

3.2.2. *Ammonia and Nitrate Removal*

Ammonia is not normally present in groundwater but may be present in surface water at concentrations of the order of 1 mg litre^{-1}, due to pollution from sewage treatment works or industry. Nitrates can occur in both surface and subsurface water and, in the UK, occasionally exceed the concentration of 45 mg litre^{-1} specified by the WHO. It may arise from a well oxidised effluent from sewage treatment, industrial wastes or run-off from land to which nitrogenous fertilisers have been applied.

Ammonia can be removed by chlorination but the chlorine demand, about 9 mg litre^{-1} for each mg litre^{-1} of ammonia, leads to an undesirable increase in chloride content, high cost and the risk of forming unwanted chlorinated organics. Both ammonia and nitrate can be removed by ion exchange processes but the lack of specific media leads to high cost and there is also the problem of disposing of spent regenerants. Both can also be removed biologically and this is now regarded as the best method.

In the most recent version of the treatment processes ammonia is oxidised to nitrate by passing the water through a fluidised bed of sand grains on the surface of which are aerobic bacteria. These use oxygen dissolved in the water to carry out the oxidation and, as 4·57 mg litre^{-1} of oxygen is needed to oxidise 1 mg litre^{-1} of ammonia, it is essential that the water is well aerated. If necessary some of the treated water may be aerated and recycled. The resistance time of the water in the bed is of the order of a few minutes.[6]

The nitrate formed, and that originally present, may be removed in another fluidised bed in which the bacteria use the nitrate to oxidise a carbon substrate added for the purpose. Methanol is commonly used and the quantity needed has been determined experimentally. Although experimental work is in progress, the problem of controlling the addition of methanol automatically does not yet appear to have been solved, so that hand control is necessary. Storage before treatment is, therefore, desirable, to reduce the rate of change of nitrate concentration. Other substrates which might be controlled more easily have been considered, but so far all have been found to be more expensive.

The concentration of nitrates in surface water fluctuates and treatment may not be needed for more than a few months each year. In some cases concentrations can be reduced sufficiently by adding water from a low-nitrate source. The economics of this solution depend on the amount of water needed, the distance it has to be conveyed and the pumping costs. In most cases biological treatment is cheaper.[7]

3.2.3. *Softening*

The fluidised bed system has also been used to advantage in the softening process developed first in Germany and latterly by the Fylde Water Board, now part of the North West Water Authority.[8]

A vertical cylindrical reactor is used, the raw water and the lime water is injected at the bottom and flows upwards through a bed of calcium carbonate pellets. These grow by accretion of the calcium carbonate formed during the softening process and the larger ones are eventually removed. Some are crushed and returned to the process, the remainder are used for agricultural purposes. One of the main advantages of the process is that it does not produce sludge.

The effects of hardness can be reduced by the addition of polyphosphates, such as sodium hexametaphosphate (Calgon), which form soluble compounds with calcium and magnesium.

With the requirement for a minimum hardness the addition of lime to soft waters may be necessary. Carbon dioxide is also added to adjust the pH to the required level and provide a degree of buffering.

3.2.4. *Removal of Organic Matter*

As far as possible this process is avoided by selecting sources low in organics. The presence of dissolved organics is generally due to pollution although they are present naturally in moorland waters. Slow sand filtration will remove some organic matter and it may be oxidised by chlorination. A little may also be oxidised during ammonia and nitrate removal.

Activated carbon is the method principally used for the removal of organics, either in granular or powdered form. It has been made experimentally from a wide range of materials, even waste plastics, but commercially transport costs limit the choice to those containing a high proportion of carbon, such as coal and wood, or those with special properties, such as nut shells.

The raw material is first carbonised, crushed and sometimes briquetted. Inorganic salts may also be incorporated. It is then activated by heating to about 800 °C under carefully controlled conditions in the presence of steam, and then cooled and screened. The adsorptive characteristics can be controlled by adjustment of the activation conditions.

Granular carbon, i.e. that coarser than about 50 mesh is used in beds, either open or under pressure in closed vessels, through which the water may flow upwards or downwards. In the latter case periodic backwashing is required. Organic matter is adsorbed by the carbon but the process is reversible and the residence time in the bed is normally too short to allow an equilibrium to be established. Low molecular weight compounds are adsorbed more quickly than high molecular weight ones but the carbon will adsorb a greater weight of the latter. Biological growth is likely to occur in the bed and the water to be treated must contain an adequate level of dissolved oxygen to avoid the development of anaerobic conditions.

When the adsorptive capacity of the granular activated carbon is no longer sufficient to maintain an appropriate standard of treated water it can be regenerated by heating in a controlled atmosphere to a temperature slightly lower than that originally used for activation. Some carbon is lost by oxidation and attrition so that an addition of 10 % or so of fresh carbon may be needed. The process is relatively expensive, the granular activated carbon alone now (1980) costing more than £1000 t^{-1}, and it is only used in special circumstances. Nevertheless the process is now in continuous operation at some works[9] and is likely to become more widespread as high quality water sources become fully utilised.

The price of powdered activated carbon is of the order of that of granular activated carbon but it is much more difficult to regenerate. It is added to the raw water in the initial stages of treatment and removed by the filters, to be discharged with the other solids in the backwash stream. It may be used continuously but more commonly it is used in emergency when undesirable tastes or odours occur unexpectedly in the water.

It is sometimes difficult to judge the practical success of the process, other than by an obvious reduction in taste and smell, in view of the difficulty in identifying the large number of organic compounds likely to be present in low concentrations and lack of knowledge of their practical significance.

3.2.5. *Membrane Processes*

These include ultrafiltration, reverse osmosis and electrodialysis. All will reduce concentrations of organic matter and the second and third dissolved solids also. All are relatively expensive when compared with other water treatment processes, the membrane life being a critical factor.

The processes work by forcing water through a specially manufactured membrane, by pressure in the case of ultrafiltration and reverse osmosis and under the influence of an electrical current in the case of electrodialysis, the passage of other molecules being hindered. The efficiency of each process falls as the concentration of contaminants increases and the proportion of feed rejected can be high. They are, therefore, best suited to the production of relatively small volumes of water for special purposes rather than bulk supplies. Typical applications for reverse osmosis and electrodialysis would be the provision of a drinking water supply from a brackish source for a dual supply system, the reject stream being used for the less critical applications. They are also used industrially for the production of water of a particular quality, using towns' water for the feed. Figure 5 shows typical units.

Reverse osmosis and electrodialysis can be used to provide potable water

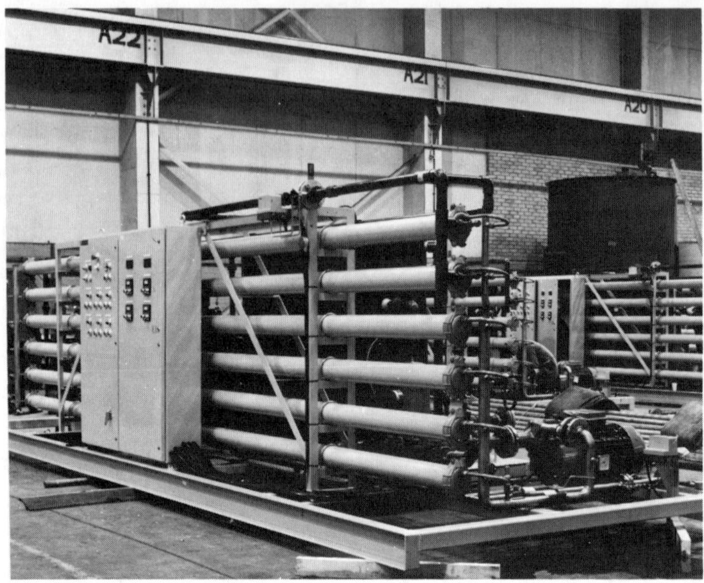

FIG. 5. Reverse osmosis units during assembly. (By courtesy of Ames Crosta Babcock Ltd.)

from sea water but are not efficient at the high concentrations of salts present. The most common process for this purpose is now multi-stage flash distillation. The cost of supplying water in this way is several times that of the treatment of fresh water and it is only used as a last resort. The cost may be reduced to some extent if the desalination plant is combined with a thermal power station generating steam at high pressure and extracting energy from it before it is passed to the desalination plant.

Distilled water can be produced on a small scale by a solar still, as at Patmos.[10] The heat of the sun evaporates water contained in glass covered concrete troughs lined with butyl rubber. The water vapour condenses on the under side of the glass to run into collecting channels. Rain falling on the upper surface is also collected. Whilst requiring a relatively large land area, $9000 \, \text{m}^2$ for $27 \, \text{m}^3 \, \text{day}^{-1}$ in the above case, running costs are low.

3.3. Disinfection

Disinfection is necessary both to kill bacteria present in the raw water supply and to discourage the growth of bacteria in the distribution system. Bacteria capable of causing disease should be completely absent and others which are harmless but likely to lead to corrosion, tastes or odours should be kept to a very low level. The types of bacteria and their significance are shown in Table 3.[11] The number of bacteria present in the raw water varies widely with the source; deep spring and borehole water are likely to contain very few, whilst a lowland river may contain relatively large numbers. The main developments in this area have been a better understanding of the requirements, the mechanism of disinfection and improvements in measurement and control techniques. The agents mainly used for disinfection are chlorine or chlorine-containing compounds and ozone. Ultra-violet light may be used in particular situations.

3.3.1. *Chlorination*

The action of chlorine is complex and depends on substances, such as ammonia and organic compounds, already in the water which react with it. Sufficient chlorine must be added to allow for this and leave a residual level, usually up to about $0.5\,\text{mg litre}^{-1}$. Ammonia reacts with chlorine to form chloramines. These are not as powerful disinfectants as chlorine but are more persistent. In some circumstances ammonia may be added after chlorination, in order to take advantage of this property.[12]

The quantity of chlorine added may be controlled automatically, using a gold/copper electrode system to measure the residual chlorine present after a given contact time. In some cases a heavy dose of chlorine is used in the first instance, followed by partial dechlorination, using sulphur dioxide or a sulphite, to yield the desired level of residual chlorine.

Ideally, residual chlorine should be present at all points in the distribution system and the level of chlorine in the water entering the system controlled accordingly. In practice it may be difficult to achieve this without complaints of chlorine taste if some consumers receive the water shortly after treatment. The problem may be made worse by the presence of some organic compounds, such as phenol, which form strongly tasting compounds with chlorine. In this case break-point chlorination or other reagents, such as chlorine dioxide or ozone, may be used.

The quantity of chlorine required varies both with the flow and chlorine demand of the water. If both remain relatively constant, or are subject only to slow variations, a simple type of controller can be used. In other circumstances a ratio controller may also be needed. In this case the ratio controller ensures that chlorine is added as a proportion of the flow of water and the chlorine residual controller sets the value of the proportion.[13]

In the past and in many cases at present, chlorine has been supplied for large installations as a liquid under pressure in steel tanks and rigorous

TABLE 3

MICROBIOLOGICAL DETERIORATION OF WATER QUALITY IN SUPPLY

Stage of supply	Problem	Organisms concerned	Significance
Final water	Organisms surviving treatment	Spore-forming bacteria (including *Bacillus cereus* and *Clostridium perfringens*)	Metabolically active in nitrate-reduction and putrefaction / These two species can form enterotoxins if allowed to contaminate and grow in food
		Flavobacterium spp. / Yeasts	Spoilage in food processing
		Mycobacterium spp. / *Klebsiella*	Some species are potential pathogens
		Amoebic cysts: *Entamoeba histolytica* / *Naegleria* spp.	Amoebic dysentry / Amoebic meningitis—especially in the context of heated swimming pool waters
		Giardia lamblia	Intestinal disorders
Distribution pipelines	Corrosion	(a) Sulphate-reducing bacteria *Desulfovibrio vulgaris* *Desulfotomaculum nigrificans*	Internal pitting and nodule formation in iron mains
		(b) Nitrate-reducing bacteria *Micrococcus* spp. *Bacillus* spp. *Pseudomonas* spp.	Loss of carrying capacity / Hydrogen sulphide odours
		(c) Bacteria which alter pH and redox	Loose iron deposits

Discoloured water	(a) True iron bacteria
	    Gallionella spp. and
	    Leptothrix spp.
	(b) Organisms which adsorb
	    ferric iron—most
	    micro-organisms
	(c) Organisms which utilise
	    iron/humic complexes
	    Arthrobacter spp.
	    Siderocapsa spp.
		Consumer complaints with
		laundry and sanitary ware
		Blockage of filters and meters
		Deposits in drink manufacture
		Formation of iron/organic slimes
		with loss in carrying capacity
		Entrainment of algae
		Animals graze any slime or deposit

	Depletion of oxygen	Many common heterotrophs, e.g. plate count bacteria	Putrefaction leading to offensive taste and odours
	Reduction of nitrate	Denitrifying bacteria	Nitrite formation Ammonia formation with the possibility of odorous chloramines in supply
	Biodeterioration of materials	Many species of bacteria *Nocardia* spp.	Biodeterioration of tank sealants Biodeterioration of rubber sealing rings
Domestic or industrial plumbing	Microbiological growth on materials, e.g. tap washers, fibre seals, 'O' rings, hemp yarn and sealant pastes, tallow, fluxes, joint lubricants, plastic components	Coliforms Pseudomonads, including *Ps. aeruginosa* *Mycobacteria/Nocardia* spp. Yeasts Fungi and actinomycetes High plate counts at 22° and 37°C *Flavobacterium* spp.	Complicates surveillance Potential pathogens Potential pathogen Taste and odours Deterioration of water quality Spoilage of food and manufacturing processes

TABLE 3—*contd.*

Stage of supply	Problem	Organisms concerned	Significance
Domestic or industrial plumbing	Biological slime growths in header tanks and water softeners	Various fungi, bacteria and actinomycetes derived from the water or surrounding environment and growing on volatile organic solvents	Water becomes jelly-like and unusable Bacteria in such large numbers could be harmful
Medical aspects	Biological slime growths in medical and ancillary equipment, e.g. (a) Dentist drills	Non-specific heterotrophic bacteria	(a) Direct application to open wound, therefore potentially dangerous
	(b) Renal dialysis units		(b) Danger of toxin formation and leakage to bloodstream when large volumes of tap water are incubated at 37°C in the presence of organic nutrients in dialysis fluid
	(c) Air conditioning plant (d) Water softeners		(c) Can cause allergies (d) There is a danger of bacteriological contamination if not periodically sterilised

Modified from reference 11.

precautions are needed in handling it. Although the safety record of the water services is good there is nevertheless a potential danger and there is growing pressure for the substitution of available chlorine in other forms, such as hypochlorite.

Doubts have been raised to the use of chlorine where significant organic matter is present in the water, in view of the risk of forming halomethanes, albeit in very low concentrations. The problem can be avoided by using ozone, which is also of value in removing colour.

3.3.2. *Ozonation*

Ozone is a toxic irritant gas that decomposes readily, particularly in the presence of water vapour. In liquid form it is very unstable and it cannot, therefore, be stored and must be produced on-site by passing dry air or oxygen over an electrode system with a glass dielectric across which there is a silent electrical discharge. The gas stream, now containing a few percent of ozone, is passed through scrubbing towers so that the ozone is dissolved in water flowing through the towers. The vent gas from the towers is passed through activated carbon or an oxidation furnace to remove any

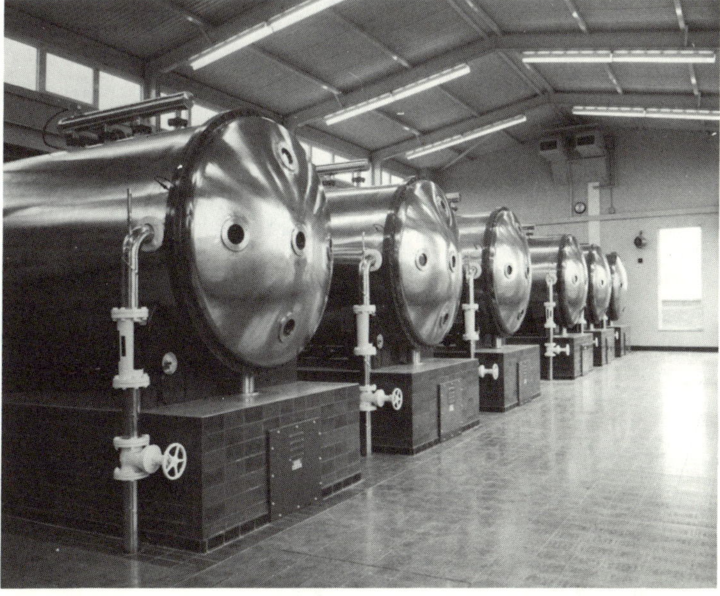

FIG. 6.   Ozonators at the Watchgate works of the North West Water Authority. (By courtesy of the North West Water Authority and Trailigaz Compagnie de l'Ozone-Procedes.)

unadsorbed ozone before it is discharged to the atmosphere. Typical units in use at the Watchgate Treatment Works of the North West Water Authority are shown in Fig. 6.

Whilst ozone is an effective bactericide it does not have the persistence of chlorine and there is some evidence that organic matter oxidised by ozone is more readily biodegraded than the original substance.[14] It is, therefore, necessary to chlorinate the ozone-treated water before it enters the distribution system.

3.3.3. *Ultra-Violet Light*

Whilst an effective sterilising agent, the use of ultra-violet light is generally restricted to special applications, such as in surgical operating theatres and in the kitchen cars of railway refreshment services.

4.   WATER DISTRIBUTION

The purpose of the distribution system is to ensure that all consumers have adequate water of appropriate quality available whenever required at the lowest cost consistent with the other criteria. The latter is important in view of the major contribution of the system, including trunk mains, to the total cost of water supplied. Table 4 shows the proportion in a typical case. The cost is influenced mainly by decisions taken at the design stage, in particular the size and location of the pipe systems, the level of service reservoirs and pumping arrangements.

In a specific case there is always a choice between different combinations of pump size and head loss, the latter in many cases reflecting pumping costs. The ideal system is one which provides the service required at

TABLE 4

PERCENTAGE APPORTIONMENT OF COSTS FOR THE FYLDE WATER
BOARD, 1972–73

Supply, i.e. catchment areas, reservoirs and boreholes	15
Treatment	18
Transmission to centres of consumption	15
Distribution	27
Rates	10
Management and general	15

From Hilson, M. A., 'Water treatment for public supply', *Chemistry and Industry*, 4 Jan., 1975.

minimum total cost for the life of the installation. The cost of the pipe and its installation is essentially a capital charge, that of pumping depends mainly on the cost of energy. Both interest rates and energy costs have changed radically during the recent past and are likely to continue to do so in the future.

The level of capital charges is imposed on the industry by external conditions. At one time $2\cdot5\%$ was considered a reasonable return on capital in a low-risk situation. During the last few years interest rates have increased greatly; lenders have expected to be compensated for the loss in value of their money as well as for lending it. The real rate of return may be considered to be the interest rate in force less the rate of inflation. An estimate made in this way[15] covering a period of about 30 years ending about five years ago indicates that the real rate of interest has not risen significantly. Nevertheless the test discount rate, a notional interest rate used for comparing the economics of different technical solutions, imposed on the water industry has been as high as 10%. At the time of writing, the industry is advised to use a figure of 5%.

When high test discount rates are used in the economic comparison of different schemes, high capital cost solutions become less attractive and there is a trend towards low capital cost solutions requiring more energy, i.e. smaller cheaper pipes with higher pressure losses. This is unfortunate at a time when a continuing rise in energy costs seems certain. It is also unfortunate that the cost effectiveness of distribution systems, with lifetimes likely to be of the order of at least 100 years, should be affected by short-term political decisions.

A water distribution system is primarily a network such that the design and performance of one portion influences that of other parts. Whilst manual methods of calculation have served well in the past for relatively simple systems it is doubtful whether they could cope with the large networks developing since reorganisation. Whilst the designer still has to provide the initiative, computer programmes have been developed which enable him to calculate the effects of design changes very much more easily than in the past. At the same time a great deal of data on the performance of existing systems has become available following the introduction of automatic and remote monitoring systems. New pipe materials, with lower friction losses, have also been introduced.

4.1. Materials of Construction

The traditional materials for water mains are cast iron, ductile iron or asbestos cement with mild steel, usually galvanised, lead or copper for small pipes. Iron is still used extensively, as is asbestos cement. Although doubts have been expressed about the advisability of using the latter, there does not seem to be any firm evidence of any harmful effects. Lead on the other hand can be attacked by soft water supplies and even though treated water is deliberately made hard enough to avoid the problem, the use of lead is being discouraged. The life of galvanised iron is limited and it is difficult to install neatly whilst the price of copper limits its use for all but the smallest sizes. This is in spite of a reduction in wall thicknesses made when metric standards were introduced.

The major development has of course been the introduction of plastic materials, particularly high density polyethylene and unplasticised polyvinyl chloride. The main difference between them is in the jointing techniques used. Unplasticised PVC pipes may be joined by cementing or solvent welding, although mechanical joints involving a flexible seal are also used, together with screwed connections for smaller sizes.

Various classes are available to suit different pressure conditions, the outside diameter being kept constant and the inside diameter being reduced to provide greater wall thickness for higher pressures. The strongest pipe generally used, class E, will withstand a sustained water pressure of 15 bar at 20 °C. The strength of PVC falls with increasing temperature and the maximum working pressure is reduced by 2 % for each 1 °C rise above 20 °C. PVC also expands about five times as much as cast iron for the same temperature rise.

Unplasticised PVC pipe is about one fifth of the weight of the equivalent iron pipe and, being slightly flexible, will take up some ground movement without breaking, particularly if mechanical joints are used. These rely on a rubber seal, for which the specified lubricant must be used. Difficulties were experienced in the early days in sterilising mains with this type of joint, because some bacteria were protected by the lubricant from the action of the chlorine. The lubricants now used are bacteriostatic. Skill is required in making solvent welded joints, the joint has to be made within a short time of applying the solvent and trapped excess solvent can lead to a point of weakness.

More care is also needed than for the older materials in bedding and backfilling trenches, since the pipe can be damaged by sharp stones. Unplasticised PVC is also more easily damaged by surge pressures than older materials.

Other plastics, such as acrylonitrile butadiene styrene (ABS) and polypropylene are also used but only to a limited extent.

Plastics are much less stable than metals under maintained stress and fittings requiring close mechanical clearances, such as valves, and pumps are normally made of metal and coupled to the plastic pipe with screwed or flanged adaptors. Valves incorporating compression fittings are available in small sizes and valves and cocks are also made in plastic for light duty in small sizes. All plastics are much more resistant than metals to attack by water although insignificant traces of stabiliser may be leached out during the first few months of use.

Plastic sheeting, especially butyl rubber, is used for lining reservoirs, either existing ones which have developed leaks, or new ones. In the latter case a prepared excavation is all that is required, although care must be taken to ensure that air or other gases trapped beneath the sheeting can escape, otherwise part of the lining may balloon to the surface.

4.2. Control of Water Distribution Systems

The supervision and control of a water distribution system requires a knowledge of the conditions at the collection and storage points and at the pumping stations and service reservoirs as well as at key points on the system. The information is needed preferably at a central point from which instructions regarding the operation of the system can be given. The relevant information can be obtained by attendants at manned stations or on inspection visits to unmanned ones and relayed by telephone or radio to a central control room. With the reduction in number of manned stations data obtained in this way is either limited or involves substantial costs in making journeys specifically for that purpose. The present trend is, therefore, towards the automatic sensing and transmission of data. This in turn can lead towards a reduction in the number of inspection visits needed.

A system based on the automatic transmission of indications of flow, level, pressure and the condition of operating plant units has been operated by the Sunderland and South Shields Water Company since 1968.[16] The information is transmitted to a control room which is continuously manned and provided with equipment which enables the staff to know what is happening at each of the 61 outstations and to operate equipment at the outstations which controls the supply and distribution of water through the system. The system cost approximately £165 000 in 1968 and supplies, based on 1976 figures, an average quantity of 127 000 m^3 day^{-1} to a total of 580 000 people.

The following operating benefits are claimed.

1.   Quicker action is possible when required by operating conditions, because information of the conditions at the outstations is continuously available to the operators.

2. Energy has been saved in pumping and costs reduced as a result of better knowledge of conditions in the pumping systems.
3. More effective use of the existing system has saved the construction of a new service reservoir.
4. Consumers have experienced fewer variations in water pressure and interruptions in supply have been detected more quickly. Staff carrying out repairs can be used more effectively.
5. Records are kept mechanically and centrally, requiring less clerical effort and fewer visits to outstations.
6. The detailed knowledge now available of the performance of the system has helped in planning and development.

The system is maintained by the company's own staff and has proved to be very reliable.

A system of rather smaller capacity and with fewer outstations was installed by the East Worcestershire Waterworks Company in 1971.[17] This system is controlled by an on-line computer and uses UHF radio links as well as cable circuits.

Besides providing better control, centralised systems of these types reduce the number of people required to work unsocial hours and enable the staff to work more effectively. On the other hand additional maintenance, requiring a high standard of skill, is needed. Special care has to be taken in the mechanical maintenance of remotely controlled plant to ensure that the plant does not operate unexpectedly whilst it is being maintained and is restored to normal control on the completion of maintenance. Provision also has to be made for manual operation in the event of a failure of the automatic control system.

5. ADMINISTRATIVE DEVELOPMENTS

A major development in water supply in the UK took place in 1974. Prior to that time water supply was the responsibility of local authorities, water boards and water companies supplying areas, the boundaries of which were largely the results of historical accident. On reorganisation of local government the opportunity was also taken to reorganise the water services so that a single authority became responsible for all aspects of water supply and wastewater disposal in a particular area, as well as river quality, flood control and leisure uses.

One of the aims of reorganisation was that water resources and water use should be developed more rationally than previously, when different aspects of water use in an area had been controlled by several authorities, often with very different outlooks. To this end, the Regional Water Authorities were based on river basins, or groups of river basins, the boundaries being along watersheds. The whole of England is covered by nine Authorities and Wales by one. The arrangements in Scotland, introduced a year later, are rather different. The water companies have been retained but work under the aegis of the RWAs.

The formation of the Regional Water Authorities has allowed the implementation of water supply schemes covering wide areas and using a variety of sources more easily than would have been the case previously. The Lancashire Conjunctive Use Scheme is a case in point, although the first steps had been taken by the water undertakings in the area prior to reorganisation.

The water authorities are required to treat consumers equally as far as possible and to recover their costs by levying charges. This has led to some levelling of the prices charged, there being balancing payments—those areas in which water would be more expensive, generally areas of low population density, are subsidised by those in a better economic situation. This has not always been welcomed. There are cases of village supplies where, prior to reorganisation, an annual levy on ratepayers of less than one pound each sufficed to provide an honorarium for a local farmer to look after a small service reservoir fed by a deep spring. The ratepayers are now each faced with an annual bill of tens of pounds for what is essentially the same service.

The cost of water to the community has risen sharply but this cannot wholly be ascribed to reorganisation. The price of water prior to reorganisation was, in many cases, very low, supply installations having been built a long time previously, at prices much lower than today's, and almost or completely written off. With inflation, the current cost of replacement is many times that of the original; a life of 60 years is not unusual for many items in water supply and the pound is worth only about one fifteenth of its value in 1920.

The extra cost of the new administrative structure must be offset by the reductions in cost made possible by shared services and the reduction in numbers of small units. There has, however, been a strong trade union development and wage rates have increased sharply, approximately 20 % in each of the last two years (1979 and 1980). Whilst from a technical standpoint the reliability of the water supply has improved, this must be set against the unfortunate fact that in 1979, for the first time, some consumers were without water for several weeks, as a result of unofficial industrial action by maintenance workers, and other stoppages have been threatened.

Following reorganisation the research establishment concerned with water supply, the Water Research Association at Medmenham, was merged with the Water Pollution Research Laboratories at Stevenage to form the Water Research Centre. Shared services have led to economies and the laboratories have carried out a number of joint operations. Amongst these has been the production of Technical Report No. 61.[18] The report provides a means of estimating, primarily for planning purposes, the cost of the elements of water supply and wastewater disposal systems, based on the cost of works completed in the years between the early sixties and the mid seventies, adjusted for inflation to prices obtaining in the third quarter of 1976. The data is presented in the form of equations for individual items such as water mains, boreholes, dams and reservoirs, pumping systems and treatment works, relating the cost at the third quarter of 1976 to outline process parameters such as flow, head, detention period and superficial area of tanks. The statistical basis and a review of the probable limitations in accuracy are also included in the report.

The use of computers has resulted in many changes in the water services. As well as enabling the more efficient control of water distribution computers are used for the storage of technical data, for technical calculation, for the keeping of commercial records, for salary payments and the production of customers' accounts. These developments are, however, not dissimilar from those elsewhere in industry and commerce, although on a somewhat larger scale. The use of closed circuit television for surveillance is also similar.

6. THE FUTURE

The scope for enlargement of the water supply system in the UK is now limited. Almost all habitations now have a supply of piped water. The demand for water has temporarily stopped increasing. Whilst this may be the result of the economic situation, both may have arisen from the same cause, the rise in the cost of energy. A fall in the cost of energy does not seem likely at the present time. Industrially, the price of water has reached a level where economy in use can lead to significant economies.

Further developments in treatment are likely to take place in order to meet EEC regulations, as and when imposed. In addition the discharge of some specific pollutants to rivers from which water for potable supplies is subsequently taken may be severely restricted. The RWAs have the means and the authority to do both.

New forms of pollution are likely to occur and some existing forms may become more significant. Radioactive substances have always been present naturally in water supplies but are likely to increase with the wider use of nuclear energy. Fortunately they can be detected in very low concentrations. Use is in fact being made of their presence, in hydrological studies.[19]

There is still considerable scope for technical development in the automatic remote control and monitoring of sources and treatment and distribution systems. Such developments will have to take account of, or may even be initiated by, the changing attitudes of the labour force.

Microprocessors are already used for local control, monitoring and alarm indications but there appears to be a limitation in the form of the accuracy and reliability of the sensor elements and there is still much work to be done in this area.

Overseas the scope for development is considerably greater. The situation varies widely between the western countries, where problems similar to those encountered in the UK may be found, to the developing countries, where there is still a need, in many places, for basic installations and even hospitals may be without piped water. The problems are mostly economic rather than technical but the technologist can help by developing systems and equipment which make the best use of what is available locally at a price the community can afford. The aim must be to ensure that all can have access, without undue physical effort, to a piped supply of wholesome water adequate for their needs. This does not mean that western practices, with a water usage of upwards of 200 litres/day will always be appropriate. Many of the developing countries are in areas where there is insufficient water available to meet such a demand. The cost also rises sharply when water usage reaches the point at which it entails the construction and operation of a wastewater disposal system.

ACKNOWLEDGEMENTS

The author thanks his friends and colleagues at Howard Humphreys and Partners, the North West Water Authority, Water Research Centre and manufacturers for their help and for providing illustrations.

REFERENCES

1. CLOUGH, G. F. G. Making water fit for use, *Proc. 9th Public Health Engineering Conf.*, Pickford, J. (Ed.), Loughborough University of Technology, UK, 1976.

2. World Health Organisation. *International standards for drinking-water*, WHO, Geneva, 1971.

3. JENKINS, S. H., SANE, M. and WALLBANK, T. Physico-chemically aided biological treatment of sewage, *Chem. Ind.*, Oct. 1977, p. 821.

4. WRC. Analytical quality control in the British water industry, *Notes on Water Research* No. 17, Water Research Centre, Medmenham, UK, Aug. 1978.

5. MORGAN-JONES, M., FLAVIN, R. J. and HOARE, M. J. A review of past and present values of nitrate in groundwater sources in the Thames Water Authority catchment, *Pub. Health Engnr*, Apr. 1980, **8**(2), 49.

6. GOODALL, J. B. and GAUNTLETT, R. B. Removal of ammonia and nitrate in the treatment of potable water, *Proc. Conf. on Biological Fluidised Bed Treatment of Water and Wastewater*, Paper No. 3, Water Research Centre, Medmenham, UK, Apr. 1980.

7. GREGORY, R. and SHEIHAM, I. Biological denitrification of surface water—economics of a remedy for nitrate in drinking water, *Proc. Conf. on Biological Fluidised Bed Treatment of Water and Wastewater*, Paper No. 19, Water Research Centre, Medmenham, UK, Apr. 1980.

8. MILLER, D. G. Fluidised beds in water treatment—a short historical introduction, *Proc. Conf. on Biological Fluidised Bed Treatment of Water and Wastewater*, Paper No. 2, Water Research Centre, Medmenham, UK, Apr. 1980.

9. SCHALEKAMP, M. and BAKKER, S. P. Use and thermal regeneration of activated carbon in Switzerland, *Effluent Water Treatment J.*, Jan. 1978, p. 28.

10. OVERMAN, M. *Water*, Aldus Books, London, 1968, p. 142.

11. WRC. Deterioration of bacteriological quality of water during distribution, *Notes on Water Research* No. 6, Water Research Centre, Medmenham, UK, Oct. 1976.

12. HILSON, M. A. Water treatment for public supply, *Chem. Ind.*, Jan. 1975, p. 4.

13. MORROW, J. J. and MARTIN, J. B. Effective measurement of chlorine residual, *Effluent Water Treatment J.*, May 1977, p. 217.

14. LIVESEY, R. J. The ozonation of potable water supplies, *Water Services*, Nov. 1975, p. 460.

15. CLOUGH, G. F. G. Implications of the energy crisis on sewage treatment, *Wat. Pollut. Control*, 1975, **74**(3), 328.

16. NWC/DOE Working Party on Control Systems for the Water Industry. *First Interim Report*, Natl. Water Council, London, Jun. 1978, p. 11.

17. NWC/DOE Working Party on Control Systems for the Water Industry. *First Interim Report*, Nat. Water Council, London, Jun. 1978, p. 10.

18. WRC. Cost information for water supply and sewage disposal, *Technical Report* No. 61, Water Research Centre, Medmenham, UK, Nov. 1977.

19. WHITE, K. E. Hydrological studies possible with radionuclides of bomb test, primordial and natural origin to complement investigations using manufactured radiotracers, *Paper presented to the NW Branch, Inst. Wat. Pollut. Control*, Water Research Centre, Medmenham, Feb. 1979.

Chapter 8

ENVIRONMENTAL MONITORING BY BIOLOGICAL MEANS

E. G. Bellinger, B.Sc., Ph.D., M.I.Biol., F.I.W.E.S.

*Assistant Director, Pollution Research Unit,
University of Manchester, UK*

SUMMARY

The processes by which pollution is generated and the main types of pollutant are outlined. The movement of pollutants through the environment is also discussed together with the range of variations in concentration that might be expected at a given location. The problems to monitoring programmes arising from this are indicated and the advantages and disadvantages of using biological methods of environmental assessment are outlined. Specific examples of such biological methods are described including ones for the atmosphere (moss bag technique for heavy metals), aquatic systems (algal bioassays for nutrients and the 'Mussel Watch' programme for general contaminants) and terrestrial systems (small mammals and plant material for metal and other contaminants). The benefits of using biological monitoring, together with the ways in which it complements other methods, are summarised.

1. INTRODUCTION

During his early history man existed in relatively small populations which, although they utilised natural resources and created some waste products, probably had little impact on the environment as a whole. Their wastes and activities had only local effects.[1,2] Changes in agricultural practice and, in more recent decades, industrialisation have greatly increased man's

E. G. BELLINGER

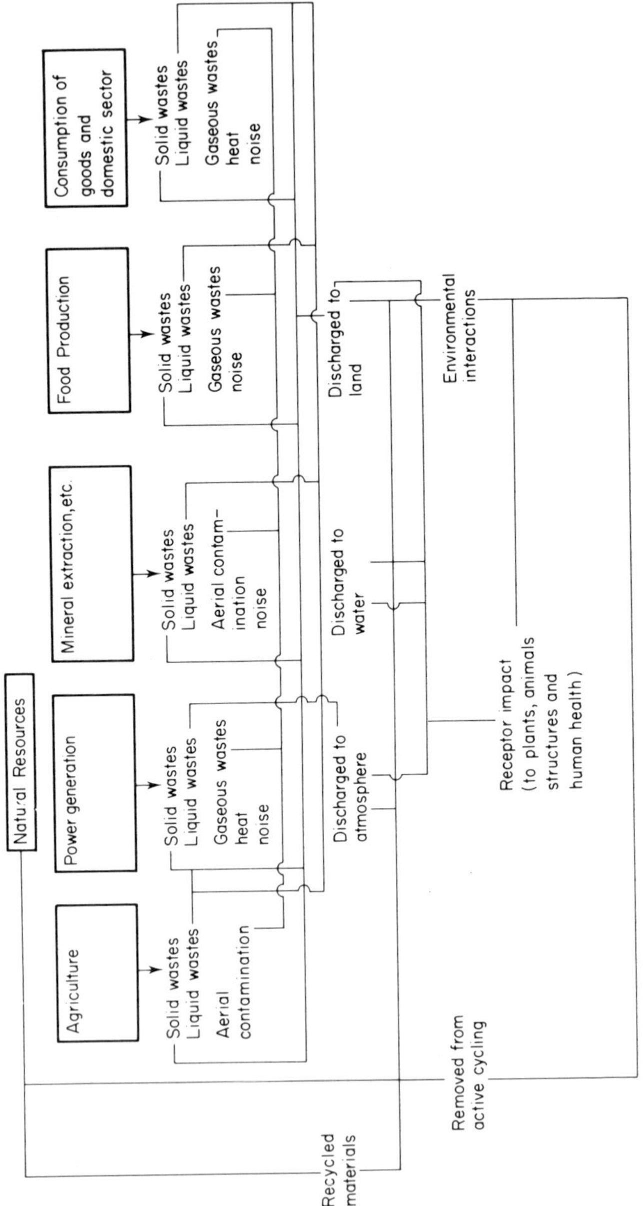

FIG. 1. Waste creation through man's activities.

environmental impact, both by using more of the Earth's resources and by creating more waste.

The growth of the industrial society with the parallel increase in urbanisation creates environmental problems which are different from those caused by agriculture and other activities. These problems arise from a range of man's activities such as power generation and manufacturing industries[3] (see Fig. 1) and produce wastes and pollutants which are discharged into the environment in large quantities. These substances may be very diverse ranging from heat energy to plastic bags. Indeed many of the chemicals concerned were previously unknown. Because of this their true biological impact was not known at the time of their creation and use; this sometimes gave rise to severe ecological perturbances. Even chemicals that are found in nature and are produced by natural phenomena, e.g. SO_2 from volcanoes, have now been produced by man's industrial activities in very large quantities which too have had adverse ecological effects. These products of man's activities will always be with us and are likely to increase in amounts unless society itself changes.

Figure 1 shows that the results of these activities may be discharged into various media, i.e. onto land, into the air or into water. Whilst it is possible to define pollutants according to other criteria, e.g. the nature of the pollutant (chemical composition or physical state), source of the pollutant (fuel combustion, agriculture, etc.) or by target and effect (affecting crops, affecting wild animals, etc.), it is convenient here to define pollutants according to the medium of discharge.

Table 1 outlines the main pollutants in the three categories land, air and water, with some examples of each. Some of the pollutants are peculiar to one industry or activity, others are produced from a wide range of activities. It should also be noted that the type of source can vary as well. Sulphur dioxide produced as a result of coal burning in a power station and emitted through a chimney can be regarded as coming from a point source. Other point sources include liquid effluent discharges from treatment works and noise from factories. Other pollutants arise over a wide area as the exact location of a discharge cannot be pin-pointed. Such sources are said to be diffuse and include pollutants like vehicle exhausts or run-off from agricultural land. Pollutants in the former category are usually regarded as being easier to quantify and easier to legislate against.

The source of a pollutant does not necessarily determine its ultimate fate, geographical or biological distribution. Some pollutants may undergo chemical reactions, interactions or breakdown which change their nature (e.g. some oxides of nitrogen). Others may be persistent and remain

TABLE 1

THE NATURE OF POLLUTANTS IN VARIOUS MEDIA

Physical state	Medium		
	Air	Water	Land
Gaseous or dissolved	CO_2, CO, NO_x, SO_2: from nature and fuel combustion. Aldehydes, fluorides, organics and acids: from industrial processes.	NO_3, PO_4, pesticides: from domestic, industrial and agricultural sources and (except the latter) nature. Detergents, oils, pharmaceuticals: from domestic and industrial sources. Metal salts, etc.: from industrial sources.	Wide range of liquid wastes: from industrial sources, but some from agriculture.
Particulate	Smoke, grit, dust, metallic particles: from fuel combustion, industrial processes and nature.	Organic and inorganic particles: from agriculture, industry, domestic and natural sources.	Polythene, metals, refuse, sludge, pesticides, etc.: from industry, domestic, agriculture and some particulates from natural sources.
Energy	Heat, noise, radiation: from industrial, domestic and natural processes.	Heat, radiation, noise: from industrial and natural sources.	Radiation and noise: from industrial and natural sources.

unchanged for many years (e.g. DDT). The geographical distribution of a pollutant, i.e. whether it will be local, national or global in its distribution, depends upon the medium into which it is dispersed, its diffusion coefficients in that medium, its solubility and its settlement rates. All of these factors must be taken into account when attempting to determine the potential toxicity of a substance.

As an example, DDT can inhibit photosynthesis in planktonic algae and if this were to happen on a large scale could pose a threat to marine ecosystems and global oxygen and carbon cycles. It has been found, however, that solubility of DDT in water is so low that the concentrations required for such inhibition are unlikely to be attained.[4] There is also a great deal of variation amongst pollutants as to whether or not they accumulate in biological systems. A tendency to accumulate in organisms is often associated with pollutants that are persistent but this is not necessarily so. Fat soluble materials and metal ions do, for example, tend to be accumulated.

Referring back to Fig. 1, we can see that pollutants are generated by different processes before discharge into the environment. Once in the environment the polluting substances often move through various media. They may eventually reach a final destination where their residence time can be measured in thousands or millions of years, e.g. deep ocean sediments, or they may be more or less continually recycling. The amount of movement depends on the environmental reactivity of the substance, and this in turn depends upon such things as solubility, chemical reactivity, biological absorption, etc., and the properties of the medium, e.g. current flow in rivers, turbulent mixing in the atmosphere, etc.

These movements within the environment are termed pathways. The most important of these are from source to target organism. An example of the various pathways of one element of environmental importance, carbon, is given in Fig. 2. Carbon is cycled naturally as well as being introduced as a pollutant so the pathways followed are numerous and complex. Figure 2 gives a simplified view of the situation.

Where organisms are concerned the pathway from source to target is in two main sections. The first concerns the passage of the substance through the environmental medium, i.e. air, water or land and the second is the passage through the target or receptor organism to its point of impact.

The accumulation of a pollutant within an organism is a function of its rate of uptake and rate of excretion. As both of these processes proceed simultaneously a plateau of concentration is usually attained in the tissue, the level of which is determined by the rates of the two processes.[5,6]

E. G. BELLINGER

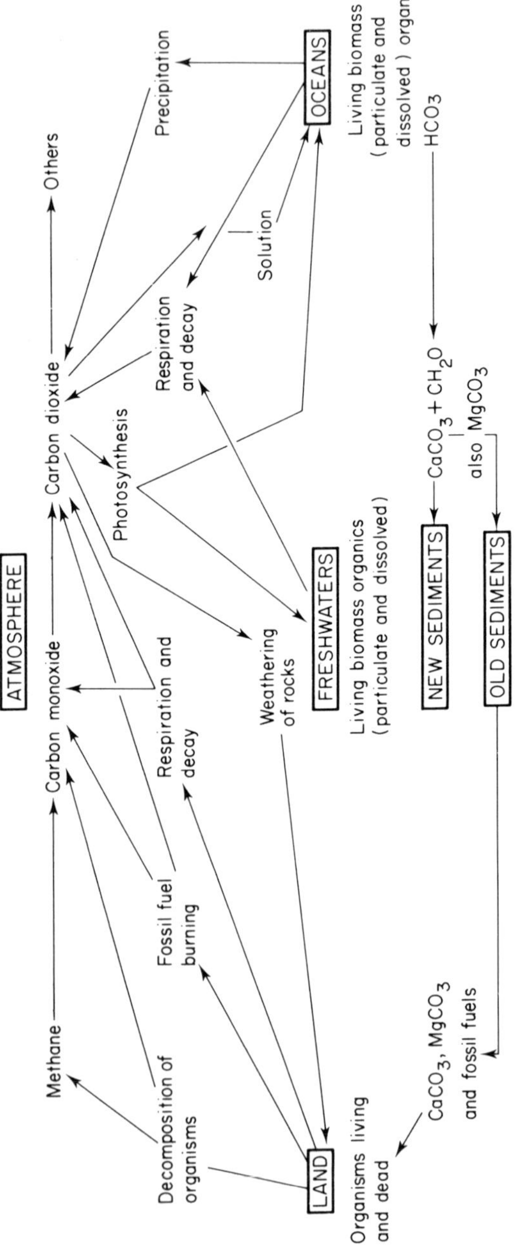

FIG. 2.   The carbon cycle.

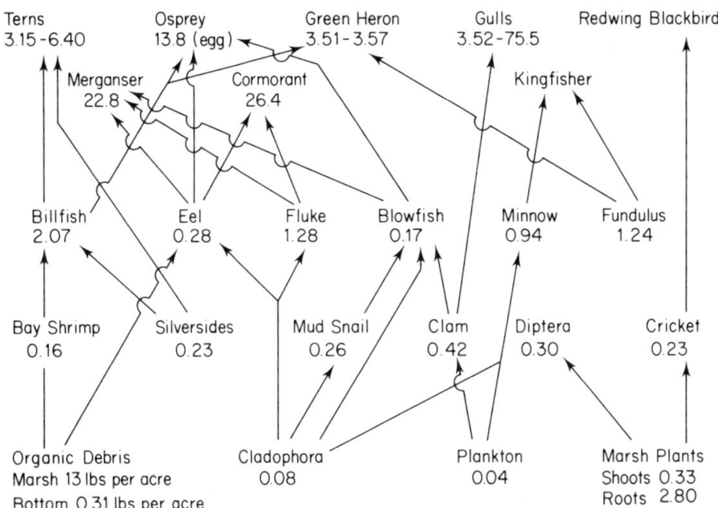

FIG. 3.   A food web in the Long Island Estuary. (Figures in ppm dry weight DDT.)[7]

Conditions in nature do tend to be more complex so that the relatively simple situation often does not exist.[4]

Pathways in the environment do not only exist from the various media to organism, they also exist from one species of organism to another because of their feeding relationships. Thus pollutants may be handed on from one organism to another through food chains. Because of the relatively inefficient energy conversion factors between one stage in a food chain and another accumulations of pollutants through food chains may arise (see Fig. 3). Thus although passage of chemicals along non-biological pathways often leads to dilution, accumulation through food chains acts in reverse of this.

2. BIOLOGICAL METHODS FOR ESTIMATING CONCENTRATIONS OF ENVIRONMENTAL CHEMICALS

Whilst it is true that major acute environmental polluting incidents do occur at the present time, e.g. large oil spillages, most discharges are of a chronic long term nature. Because of this, and because of the range of ways in which substances can behave in the environment (see Section 1.), the effects may be quite difficult to recognise and assess.

Apart from the damage done to structures by pollution most environmental monitoring is concerned, ultimately, with effects on living systems. Over the past century many systems of environmental monitoring have been developed based on chemical and physical measuring systems. Typical examples of these include smoke and SO_2 measurements in the atmosphere, temperatures and metal concentrations in waters and nutrient concentrations in soils. In all cases a technique is chosen to measure a particular parameter as accurately and precisely as possible within the context of the exercise. You thus end up with a number representing the level or concentration of that parameter. Are these numbers or concentrations exactly what one needs? To answer this question we must not only consider the target organism or receptor but also the behaviour and pathways of a chemical or substance in the environment.

Chemicals or energy forms are seldom discharged into the environment at a constant rate. Discharges from industry and power generation often, for example, vary in both concentration and volume from day to night and

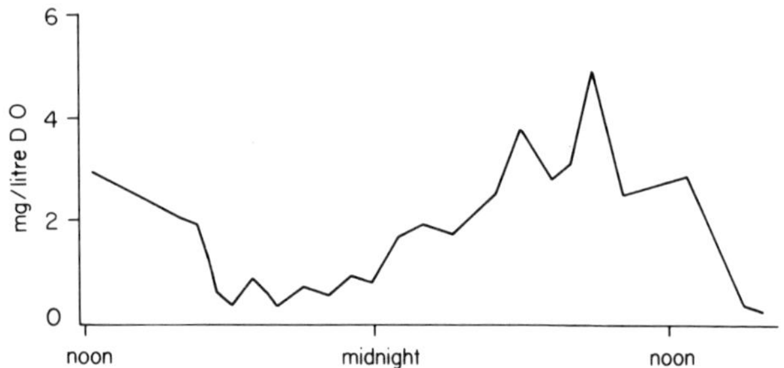

FIG. 4.   The daily variation in dissolved oxygen over a 24 hour period in the River Tame Orton.

from one time of year to another. Figures 4 and 5 show typical variations for two selected parameters. Thus a single sample collected from the R. Tame on the date represented in Fig. 4 would not give the true oxygen picture for that site. It would probably not give the maximum or the minimum concentrations or the time for which a concentration exists. Similar problems exist when daily or weekly averages are taken over a whole year as with SO_2 (Fig. 5). Although seasonal variations are taken into account, hourly or daily ones are not, neither is the maximum and minimum concentration and duration of exposure for those recorded.

Predictions of toxicity can be awkward if there is imprecise knowledge of the bio-availability of the substance. The presence of humic acids or other

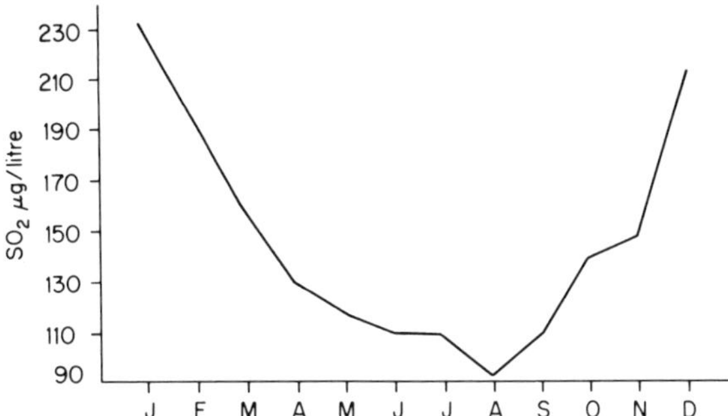

FIG. 5.   The daily variation of sulphur dioxide in the atmosphere of Manchester over the period of one year.

complexing agents can render some metals in water unavailable to organisms, leading to erroneous conclusions if only chemical determinations are being used.

All of these factors could potentially affect an organism's response to an environmental factor or contaminant. Because of these unknowns, as well as our imperfect knowledge of the nature and recycling of biologically important elements and their compounds, chemical and physical measurements on their own do not always give us all of the information we require.

As most environmental monitoring is ultimately for assessing the effects of factors on living organisms, why not then, where possible, use living organisms for the monitoring?

Organisms have long been used as indicators of prevailing conditions, e.g. Shantz[8] used plants as indicators of water and soil conditions, Merriam[9] used vertebrates as indicators of temperature zones and Kolkwitz and Marsson[10] used invertebrates as indicators of organic pollution in water. More recently bivalve molluscs have been used to monitor metal concentrations in the seas.[11,12,13] This approach has been steadily broadened over the years and its usefulness is in the fact that the response of an organism integrates a range of environmental factors.

Not all organisms are suitable as indicators. The organism chosen must be able to give a good indication of the relative levels of whatever environmental factor we are interested in. Some of the ideal characteristics of such an indicator were outlined by Butler et al.[14] as follows.

1.   The organism should accumulate the pollutant without being killed by the levels encountered.

2. The organism should be static within the area being studied.
3. If naturally occurring species are being used they should be relatively abundant in the study area.
4. It is better if the organisms are long lived enough to allow sampling over at least one year.
5. If tissue analyses are used the organism needs to be of a reasonable size.

The first point only applies to certain types of biological monitoring. Butler *et al.* were particularly referring to marine organisms and pollution.

There are examples where presence and absence of a species can be used (e.g. with lichens and SO_2) or the organism can act as an accumulator whether it is alive or dead (e.g. moss plants and metals).

A biological reaction to a chemical does not only depend upon the chemical's concentration but also upon the rest of the chemical environment, the physical environment, as well as species of organism, age, etc. An example of this is clearly seen in the effect of certain metals on fish. Lloyd[15] found that zinc was toxic to rainbow trout, under standard test conditions, at a concentration of 5 mg litre^{-1} applied for a period of 900 min. He also found, however, that the toxicity of zinc varied depending upon the concentrations of certain other chemicals in the water. Examples are given by Lloyd[15-17] and Herbert and Vandyke.[18] It can be seen that in some cases there is an enhanced toxic effect, i.e. synergism, whilst in others there is a reduced effect, i.e. neutralising or antagonism. In undertaking environmental monitoring the effects of combinations of chemicals must be taken into account.

Concentrations may fluctuate daily, monthly or yearly (see Figs. 4 and 5) and our sampling programme may not pick up these trends or variations. An indicator organism is, however, present all the time and thus allows us to get a time integrated picture of these variations. This would usually not be possible if we relied only on chemical and physical methods because of the cost of equipment and the large number of samples that would probably need to be taken. The response of the organism will take into account the size and duration of peak concentrations whenever they occur.

By careful selection of the organisms we can be sure that we are recording a response to only biologically active parameters. This can also include the phenomenon of accumulation through food chains in which biological magnification of certain chemicals can occur leading to problems of toxicity to certain species even though environmental concentrations might be low. Examples of this effect are described in references 19 and 20. Some chemicals are present in the environment at concentrations which appear to have no obvious effects. There may be, in some cases, what is classed as hidden damage to the biota where symptoms are difficult to detect because they are obscured by other environmental factors but reduced growth (and hence, in the case of food crops, reduced yield) may result, or behavioural changes may occur in animals, which reduce reproductive capacity. Such effects can only be picked up with direct long-term observations on organisms.

Basically, biological monitoring measures any ecological imbalance caused in the environment whereas chemical monitoring measures concentrations of chemicals. Biological systems can thus be of importance not only in environmental monitoring but also in regulation and control. Discharge concentrations, conditions and quantities must take into account biological effects before threshold limit values can be prescribed. The limits selected must take into account varying sensitivities of species, acute or chronic effects, possible synergisms, etc., and variations in pathways of pollutants from source to receptor.

3. BIOLOGICAL MONITORING OF THE ATMOSPHERE

Many atmospheric pollutants which have a biological impact are often present in low concentrations. Examples of these include metals and SO_2. Biological monitoring has proved useful in this field. In particular certain groups of plants, the mosses and lichens, have been widely used. Other organisms have also been studied, however, including organs of sheep for lead,[21] tree ring analysis,[22,23] and small mammals.[24,25] In the latter case voles were suggested as being promising indicator species by which to monitor the hazards to wild life of grazing on metal contaminated vegetation. Biological monitoring is also used in industry as a check on potential hazards to human health. An example of this is in lead battery factories where airborne lead effects on human health can be assessed by blood monitoring.[26,27]

Epiphytes and plants without true root systems are particularly suitable for monitoring air pollution because their growth form naturally exposes them to the atmosphere and, in the case of mosses and lichens, they gain their nutrients from the air or, at least, from aerial precipitation. Techniques of monitoring using epiphytes are generally inexpensive and may be applied over large areas.

Lichens have long been known to be sensitive to air pollution[28] and in recent years their response to SO_2 in the atmosphere has been used to observe the distribution of this parameter. Gilbert[29,30] combining observations on lichen growth and distribution and results from standard volumetric gauges was able to draw up a scale for the biological estimation of SO_2 concentrations. This scale in its original or modified form has been used in many surveys throughout the country and has provided much detailed information on SO_2 distribution in specific areas.[31–35]

Lichens have not only been used as SO_2 monitors. They have also been used to monitor fluoride in the atmosphere[36] and metals around industrial complexes.[35,37–39] To a certain extent, however, the use of lichens is confined to specialists as they are not always easy to identify. Whist this can also be a problem with moss plants it is less true than with lichens as the most common technique does not involve the identification of numerous species.

The technique of using the ability of moss plants to accumulate metals in the form of moss bags was first conceived by Goodman and Roberts.[40] They noticed that mosses can both intercept and retain metals with great efficiency. They attempted to standardise the collecting bags into a 10 cm × 10 cm flat square containing *Hypnum cupressiforme*.[40] The great benefits of this technique over traditional ones of the time were that the construction of the moss bags was simple, quick and inexpensive so that large detailed surveys could be carried out without the use of expensive pumps, filters and electric power. Useful results using this technique were obtained.[41]

Although the flat bag of Goodman and Roberts has advantages in calculating surface areas and deposition rates, it has disadvantages in that it might, over a period of a few weeks exposure, be orientated edge-on to the wind for a reasonable proportion of the time giving completely different results. The shape has been modified by some authors to a spherical one to overcome these problems.[42–44] This design is even more cheap and easy to construct and when hung in location is less obvious and thus less prone to vandalism, although in the nesting season birds do avail themselves of the moss!

Results of a typical survey around a point source emitter (in this case a lead–acid battery factory) are given below. The bags were placed at approximately 0·5 km intervals along NE, E, SE, SW and NW radii from the point source and left exposed for 5–6 weeks. This survey was a follow-up to the one by Ratcliffe in 1975.[44]

The results from such a survey can be expressed as isopleths of lead in moss and an example is given in Fig. 6. Whilst these results do not give

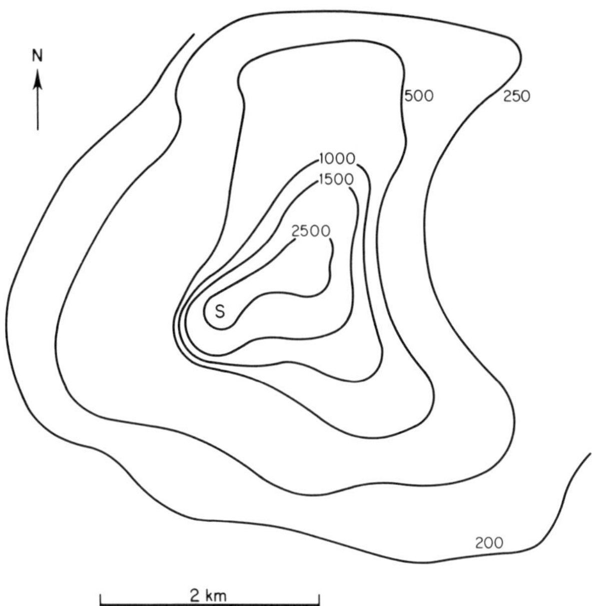

FIG. 6. Contour map of lead deposition in ppm around a point source emitter.
(Figures are ppm lead in moss bags.)

absolute concentrations they do clearly show the general distribution of atmospheric lead around the source. This effectively and cheaply allows an environmentalist to select far more detailed study zones which are of particular interest, e.g. high isopleths spanning residential areas. Because of the low cost many sampling sites can be monitored giving a comprehensive picture of an area.

Although this survey and many others have used moss bags to monitor heavy metal concentrations in the environment there are recent reports[45] that they may also be used to measure other airborne substances such as NaCl, NH_4^+, NO_x^-, SO_4^{2-}, NH_3 and radioactive fall-out. There is also increasing evidence that the sensitivity of moss bags means that in zones of high contamination such as would occur close to motorways the presence of airborne lead can be demonstrated within a period of only $\frac{1}{2}$ h.[45]

Whilst the use of moss bags, lichens and other forms of biological monitoring does offer several advantages it is often not possible to relate the results obtained to exact aerial concentrations so they tend, at best, to be semi-quantitative. It is best, therefore, to use these techniques to supplement standard methods of analysis such as deposition gauges, air filter samples and SO_2 measurement by chemical methods, and not replace them.

4. BIOLOGICAL MONITORING IN AQUATIC SYSTEMS

Water usage is very diverse, ranging from amenity through food production to drinking. Water quality criteria also vary reflecting different uses. With these different criteria have grown up sets of measurement techniques for parameters thought to be of importance for each user group. In recent years attempts have been made to adopt a less fragmented approach and to look at systems rather than just individual users.

In the past great emphasis has been placed on chemical and physical measurements with only the field of public hygiene introducing biological measurements. As the aim of many of the controlling authorities has been to conserve biological communities, this lack of biological measurements has been, perhaps, surprising. Continental countries have realised this deficiency and made attempts to redress the balance earlier than the UK. Kolkwitz and Marsson, as long ago as 1908[10] used invertebrate animals as indicators of organic pollution in German rivers. This and other works have provided a basis for more recent developments in the USA and in the UK. As in other media, biological monitoring in water does offer certain advantages over more traditional methods. The response of an organism integrates a range of environmental factors. A chemical test, however, will usually only measure one factor. It might tell us the concentration of a given chemical compound at a moment in time or even over a period of time, but we cannot always be sure that the compound we are measuring is the biologically significant one. Should we measure nitrogen in the form of nitrate, ammonium, nitrite or organic nitrogen and phosphorus in the form of orthophosphates or polyphosphates?

Concentrations may fluctuate daily, monthly or yearly and our sampling programme may not pick up these trends or variations. The biologist observing the aquatic biota is able to take all of these things into account. Thienemann[46] observed that 'a biologist can judge the composition of the water even if it (a factory discharge) is no longer there when he starts his investigation'.

Numerous systems of biological assessment of water quality have now been developed. A literature survey by Hellawell[47] indicated that various groups of organisms have been recommended as water quality indicators. Of these, 26 % of the authors chose to use algae, 27 % macro-invertebrates.

The use of these various groups of organisms has been reviewed by various authors. These include Whitton[48] for plants; Price[49] for fish and Hawkes[50] for invertebrates. One particular aspect of aquatic monitoring by biological means shows how these techniques can be used.

There is frequently a need, in aquatic situations, to obtain information as to the fertility of the water, either to assess the impact of existing industrial or other discharges, or to predict possible future impacts of proposed changes in discharges or use. An important tool in the hands of biologists for this purpose is the algal bioassay. In this, standard cultures of microscopic plants (algae) are grown in waters under investigation. Variations in algal growth rate and production reflect variations in water quality. This type of bioassay, which in one form has been fully described by the US Environmental Protection Agency,[51,52] is well suited for (a) evaluating the nutrient status of a water body; (b) enabling one to distinguish between total and biologically available nutrients and (c) to determine the potential effects of changing water quality on algal growth. The first of these points has been widely investigated using algal bioassays.[53-57]

The US Environmental Protection Agency bottle test, which is now accepted as a standard method, does suffer from several disadvantages. These have been outlined in Bellinger[58] and include accumulation of metabolites, depletion of nutrients and unrepresentative physical conditions. In an attempt to overcome these disadvantages a new cell based on the dialysis technique has been developed.

The technique using dialysis membrane has been used in fairly simple arrangements in the laboratory.[59,60] It has the advantages that (a) high cell densities can be obtained in small volumes; (b) local nutrient depletion does not take place because of replacement across the membrane and (c) by-products do not accumulate. The technique developed by the present author has the further advantage of being suitable for field or laboratory use. The essential difference to previous techniques which used a dialysis bag[57] is the use of a rigid dialysis cell (see Fig. 7). This has been developed from one previously described and developed by the author.[58] The procedure for use is as follows. The test sample was first prepared according to Lund.[61] The dialysis cell was then filled with both taps open so that no air was trapped inside. Each cell was then inoculated with an algal culture (*Selenastrum capricornum*) to give an approximate concentration of 10^3 cells ml^{-1}.[51] The initial cell concentration was also estimated by determining the chlorophyll-a concentration as a check.[62]

For field exposures the cells were suspended vertically in the

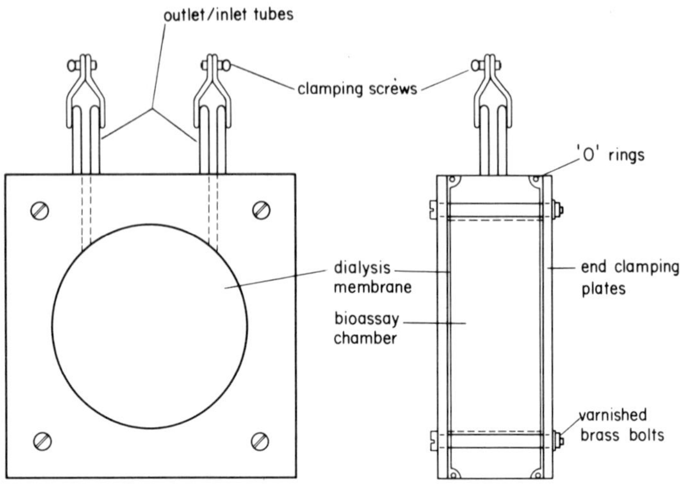

Fig. 7. Bioassay dialysis cell.

lake/reservoir for the appropriate period (usually 5–7 days). At the end of the exposure the entire contents of the cell were filtered, extracted in hot methanol, and the chlorophyll-a content measured. For laboratory exposures the cells were suspended in a 15 litre tank the contents of which were gently stirred. The period of exposure was either 4 or 7 days and the sample water in the tank was changed by means of a continuously pumped inflow and outflow. The flow rate through the tank was arranged so that the entire contents were replaced every three days. Up to six dialysis cells could be placed in each tank at a time. The lighting was arranged to give 4000 lux for a 16 h day. An 8 h dark period was used to give a better comparison with the field exposures. The temperature was $20\,°C \pm 1\,°C$. All exposures were carried out in duplicate for field and triplicate for laboratory tests and analysed statistically according to the USEPA.[51]

This bioassay (and the standard USEPA bottle test) can provide useful information in predicting changes which might occur in waters. One case investigated was the effect on biological productivity of mixing waters of different chemical composition from different catchments. A Regional Water Authority had proposed to pump either different river waters (either the R. Wharfe or R. Ouse) into a reservoir (Eccup), in order to increase their storage capacity. Both of these rivers are considerably richer, chemically, than the reservoir (Table 2) so a change in productivity might be expected.

This potential change can be assessed in two ways: (a) by growing the

TABLE 2

AVERAGE CHEMICAL COMPOSITION OF ECCUP RESERVOIR, THE RIVER WHARFE AT ATHINGTON AND THE RIVER OUSE AT NETHER POPPLETON

	$NH_3.N$ $(mg\,litre^{-1})$	$NO_3.N$ $(mg\,litre^{-1})$	$PO_4.P$ $(mg\,litre^{-1})$	Ca $(mg\,litre^{-1})$	Mg $(mg\,litre^{-1})$
Eccup Reservoir	0·039	0·730	0·020	18·0	3·25
R. Wharfe	0·090	1·020	0·480	49·0	6·50
R. Ouse	0·079	2·390	0·189	79·0	17·00

bioassay organisms in various combination of the waters, or (b) by taking the reservoir water and adding various concentrations of nutrients to find if one in particular is limiting, and thus, if increased, would enhance productivity. Such tests were carried out and the results are given in Figs. 8 and 9. Additions of phosphorus or nitrogen plus phosphorus produced significant increases in growth in reservoir waters. There was also a progressive increase in yield as more river water was mixed with the reservoir water. For control purposes, however, it can be seen that at 1 % mixture of the river and lake water there was no significant change. If the mixing proportions were kept well below 10 % river: 90 % reservoir, whilst there would be an increase in productivity this would still be lower than with 25 % river water. Also mixtures containing Wharfe water did not enhance productivity as much as those containing Ouse waters.

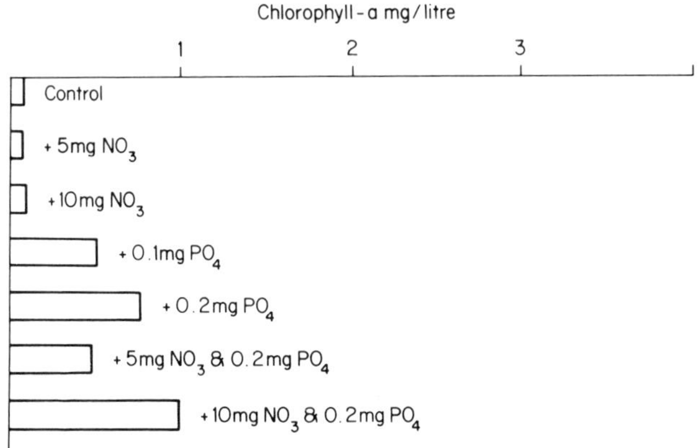

FIG. 8.   The effect of nitrogen and phosphorus additions on maximum standing crop measurements in Eccup Reservoir. (Figures for all additions are in mg litre^{-1}. Standing crop as measured by chlorophyll-a used as biomass estimate.)

 E. G. BELLINGER

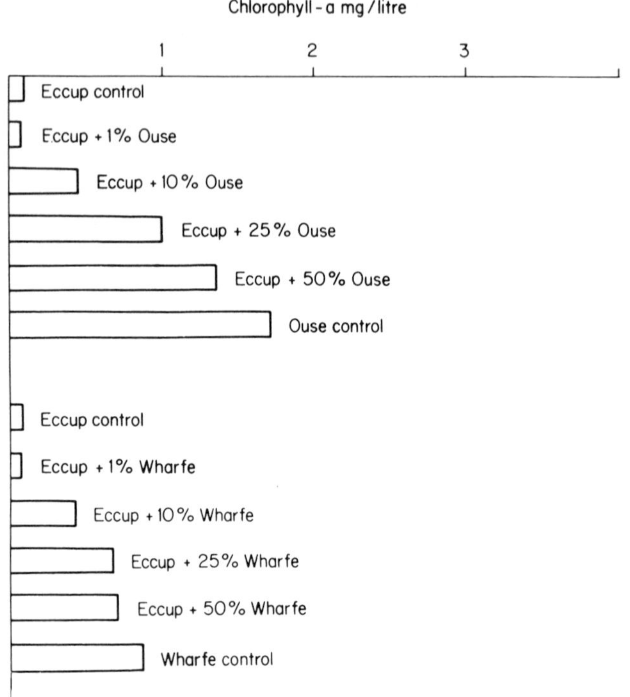

FIG. 9. The effect of additions of River Ouse and River Wharfe waters to the maximum crops in the Eccup Reservoir.

Thus it would be possible to formulate a programme of operation involving pumping from different rivers in different proportions. The bio-assay could also be used to continuously monitor the situation as water transfer took place. This type of approach could equally well apply to existing or even potential factory discharges into rivers as well as straight forward nutrient and toxic evaluations of any waters.

Metal and other contaminant concentrations within the tissues of organisms, especially in the marine environment, have long been recognised as reflecting those in the environment.[1-3] This can be equally true for organic and inorganic contaminants, e.g. pesticides and petroleum hydrocarbons.[4] It has thus been realised that carefully selected species could be used to give an indication of the degree of environmental contamination at a particular location.

In the inshore environment in particular, although this does also apply to other sections of the environment, organisms offer distinct advantages over other methods for environmental monitoring. Most environmental contaminants in sea water are present in concentrations of parts per million or parts per billion (10^{12}). This is especially true of areas where there is vigorous water movement due to tides or currents when effluents, etc., tend to be fairly well diluted but still potentially hazardous. Whilst techniques are being developed to measure these low levels they are seldom in routine use. They are also based on a single, large volume sample making collection of material a bulky exercise representing only a single moment in time. This type of sample collection, preparation and analysis would involve considerable expense if performed on a regular routine basis. Organisms, however, often have the ability to greatly concentrate substances over a period of time above the levels present in the environment. Examples of this are given in Table 3.

Thus, after a suitable period of exposure one might expect an organism to have a greatly elevated concentration of pollutant in its tissues, which is proportional to the concentrations in the environment. If one analyses the organism instead of the surrounding medium it lessens the demands on

TABLE 3

CONCENTRATIONS OF CAESIUM-137 IN SEVERAL WATER ORGANISMS (CONCENTRATION OF CAESIUM-137 IN SURROUNDING WATER = 1 UNIT)

Organism	Units of Caesium-137
Algae	
Rhizoclonium	900–4 000
Spirogyra	100–400
Higher plants	
Elodea	300–1 000
Lemora	400–600
Bullrush	50–400
Herbivores	
Snail	600
Tadpole (bullfrog)	2 600
Tadpole (toad)	6 000
Carnivores	
Pumpkinseed	1 000–11 000
Bluegill	6 500
Carp	1 000–3 000
Bullfrog	8 000–11 000

Taken from Pendleton (1962).[19]

analytical techniques and alleviates the problems of transporting large volumes of water or sediment. Carefully selected species of marine organisms could greatly aid the monitoring of environmental pollutants. Such a technique of monitoring has been introduced by Goldberg *et al.*[63] in the USA and has been extended to many other countries.

Specimens of mussels (*Mytilus*) and oysters (*Ostrea* or *Crassostrea*) are collected from a number of sites in coastal regions representing areas of suspected high and low contamination. These are then frozen and returned to the laboratory where their tissues are analysed for contaminants of

TABLE 4

CONTAMINANT CONCENTRATIONS IN MUSSELS (*Mytilus edulis*) COLLECTED FROM VARIOUS COASTAL SITES IN THE USA[63]

| | Contaminant (ppm dry weight) | | | | |
Sample location	*Cd*	*Cu*	*Pb*	*p,p'-DDE*	*PCB*
Sears Island, Maine	1·1	6·3	2·2	0·005 48	0·079 2
Portland, Maine	0·9	6·1	5·0	<0·007 88	0·094 6
Cape Cod	1·9	4·3	3·5	<0·010 5	0·215 0
Savannah River	3·7	192·0	0·2	0·006 61	0·033 1
St Augustine Fla.	1·8	25·0	0·1	<0·010 1	0·149 0

interest. Variations in contaminant concentration are taken to reflect variations in environmental concentrations for that chemical. Examples from the USA survey are given in Table 4.

These results, which represent only a small part of a typical survey, show changing patterns of contamination with location.

For accurate comparisons, the organisms collected from different sites should be the same age and have had the same period of exposure. This is not always possible as the ages of mussels are not easy to determine. An attempt should be made, however, to meet this point. As well as being potentially cheaper to operate than many other methods this technique also offers the potential, for certain contaminants, of building up a library of frozen specimens from certain locations for reference purposes. This would be difficult, if not impossible, to do with bulky water samples.

Similar surveys are taking place in other countries and the potential of species other than mussels investigated. This could potentially extend the geographical range of sites capable of investigation and possibly the number of contaminants capable of being assessed.

5. BIOLOGICAL MONITORING IN TERRESTRIAL SYSTEMS

Pollution on land can arise from many sources such as industrial discharges, municipal refuse, mining activities, disposal of sewage sludge, motor vehicles and also deposition from the atmosphere and water. We are thus concerned with a wide range of substances. Many of these are difficult to detect but others, such as heavy metals, can be monitored using biological means. As with aquatic systems monitoring on land has often centred around land usage, e.g. cereal or crop growth, amenity or wild life preservation.

Many terrestrial organisms are affected by air as well as land pollutants. For example, a tree will be affected by soil-based pollutants through its roots and air-based pollutants through its leaves. One must always, therefore, be careful in one's interpretation of the concentrations of pollutants present in an organism in these situations. Chlorosis (yellowing) of the leaves in plants is an example which could be due either to soil nutrient deficiency or SO_2 contamination of the atmosphere.

Plants and animals can be used to monitor pollution on land. Vascular, or higher, plants often require a specialist knowledge to recognise pathological changes due to pollution, however.[64] Perhaps a better way to use them is to take advantage of their capacity to absorb contaminants, as will be seen later. In recent years there has been an increasing number of surveys using small animals for monitoring[65] pollution, e.g. metals, especially around industrial sources and roads. Many species of small mammals are common in rural areas in many countries. These can often be easily caught by means of Longworth traps[66] and their tissues analysed. This technique is attractive in that one is using an animal not too different to man in its physiology or in its position in a food chain especially when compared with plants or invertebrates. This approach has been used by a number of authors with varying success at sites ranging from the sides of busy roads to fields and woodlands.[65–69] It has been generally found that useful additional information can be obtained by collecting vegetation from the sites for comparison. Examples of the type of results obtained are given in Table 5.

These results, especially from USA, show that small mammals do exhibit increased body burdens of contamination near to pollution and that this changes with source intensity and distance.[67] To be of any use in monitoring, the response of the indicator should be quite definite and, if possible, graded. Small mammals can show these types of response but various authors have found considerable variation between individuals at

TABLE 5

CONCENTRATION OF POLLUTANTS IN SMALL MAMMALS COLLECTED FROM VARIOUS LOCATIONS

Location	Ref.	Source	Lead	Contaminant (ppm) Mercury	Copper	DDE
Main road	66	*Microtus*[a]	3·31	—	—	—
		Apodemus[a]	1·37	—	—	—
		Vegetation[a]	226·00	—	—	—
Field	69	*Apodemus*[a]				
		whole	—	0·85	13·3	1·02
		liver	—	1·35	5·0	—
Roadside						
light traffic	67	*Peromyscus*[b]	0·70	—	—	—
heavy traffic			4·60			
light traffic		Soil	approx. 900			
heavy traffic		Soil	approx. 1 100			

[a] Wet weight.
[b] Dry weight.

the same site, which can make interpretation of small differences in pollution loadings difficult.[25]

For straightforward monitoring purposes on land evidence suggests that herbage may exhibit a greater and better response to pollution. This is particularly true for metals. This is shown well with collections of plants at varying distances from roads in order to assess the extent of lead pollution. One has to be careful to collect only the same species of plant at each site as there can be variation from one species to another. Examples of such a survey are given in Table 6.

TABLE 6

CONCENTRATIONS OF LEAD IN PLANT LEAVES AND SOIL

Site	Dock	Vegetation type Rhubarb	Elder	Soil
Near battery factory	1 474·0	1 807·0	1 219·0	4 570·0
Busy road				
at road verge	83·0	—	72·0	625·0
10·0 m distance	60·4	25·0	53·0	340·0
20·0 m distance	42·0	19·0	36·0	120·0

Concentrations in ppm dry weight.

These results show that both vegetation and soils respond to environmental contamination in a graded way. Pollutant concentrations are higher in the soil samples in the case shown although this is not always so. The concentrations in the soil do not necessarily represent what is biologically available as the lead, in this case, may be bound chemically in an insoluble form.

It has been found that for many pollutants broad leafed plants give a better indication than narrow leafed ones. Also, if one is interested only in the pollutant that is absorbed into the plant it is a good idea to wash the outside to remove surface contamination as this represents aerial pollution rather than that truly in the soil.

6. CONCLUSIONS

1. Biological monitoring can, thus, be of considerable use in environmental control inside and outside the work place.

2. Properly selected methods can be used to gain information on the amounts of biologically active substances in the environment rather than just the total chemical concentrations.

3. Because most biological monitoring techniques are relatively inexpensive they can be used for longer periods of time if required giving an integrated picture of polluting events with time.

4. Biological monitoring techniques also enable the environmentalist to 'see' many types of pollution even when he is not present at the sampling point.

5. Their cheapness of operation enables biological monitoring techniques to be used over a wide geographical area, monitoring at many dozens of sites simultaneously. They are also often free from requirements such as power supplies in the field.

6. Although biological monitoring techniques will not usually tell you the absolute environmental concentration of a given chemical they can give relative concentrations and allow 'hot spots' to be identified.

7. The areas of high contamination identified by biological methods can then be investigated in detail using more traditional chemico/physico/mechanical techniques. Less of this more expensive, and often power dependent, equipment is then needed than for a purely general survey.

8.   Certain biological techniques can be used for predictive work as well as for present time monitoring. This enables the environmentalist to more accurately assess the potential impact of future changes of industry, etc., in the environment.

9.   Schemes of biological assessment where organisms are used *in situ* enable the impact of a number of pollutants to be monitored at once, e.g. dissolved oxygen, temperature and metals in water. Thus synergistic, neutralising and additive effects can be taken into account.

REFERENCES

1. SVENSSON, B. H. and SODERLUND, R. (Eds.). Nitrogen, phosphorus and sulphur: global cycle, *SCOPE 7, Ecological Bull.*, No. 22. Stockholm, Swedish Natural Science Research Council, 1976.

2. LE CREN, E. D. and HOLDGATE, M. W. The exploitation of natural animal populations, *Brit. Ecological Soc. Symp. No. 2*, Blackwell, Oxford, 1962.

3. LEE, N. and LUKER, A. J. An introduction to the economics of pollution, *Economics*, 1971, **9**, 19–32.

4. HOLDGATE, M. W. *A Perspective of Environmental Pollution*, Cambridge University Press, Cambridge, UK, 1979.

5. MORIARTY, F. (Ed.). *Organochlorine Insecticides: Persistent Organic Pollutants*, Academic Press, New York and London, 1975.

6. MORIARTY, F. *Pollutants and Animals. A Factual Perspective*, George Allen & Unwin, London, 1975.

7. WOODWELL, G. M. Toxic substances in ecological cycles, *Scientific American*, 1967, **216**, 24–31.

8. SHANTZ, H. L. Natural vegetation as an indicator of the capabilities of land for crop production in the Great Plains area, *US Dept Agr. Bureau of Plant Industry*, Bull. 201, 1911.

9. MERRIAM, C. HART. Laws of temperate control of the geographic distribution of terrestrial animals and plants, *Natl. Geog. Mag.*, 1894, **6**, 229–38.

10. KOLKWITZ, R. and MARSSON, M. Okologie der pflanzlichen saprobien, *Ber. Dt. Botan. Ges.*, 1908, **261**, 505–19.

11. FOLSON, T. R., YOUNG, D. R., JOHNSON, J. N. and PILLAI, K. C. Manganese-54 and zinc-65 in coastal organisms of California, *Nature*, 1963, **200**, 327–9.

12. BRYAN, G. W., PRESTON, A. and TEMPLETON, W. L. Accumulation of radio nuclides by aquatic organisms of economic importance in the United Kingdom, in *Disposal of Radioactive Wastes into Seas, Oceans and Surface Waters*, International Atomic Energy Agency, Vienna, 1966, 623–37.

13. YOUNG, D. L. and FOLSOM, T. R. Loss of Zn^{65} from the California sea-mussel *Mytilus californianus*, *Biol. Bull. Mer. Biol. Lab. Woods Hole*, 1967, **133**, 438–47.

14. BUTLER, P. A., ANDREN, L., BLONDE, G. J., JERRNELOV, A. and REISCH, D. J. Monitoring organisms in food and agricultural organisations, *Tech. Conf. on*

Marine Pollution and its Effects on Living Resources and Fishing, Rome 1970, Supplement I, Methods of detection. measurement and monitoring of pollutants in the marine environment, Ruivo, M. (Ed.), Fishing News (Books) Ltd, London, 1971, 101–12.

15. LLOYD, R. The toxicity of zinc sulphate to rainbow trout, *Ann. Appl. Biol.*, 1960, **48**, 84–94.

16. LLOYD, R. The toxicity of mixture of zinc and copper sulphates to rainbow trout (*Salmo gairdnerii*, Richardson), *Ann. Appl. Biol.*, 1961, **49**, 535–8.

17. LLOYD, R. The effect of dissolved oxygen concentrations on the toxicity of several poisons to rainbow trout (*Salmo gairdnerii*, Richardson), *J. Exp. Biol.*, 1961, **38**, 447–55.

18. HERBERT, D. W. M. and VANDYKE, J. M. The toxicity to fish of mixtures of poisons, *Ann. Appl. Biol.*, 1964, **53**, 415–21.

19. PENDLETON, R. C. Accumulation of caesium-137 through aquatic food chains, in *Biological problems in water pollution*, 3rd Seminar in the Environmental Health Series, Water Supply and Pollution Control, US Department of Health, Education and Welfare, 1962, 355–63.

20. HUNT, E. G. and BISCHOFF, A. I. Inimical effects of periodic DDD applications to Clear Lake, *California Fish Game*, 1960, **46**, 91–106.

21. WARD, N. I., BROOKS, R. R. and ROBERTS, E. Lead levels in sheep organs resulting from pollution from automotive exhausts, *Environ. Pollut.*, 1978, **17**, 7–12.

22. WARD, N. I., BROOKS, R. R. and REEVES, R. D. Effect of lead from motor vehicle exhausts on trees along a major thoroughfare in Palmerston North, New Zealand, *Environ. Pollut.*, 1974, **6**, 149–58.

23. LEPP, N. W. The potential of tree-ring analysis for monitoring heavy metal pollution patterns, *Environ. Pollut.*, 1975, **9**, 49–61.

24. JEFFERIES, D. J. and FRENCH, M. C. Lead concentrations in small mammals trapped on roadside verges and field sites, *Environ. Pollut.*, 1972, **3**, 147–56.

25. BEARDSLEY, A., VAGG, M. J., BECKETT, P. H. T. and SANSON, B. F. Use of the field vole (*M. agrestis*) for monitoring potentially harmful elements in the environment, *Environ. Pollut.*, 1978, **16**, 65–71.

26. ELWOOD, W. J., CLAYTON, B. E., COX, R. A., DELVES, H. T., KING, E., MALCOLM, D., RATCLIFFE, J. M. and TAYLOR, J. F. Lead in human blood and in the environment near a battery factory, *Brit. J. Preventive Social Medicine*, 1977, **31**, 154–63.

27. Department of the Environment. *Lead in the environment and its significance to man*, HMSO, London, 1974.

28. JAMES, P. W. in *Air Pollution and Lichens*, Ferry, B. W., Baddeley, M. S. and Hawksworth, D. L. (Eds.), Athlone Press, London, 1973.

29. GILBERT, O. L. Bryophytes as indicators of air pollution in the Tyne Valley, *New Phytol.*, 1968, **67**, 15–30.

30. GILBERT, O. L. A biological scale for the estimation of sulphur dioxide pollution, *New Phytol.*, 1970, **69**, 629–34.

31. HAWKSWORTH, D. L. and ROSE, F. *Lichens as Pollution Monitors*, Inst. of Biology, Studies in Biology, No. 66, Edward Arnold, London, 1976.

32. FERRY, B. W., BADDELEY, M. S. and HAWKSWORTH, D. L. *Air Pollution and Lichens*, Athlone Press, London, 1973.

33. HAWKSWORTH, D. L. and ROSE, F. Qualitative scale for estimating sulphur dioxide air pollution in England and Wales using epiphytic lichens, *Nature* (London), 1970, **227**, 145–8.
34. PYATT, B. F. Lichens as indicators of air pollution in a steel producing town in South Wales, *Environ. Pollut.*, 1970, **1**, 45–56.
35. PILEGAARD, K. Airborne metals and SO_2 monitored by epiphytic lichens in an industrial area, *Environ. Pollut.*, 1978, **17**, 81–92.
36. GILBERT, O. L. in *Air Pollution and Lichens*, Ferry, B. W., Baddeley, M. S. and Hawksworth, D. L. (Eds.), Athlone Press, London, 1973.
37. BURKITT, A., LESTER, P. and NICKLESS, G. Distribution of heavy metals in the vicinity of an industrial complex, *Nature* (London), 1972, **238**, 327–8.
38. SEAWARD, M. R. D. Lichen ecology of the Scunthorpe Heathlands. 1. Mineral accumulation, *Lichenologist*, 1973, **5**, 423–33.
39. LAAKSOVITRA, K., OLKKOMEN, H. and ALAKVYALA, P. Observations on the lead content of lichen and bark adjacent to a highway in Southern Finland, *Environ. Pollut.*, 1976, **11**, 247–55.
40. GOODMAN, G. R. and ROBERTS, T. M. Plants and soils as indicators of metals in the air, *Nature* (London), 1971, **231**, 287–92.
41. ROBERTS, T. M. Plants as monitors of airborne metal pollution, *J. Environ. Plan. Pollut. Control*, 1972, **1**, 43–54.
42. LITTLE, P. *Airborne Zn, Pb and Cd pollution and its effects on soils and vegetation*, Ph.D. Thesis, University of Bristol, 1974.
43. LITTLE, P. and MARTIN, M. H. Biological monitoring of heavy metal pollution, *Environ. Pollut.*, 1974, **6**, 1–20.
44. RATCLIFFE, J. M. An evaluation of the use of biological indicators in an atmospheric lead survey, *Atmos. Environ.*, 1975, **9**, 623–9.
45. LITTLE, P. Personal communication, 1980.
46. THIENEMANN, A. Einfurung in die biologischen Probleme der Limnologie, *Das Leben in Susswasser*, Verlag Ferd. Hirt. Breslau, 1926.
47. HELLAWELL, J. M. *Biological surveillance of rivers*, Water Research Centre publication, Stevenage Laboratory, UK, 1978.
48. WHITTON, B. A. Algae and higher plants as indicators of river pollution, in *Biological Indicators of Water Quality*, James, A. and Evison, L. (Eds.), J. Wiley and Sons, London and New York, 1979.
49. PRICE, D. R. H. Fish as indicators of river water quality, in *Biological Indicators of Water Quality*, James, A. and Evison, L. (Eds.), J. Wiley & Sons, London and New York, 1979.
50. HAWKES, H. A. Invertebrates as indicators of water quality, in *Biological Indicators of Water Quality*, James, A. and Evison, L. (Eds.), J. Wiley & Sons, London and New York, 1979.
51. United States Environmental Protection Agency. Algal assay procedure; bottle test, *Natl. Eutroph. Res. Prog.*, Corvallis, Oregon, USA, 1971.
52. MILLER, W. E., GREEN, J. C. and SHIROYAMA, T. The *Selenastrum capricornum* (Prinz) algal assay bottle test. Experimental design, application and data interpretation protocol, Corvallis Environmental Research Laboratory, USEPA, Corvallis, Oregon, USA, 1978.
53. FITZGERALD, G. P. Bioassay analysis of nutrient availability, in *Nutrients in Natural Waters*, Allen, E. H. and Kramer, J. R. (Eds.), J. Wiley & Sons, London and New York, 1972, 147–69.

54. TOERIEN, D. F. and STEYN, D. J. Application of algal bioassays in eutrophication analysis, *South African J. Sci.*, 1973, **69**, 79–82.
55. MALONEY, T. E., MILLER, W. E. and SHIROYAMA, T. Algal responses to nutrient additions in natural waters. I. Laboratory assays in nutrients and eutrophication, *Special Symposia I. Limnology and Oceanography*, 1972, 134–56.
56. LUND, J. W. G., JAWORSKI, G. H. M. and BUTTERWICK, C. Algal bioassay of water from Blelham Tarn, English Lake District, and the growth of planktonic diatoms, *Arch. Hydrobiol. Suppl. 49, Algological Studies*, 1975, **14**, 49–69.
57. Nordforsk. Algal assays in water pollution research, *Proc. Nordic Symp., Oslo*, Oct. 1972, Nordforsk, 1973.
58. BELLINGER, E. G. The response of algal populations to changes in lake water quality, in *Biological Indicators of Water Quality*, James, A. and Evison, L. (Eds.), J. Wiley & Sons, London and New York, 1979.
59. JENSEN, A., RYSTAD, B. and SKOGLUND, L. The use of dialysis culture in phytoplankton studies, *J. Exp. Mar. Biol. Ecol.*, 1972, **8**, 241–8.
60. JENSEN, A. and RYSTAD, B. Semi-continuous monitoring of the capacity of sea water for supporting growth of phytoplankton, *J. Exp. Mar. Biol. Ecol.*, 1973, **11**, 275–85.
61. LUND, J. W. G. Biological tests on the fertility of an English reservoir water (Stocks Reservoir, Bowland Forest), *J. Inst. Wat. Eng.*, 1959, **13**, 527–49.
62. MARKER, A. F. H. The use of acetone and methanol in the estimation of chlorophyll in the presence of pheophytin, *Freshwater Biol.*, 1972, **2**, 361–85.
63. GOLDBERG, E. D., BOWEN, V. T., FARRINGTON, J. W., HARVEY, G., MARTIN, J. H., PARKER, P. L., RISEBROUGH, R. W., ROBERTSON, W., SCHNEIDER, E. and GAMBLE, E. The mussel watch, *Environ. Conserv.*, 1978, **5**, 101–25.
64. MELLANBY, K. Biological method of environmental monitoring, in *Measuring and Monitoring the Environment*, Lenihan, J. and Fletcher, W. W. (Eds.), Blackie, Glasgow, 1978.
65. WILLIAMSON, P. and EVANS, P. R. Lead levels in roadside invertebrates and small mammals, *Bull. Environ. Contam. Toxicol.*, 1972, **8**, 280–8.
66. JEFFERIES, D. J. and FRENCH, M. C. Lead concentrations in small mammals trapped on roadside verges and field sites, *Environ. Pollut.*, 1972, **3**, 147–56.
67. WELCH, W. R. and DICK, D. L. Lead concentrations in tissues of roadside mice, *Environ. Pollut.*, 1975, **8**, 15–21.
68. MIERAU, G. W. and FAVARA, B. E. Lead poisoning in roadside populations of Deer Mice, *Environ. Pollut.*, 1975, **8**, 55–64.
69. JEFFERIES, D. J. and FRENCH, M. C. Mercury, cadmium, zinc, copper and organochlorine insecticide levels in small mammals trapped in a wheat field, *Environ. Pollut.*, 1976, **10**, 175–82.

Chapter 9

MONITORING FOR ENVIRONMENTAL PROTECTION IN THE BRITISH STEEL CORPORATION— TWO CASE STUDIES

J. J. COLLS, B.Sc., A.R.C.S., Ph.D.

Pollution Control Engineer, Scunthorpe Division,
British Steel Corporation, UK

SUMMARY

Following a review of the basic processes involved in the production of steel and their associated emissions to the atmosphere, two divisions of BSC are examined in detail. Emission and ambient measurement methods are compared and examples given of the data produced by automated and manual systems.

It is shown that although both the systems have disadvantages, they do provide the information necessary for environmental management.

1. INTRODUCTION

Two of the major iron and steel manufacturing divisions of the British Steel Corporation are located on Teesside and at Scunthorpe. The two divisions not only have a broadly similar product range and overall steel making capacity, they also produce a similar variety of emissions to the atmosphere from a wide range of plant of different ages. It is, therefore, of interest to compare the methods used by these divisions to control and monitor such emissions and to measure their effect on local air quality. This contrast will be sharpened in the case of Teesside by concentrating on the Redcar Works, a self-contained iron making development which was constructed in one go, in comparison to the more gradual evolution at Scunthorpe. Following an initial review of the iron and steel manufacturing processes involved, a more detailed summary of Redcar Works and its pollution control systems is given. The philosophy of emission and ambient monitoring leads to an outline of the automated methods installed at Redcar; examples are given of the problems found and the machinery developed to overcome them at one particular plant. A similar course is followed through the Scunthorpe Plants and their emissions, monitoring systems and data handling activities are discussed. It is shown how two rather different approaches both provide effective control and measurement of air pollution and increase our understanding of the complicated interactions between processes, emissions and the quality of the environment.

2. IRON AND STEEL PROCESSES

Before discussing air pollution aspects of the industry in more detail, it is appropriate to review the main processes involved and to highlight the points at which atmospheric emissions are of concern. The basic process route is shown in Fig. 1. Iron ore is imported from a variety of countries including Canada, Sweden and Brazil. Foreign ore makes up 100% of the burden at Redcar, while in Scunthorpe 40% of the ore is mined locally. On arrival at the ore terminal, the foreign ore is dumped in piles. If the ore is of very fine grade, entrainment from the pile may be a problem in strong winds, especially if these occur after a long dry period. In order to arrive at an ore mixture having the right constituents, ores from many sources are blended by sequential layering at a blending yard. Again, wind entrainment may be a problem if the last layer stacked out is a very fine ore.

The main pre-processing to which iron ore is subject takes place at the sinter plant. This is designed to agglomerate iron ore, iron bearing wastes and fluxes, using coke as a solid fuel, prior to loading into the blast furnace.

A degree of beneficiation is also achieved, by drying the ore and converting carbonates to carbon dioxide. The burden is fed onto a horizontal travelling grate, 2–4 m wide and 1–400 m^2 in area. It immediately passes under a gas fired ignition hood where the coke is ignited and, during the remainder of its travel down the grate, air is drawn downward through the sinter layer to sustain combustion. By the time it falls off the end into a crusher, the burden is fused into a homogeneous layer having the right physical and chemical properties for the blast furnace. There are two main sources of particulate emissions—the waste gases from the strand and the plant dedusting system. The former involves a large flow (typically 1×10^6 Nm^3 h^{-1}) at a particulate

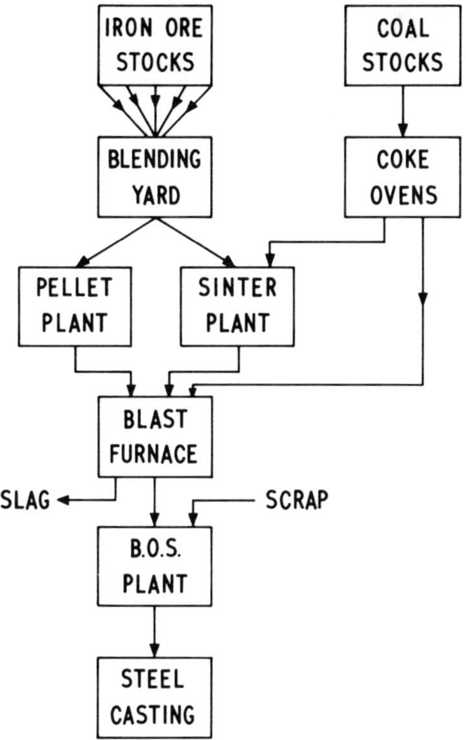

FIG. 1. The basic process route for the manufacture of steel from iron ore.

concentration of $2-3\,g\,Nm^{-3}$. The latter, which is derived from manifold dust extraction from the sinter discharge end and conveyor transfer points within the plant, involves a smaller flow of around $100\,000\,Nm^3\,h^{-1}$ containing a dust concentration of $10-20\,g\,Nm^{-3}$. The materials sintered on the grate contain a variable proportion of sulphur and about 90 % of this is released into the waste gas as sulphur dioxide. The total amount released may be calculated directly from the relative sulphur contents before and after sintering.

An alternative treatment for iron ore fines is to mix them with a binding agent such as bentonite, form the paste into balls and kiln dry the resulting pellets. There is just one such pellet plant in the UK, at Redcar, and the air pollution aspects are discussed further in Section 3.

Coke is used as a fuel both in the sinter plant and in the blast furnace. The majority of this coke is produced by BSC at its own coke ovens, where coal is held at high temperature and in the absence of air for 12–24 h, during which time the volatile oils and tars are driven off to leave essentially pure carbon. The main air pollution problems arise from charging coal into the waiting oven and pushing coke from the oven into a rail car. There are also considerable opportunities for emissions from the many doors and lids (some 500 on a large battery) although these can be reduced by intensive maintenance.

Sinter and coke (about 3:1) are processed in the blast furnace, where the coke both burns to provide high temperature and supplies carbon monoxide to reduce the iron oxide to molten iron. The blast furnace is a closed system and there are limited atmospheric emissions which mainly affect the working environment near the furnace.

The bulk manufacture of steel at Teesside and Scunthorpe involves the injection of oxygen into a molten mixture of about 200 tonnes of iron and 50 tonnes of steel scrap. The 5 % carbon in the iron burns out as carbon monoxide, and various unwanted impurities are retained in a separate slag. During the oxygen lancing, which lasts 15–20 minutes, about 1·5 % of the steel is lost as a very dense fume. Although the vast majority of this is extracted and cleaned, the escape of only a small proportion into the plant may lead to the subsequent release of fume through roof vents.

3. POLLUTION CONTROL AT REDCAR WORKS

Within the Teesside Division, on the north-east coast at Redcar, a large new iron ore terminal and iron works is nearing completion. The ore terminal, comprising berthing and unloading facilities for bulk carriers of up to 150 000 tonnes capacity, and extensive coal and iron ore stockyards and handling facilities, was commissioned in 1973. The sinter plant started in February 1978, the pellet plant, blast furnace and coke ovens in 1979. Firstly we will summarise the production capacity and air pollution control and monitoring equipment on a plant by plant basis. The data are given according to specification.[1]

3.1. Coke Ovens
There are two batteries, each of which contains 66 ovens and produces 14 500 tonnes of coke per week. The pollution control equipment includes:

1. Pipe line charging. This involves crushing and preheating the wet coal before steam injection into the ovens. The waste gas from the

preheater, which is contaminated by entrained coal dust, is cleaned by wet scrubbers handling $34\,000\,Nm^3\,h^{-1}$ and reducing the emission to $115\,mg\,Nm^{-3}$. The pipe line charging system, while installed primarily for process benefits such as reduced coking time, eliminates the black smoke emissions normally associated with charging ovens from an overhead car.

2. Oven pushing emissions are collected by Hartung Kuhn (Gneisnau-type) cars. The cars are self-contained, rail mounted units which use steam assisted venturi scrubbers to extract from around the coke as it is pushed out of the oven and to clean at a rate of $150\,000\,Nm^3\,h^{-1}$.

3. Sulphur in the coke oven gas is removed by the Stretford process before the gas is used both to heat the ovens and as a fuel elsewhere in the works. $640\,kg$ of sulphur (equivalent to $1280\,kg$ of sulphur dioxide) are removed per hour per battery, leaving the gas with a final sulphur content of $0\cdot015\,g\,Nm^{-3}$.

4. Ammonia from the by-products plant is destroyed in a purpose-built incinerator at a rate of $2\cdot9\,t\,h^{-1}\,battery^{-1}$. Oxides of nitrogen are a product of combustion and are measured continuously by a Thermoelectron 10A chemiluminescent monitor. The anticipated NO_x concentration is $50\,ppm$, and levels above $100\,ppm$ indicate mal-operation of the plant.

3.2. Sinter Plant

This plant has a production capacity of $76\,000$ tonnes sinter per week from a single strand of $336\,m^2$. The two main areas requiring air pollution control are the waste gases from the strand and dedusting extraction from the plant.

1. The main strand waste gases are exhausted via two electrostatic precipitators and a single $105\,m$ stack. The anticipated inlet gas dust burden of $2\cdot3\,g\,Nm^{-3}$ is cleaned to below $115\,mg\,Nm^{-3}$ by three of the four precipitator fields, some spare capacity being provided to allow for maintenance, outage or an increase in inlet dust concentrations. Each precipitator handles $163\,Nm^3\,s^{-1}$ at $160\,°C$, with an effective migration velocity of $4\,cm\,s^{-1}$. Particulate emissions are measured continuously by an Erwin Sick RM41 transmissometer on the stack. Sulphur dioxide, produced from combustion of sulphur in the iron ore and coke, is present at about $300\,ppm$ in the main strand gases, and is measured continuously by Hartmann and Braun non-dispersive infra-red spectrometers.

2. A great deal of dust is created in the plant both from the discharge and crushing of the sinter itself and from material conveyor transfers elsewhere. A manifold extraction and ductwork system draws all these dust laden gases out of the plant and through a single electrostatic precipitator having three fields in series, cleaning $173\,\mathrm{Nm^3\,s^{-1}}$ from $20\,\mathrm{g\,Nm^{-3}}$ down to $115\,\mathrm{mg\,Nm^{-3}}$. The particulate loading is again measured continuously by an Erwin Sick transmissometer. There is no SO_2 emission from this stack.

3.3. Pellet Plant

This is a very complex plant involving seven separate sequential operations from grinding of ore through the forming, firing and cooling of the pellets. The capacity of the plant is 9090 tonnes of pellets per day, to be used approximately 50:50 with sinter in the blast furnace. Dust and grit are produced in the rotary drier, ball mills, prewetting area, grate area and at the cooler discharge. These emissions are cleaned by one cyclone, four bag houses, five wet scrubbers and three precipitators. Particulate emissions are monitored by Erwin Sick transmissometers and SO_2 by Hartmann and Braun spectrometers.

3.4. Blast Furnace

The single blast furnace has a hearth diameter of 14 m and will produce 10 000 tonnes iron per day. The principal pollution control systems are as follows.

1. Furnace waste gas is cleaned by a Bischoff high energy venturi scrubber, which leaves a residual $9\,\mathrm{mg\,Nm^{-3}}$ particulate concentration in the gas. The gas is cleaned to these very high standards for use as a low grade fuel in the works.
2. There are two major storage bin systems for raw materials handling —one for coke and the other for ferrous materials. Each system has an independent dust extraction and cleaning unit employing bag houses. A total of 1500 terylene filament bags clean $93\,\mathrm{Nm^3\,s^{-1}}$ down to $100\,\mathrm{mg\,Nm^{-3}}$.
3. The blast furnace has two interconnected cast houses, each serving two tap holes. Two bag houses clean the fume arising from tap holes and runners, a total of 2976 polyester bags handling $276\,\mathrm{Nm^3\,s^{-1}}$ and reducing the outlet concentration to $100\,\mathrm{mg\,Nm^{-3}}$.

4. MONITORING AT REDCAR

4.1. Why Monitor?

Redcar is a scheduled works within the scope of the Alkali Act;[2] best practicable means must be used to control pollution, and certain presumptive limits on emissions have been set and must be met. Further, BSC is committed to positive and socially responsible pollution control policies, and to achieve higher standards than required by current legislation where this is economically feasible. This does not of itself imply any requirement for continuous monitoring of emissions, or for any monitoring of ambient air quality, since short-term spot measurements of particulates or gases will suffice.

The combination of these two motivations, however, has resulted in the investment of large sums of capital in a variety of pollution control equipment. This equipment has become a major item in any plant's maintenance requirements and running costs, and failure of any complete pollution control system could lead to the temporary closure of the plant. Since production from all units down the chain is interdependent, such closure would have repercussions on other plants at Redcar and on Teesside. It is thus clearly in the Corporation's business interest to monitor the performance of its pollution control equipment as conscientiously as it monitors furnace temperatures, gas flow or other important process variables. This is the internal justification for emission monitoring as an aid to plant management.

At the same time, it is clearly neither desirable nor feasible to establish a major new industrial site such as Redcar without extensive discussions between the Corporation and the local community on a wide range of topics such as employment resources or transport requirements. Redcar Works was conceived at a time of heightened environmental awareness, as a result of which there have been continuing discussions with the Local Authority to minimise the works' impact on environmental quality. In addition, the Authority will be able to request certain emission data from the Corporation under the Control of Pollution Act (1974).[3] Thus there are added inducements to BSC's own internal need for continuous measurement of critical atmospheric emissions.

Continuous emission monitoring answers the question of whether the pollution control equipment is operating within its specification. The corollary, of whether the specification gives adequate protection to the local environment, will be answered by a continuous ambient air measurement programme.

This was started four years before commissioning of the main plants at Redcar, and comparison of these measurements with ones taken after commissioning will indicate any long-term trends in air quality.

4.2. Emission Monitoring

The principal atmospheric pollutants emitted from the Redcar Works—SO_2, particulates and smoke—will be monitored continuously.

Five non-dispersive infra-red (NDIR) absorption monitors measure SO_2 on the sinter and pellet plants. NDIR was chosen for its simplicity, established technology and reputed reliability, although at the prevailing concentrations of about 300 ppm it is at the limit of its sensitivity. This means that a very long absorption gas cell has to be fitted and it is difficult to provide adequate protection against carbon monoxide cross-sensitivity. SO_2 concentrations emitted from these plants are low (3–400 ppm); stack heights are specified by the maximum design output of SO_2 in t day^{-1}.

There are five optical transmissometers on the sinter and pellet plants to measure particulate emissions. The instruments in use are the Erwin Sick RM4 and RM41, the first of which was evaluated by BSC research in 1974/5 and has since been adopted elsewhere in the Corporation. It has three switchable ranges of optical density, an hourly zero and span check and a recommended time between maintenance of three months. From the Erwin Sick outputs and the appropriate gravimetric calibration relationships the weekly average loadings and percentage time over the presumptive limits will be compiled.

Smoke density meters are used to monitor smoke emissions from the power station (three-flue stack), package boilers (four-flue stack) and coke ovens (two stacks). The general limit on emissions will be Ringelmann No. 1, apart from short periods permitted for boilers under the Dark Smoke Regulations (1958).[4]

Signals from all these continuous monitors are brought back to the appropriate plant control rooms where they are indicated or recorded. The signals will ultimately be processed by the Works Energy Distribution System computer network to produce hourly, shift, daily and weekly average values, time spent over limits and a VDU update of relevant statistical indices.

4.3. Ambient Air Monitoring

Three field stations were established in 1974 (Fig. 2) to obtain continuous data on ambient SO_2 and particulates for a reasonable period before commissioning of the Redcar Plants. SO_2 is measured by flame

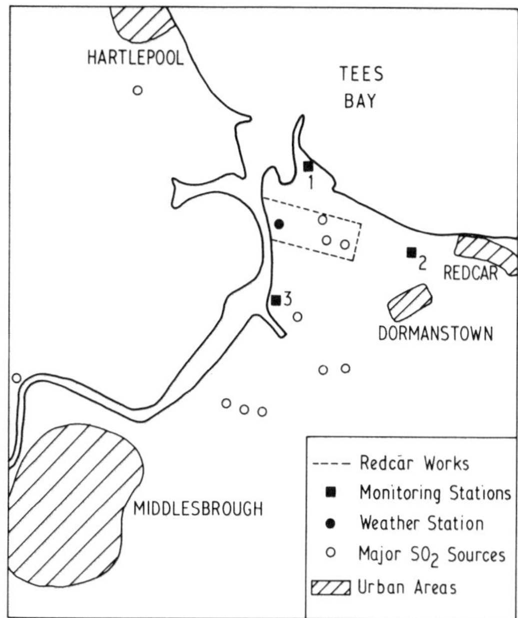

FIG. 2.   The location of BSC air pollution monitors round Redcar Works and their relationship to the Tees estuary.

photometry, suspended particulates by β-attenuation. Both techniques have proved reasonably reliable over a four year period. The outputs at each field station are logged every five minutes on to paper tape. In addition, meteorological parameters measured at a comprehensive automatic weather station are recorded every 15 minutes.

These parameters include atmospheric extinction coefficient (and thus, visibility) and temperature difference up a 50 m tower as well as more conventional wind and humidity information. After processing, a week-by-week record of pollution variation and meteorological conditions is available for detailed examination and statistical analysis. Coarse dust is measured by a network of 15 directional dust gauges, and information on atmospheric dispersion is provided by an acoustic sounder.

In Fig. 3, from reference 5, examples are given of the variation of three parameters during the week 19–25 February 1979. It can be seen that there is a degree of correspondence between the variation of SO_2 and particulates as the wind direction changes. After light and variable winds on 19 February, the wind direction settled down just west of south during 20

J. J. COLLS

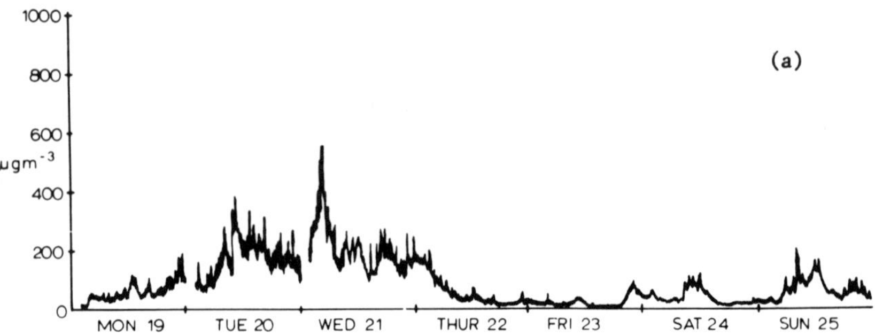

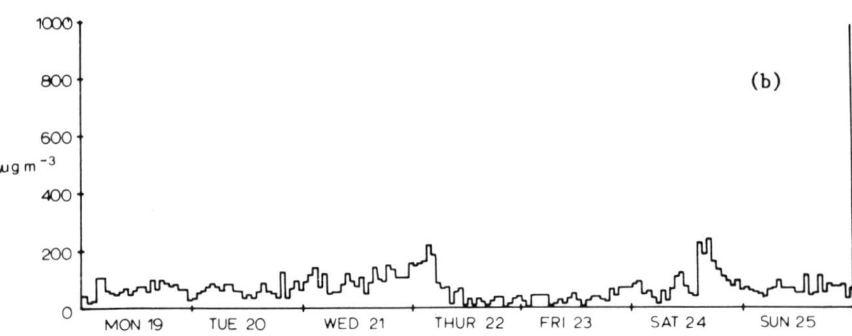

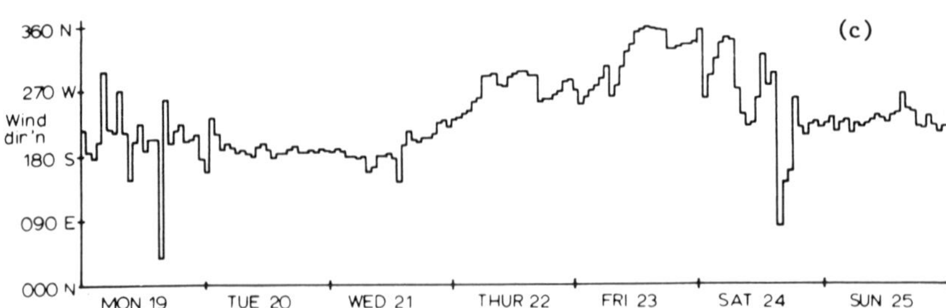

FIG. 3.   Temporal variations in (a) SO_2, (b) particulates and (c) wind direction during the period 19–25 February 1979.

February. With the wind from this direction, the field station concerned is downwind of the Teesside industrial conurbation, and consequently the SO_2 and particulate concentrations increase. As the wind veers through west to north on the Friday, bringing relatively clean air from East Durham and the North Sea over the station, SO_2 and particulate levels both fall, before increasing again at the end of the week as the wind backs to the south west. This clearly defined and repeatable qualitative behaviour will be of advantage in the future analysis of ambient pollutant measurements.

It means, for example, that any substantial increase in concentrations from a sector which contains the Redcar Works, but which was pollution-free before the works start-up, may be clearly assigned to emissions from new plants. As part of the original design study for the Redcar Works, calculations were made, both by BSC and an outside consultant, of the increase in ground level SO_2 concentrations and dustfall to be expected in the vicinity. Such calculations predict very small increases in the prevailing average pollution levels. Figures 4–6 show the types of analyses which will be used to evaluate the long term impact of the Redcar Works on air quality. Figures 4(a) and 4(b) are the cumulative probability distributions for SO_2 and suspended particulate averaged over the three field stations. With respect to SO_2, the average concentration for the period concerned (January 1975–June 1977) was $35\ \mu g\,m^{-3}$, with 50% of the daily means less than $37\ \mu g\,m^{-3}$ and 98% less than $195\ \mu g\,m^{-3}$. These compare with the World Health Organisation long term goals of $60\ \mu g\,m^{-3}$ (annual) and $200\ \mu g\,m^{-3}$ (98%). In the case of particulates, the WHO recommends that 98% of the daily mean concentrations should be below $120\ \mu g\,m^{-3}$ for the period analysed. Thus Redcar air pollution levels have been quite low for an industrial area by world standards.

Figures 5(a) and 5(b) show SO_2 and particulate pollution roses which support the behaviour discussed for Fig. 3. In both cases the background concentrations from seaward are low, with increasing levels from the Teesside sector. Figures 6(a) and 6(b) show the variation with windspeed of hourly-mean SO_2 and particulate concentrations. The gaseous component falls steadily as the wind speed, and thus, dilution, increases. Although similar behaviour is seen for particulates at moderate windspeeds, erratic high concentrations are found at high windspeeds as more dust is produced from ground level, stock piles, ore shipment or vehicle movement.

As we have seen, two predominant factors that affect the influence of emissions on the environment are wind direction and speed. A third factor, the atmospheric stability, is investigated at Redcar by an acoustic sounder. This instrument detects acoustic back-scatter from fluctuations in air

J. J. COLLS

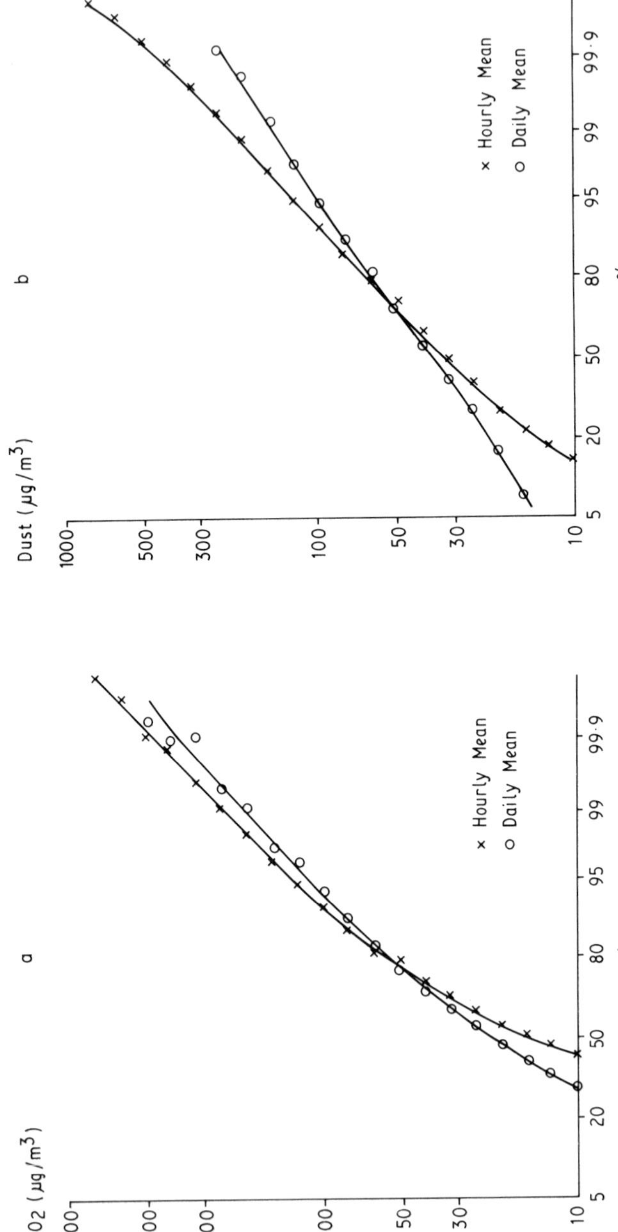

FIG. 4. Cumulative probability of the (a) SO$_2$ or (b) particulate concentrations, averaged over three monitoring stations, being less than a given value.

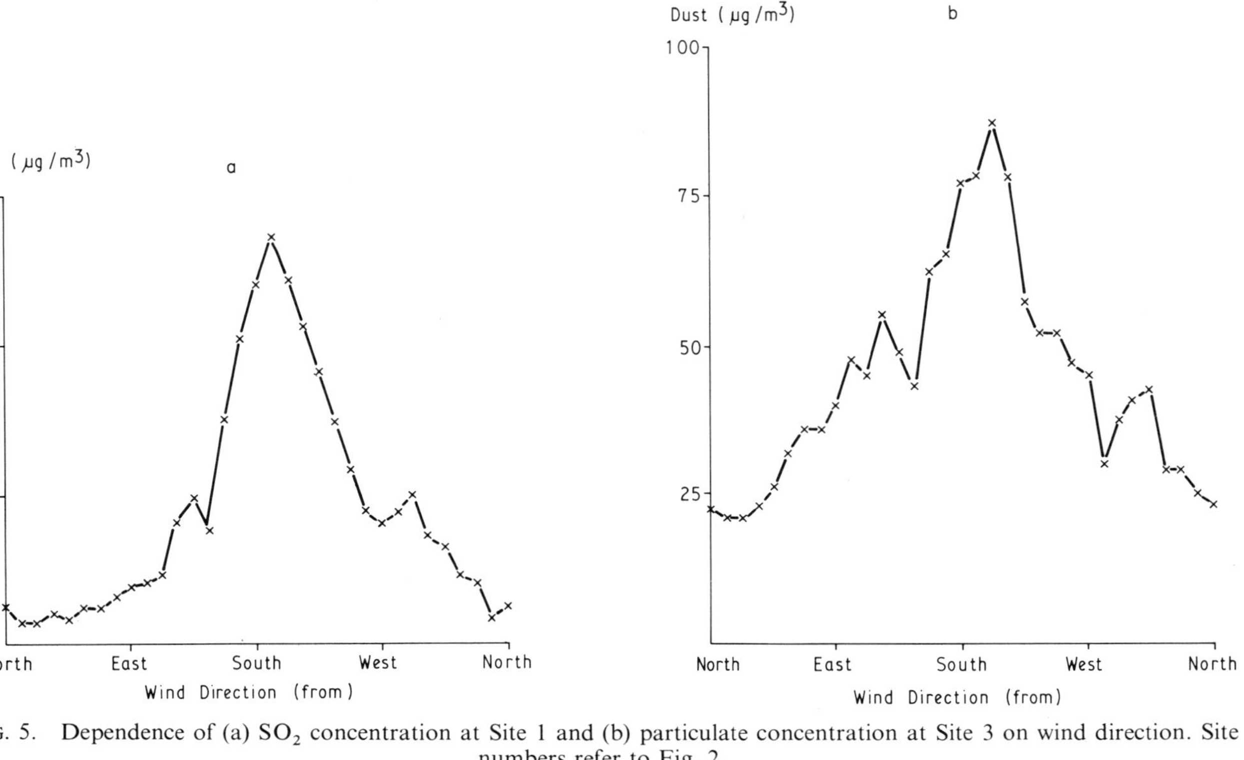

FIG. 5. Dependence of (a) SO_2 concentration at Site 1 and (b) particulate concentration at Site 3 on wind direction. Site numbers refer to Fig. 2.

J. J. COLLS

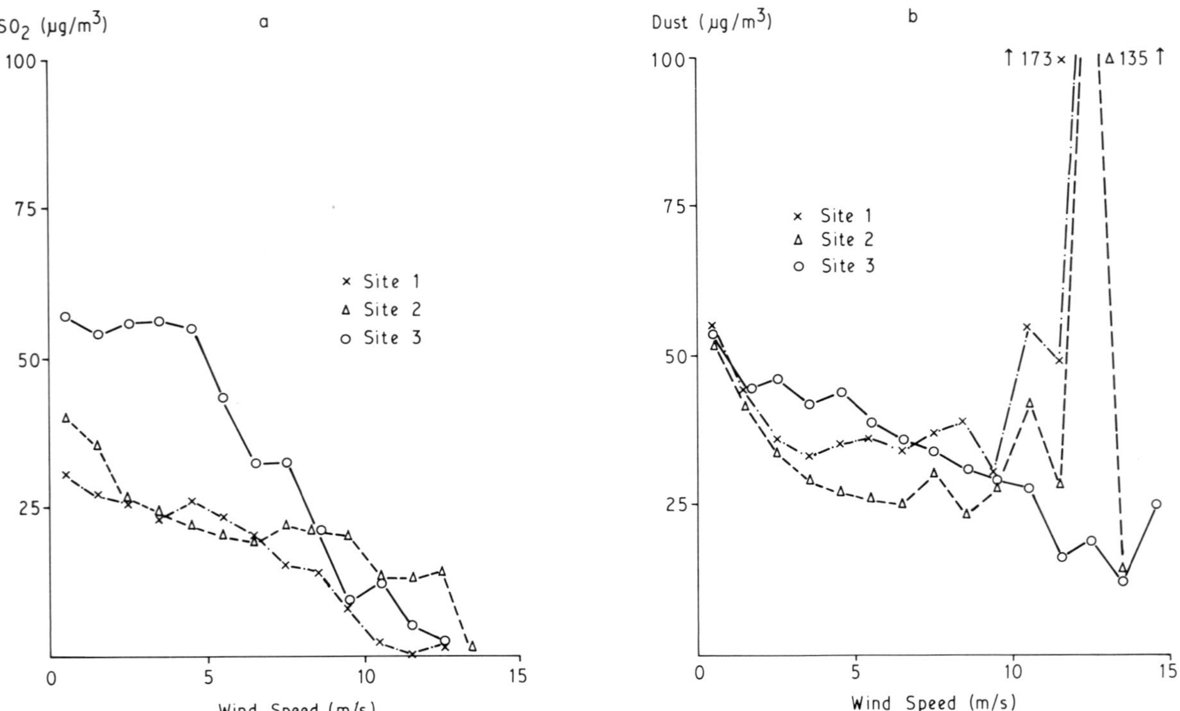

FIG. 6. Dependence of (a) SO₂ concentration and (b) particulate concentration on wind speed. Site numbers refer to Fig. 2.

refractive index which are associated with temperature variations. When these are plotted out on a facsimile recorder, a real-time picture of atmospheric stability is built up, giving a clear indication of inversion layering, neutral profile or convective thermals. Not only has this been a real asset for our understanding of the day-to-day pollution variations, but it provides another tool for long term statistical analysis.

One of the Local Authority planning consent conditions for the Redcar Development was concerned with the possible impact of process noise emissions on the nearby towns of Redcar and Dormanstown. The condition limits the average noise level along a defined line between the works and the communities to 65 dB(A). Noise levels are being measured at a field station to confirm compliance with this condition.

The main equipment is a CEL environmental noise analyser. This summarises long-term noise measurements in the form of a small number of statistical parameters, such as L_{eq}, L_{10} and L_{90}, these being the noise levels exceeded for 50, 10 and 90 % of the time, respectively. These parameters are calculated on an hourly basis, and on a cumulative basis reset at midnight, 0700 and 1900 hours. The values recorded to date indicate L_{90} (background) of 40–45 dB(A), and L_{eq} of 50–55 dB(A), well below the compliance condition. This information will shortly be enhanced by a control amplifier, which will activate chart and tape recorders when a preset threshold noise level is exceeded. This will show the true nature of high noise levels, and improve interpretation of the statistical parameters.

4.4. Sinter Plant Particulate Emissions

The application of particulate monitoring to one of the Redcar unit operations will now be discussed in more detail.

The sinter plant was the first of the major plants to be commissioned, in February 1978. Following a period of building-up to the specified production, a first calibration of the two Erwin Sick transmissometers on the main and dedust stacks was made. It should be understood that an optical dust monitor will give an output proportional to mass loading only if the particle properties (size distribution, chemical composition, shape) remain constant. Thus, direct calibration by comparison of the output with simultaneous gravimetric samples is an essential preliminary. Ideally this calibration should extend over the dynamic range of the instrument, although this is often difficult in practice without setting up false conditions such as a temporary reduction in the efficiency of a precipitator. It was found from these calibrations that the presumptive limit of 115 mg Nm^{-3} corresponded to less than 30 % obscuration on the dedust stack but to more than 80% on the main stack. Analysis of size distribution by cascade impactor has confirmed that this difference is caused by a large proportion of fine particles, which have greater obscuration per unit mass, in the main stack gases.

Thus a working system for continuous particulate monitoring, with little manual involvement other than infrequent instrument maintenance, has been established. But what of process changes? A single plant such as that at Redcar, uses a range of ores from different parts of the world, which are carefully blended to arrive at a sinter mix having appropriate properties,

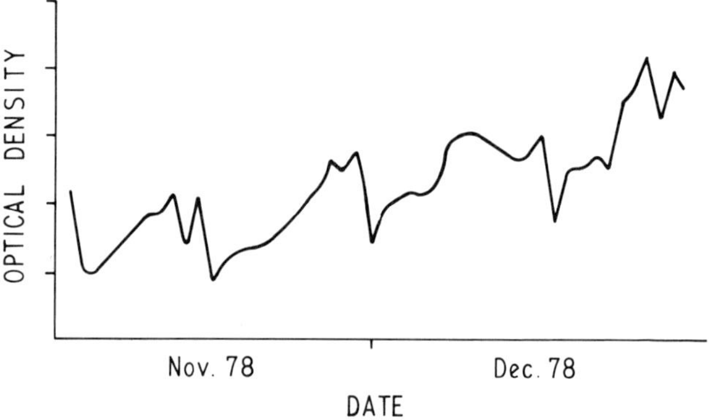

FIG. 7.   The variation over a two month period of the daily average output from the Redcar sinter plant main stack transmissometer.

for example basicity. Basicity is the ratio of the predominant basic minerals $(CaO + MgO)$ to the predominant acid minerals $(SiO_2 + Al_2O_3)$ and is one of the key parameters determining the chemical reactions that occur at every stage of iron production. Changes in this specification may change the properties of the emitted particulates and invalidate the Erwin Sick calibration. The results of such process changes are shown in Fig. 7. This is a plot of the main stack Erwin Sick output during a period of seven weeks. The plant was restarted after a two week shutdown, and low obscuration values were recorded initially. However, a strong rising trend increased the one-week average by a factor of more than two during the following seven weeks. During this period there were changes in plant variables such as output rate, bed depth, basicity and the proportion of an ore high in chloride. The latter volatilise off the strand and condense out as a fine fume which scatters light efficiently. Thus, it cannot be said that the increased output from the Erwin Sick is due entirely to increased mass loading without a recalibration at the new plant conditions. In practice, such severe short-term effects will be infrequent since the plant will be dedicated to producing a constant quality of output. Nevertheless, it does demonstrate that continuous monitors require continuous consideration if their output data are to be of full value to the works. Gravimetric measurements are taken routinely on a quarterly basis and comparison of these mass loadings with the Erwin Sick values should indicate any substantial drift away from the calibration condition. When these periodic samples are taken, they should be accompanied, if possible, by a size distribution, chemical analysis and comparison with plant conditions. Although this is all necessary to build up a picture of cause and effect, it clearly results in a conflict—having installed continuous monitors to provide information without a large manpower requirement, one is reluctant to spend a lot of effort continuously to find out whether the information is valid.

4.5. Sinter Plant Liaison

The great danger with continuous monitoring and computerised data handling is that instrument signals will be processed into a neat and easily digestible format for management appraisal without, in fact, being correct. The previous example of the effect of changes in burden practice has shown this already. On Teesside there are three groups within BSC that have air pollution roles. All routine measurements and calibrations are carried out by a section attached to the works; engineering specification, tender selection and purchasing are done by divisional department; the research organisation is involved, to a varying degree, depending on requirements. All of these groups have been involved with the establishment of the Redcar monitoring system at some stage. A working party has been set up at which representatives from each group meet regularly with plant management to examine the data from monitors, to establish criteria for assessing results and to organise the dissemination of these results to external bodies such as the Local Authority and the Alkali Inspectorate. This is a pragmatic arrangement, at which a wide range of topics is discussed.

For example, the problem arose at the start of defining the working period of the sinter plant over which results from the monitors should be averaged. Signals are fed continuously to the data handling system but there is a variety of possible sinter plant conditions which will result in a change in emissions. More specifically, the sinter grate may be stopped with or without the fans being stopped, with or without the ignition hood being lit.

It was decided that the 'fan on' condition would be the criterion for 'real' results, so that the week-long average result is divided by the proportion of the week that the main extraction fans are operating. Another question to be resolved concerned the interaction of measurement uncertainties in the calibration procedure with interpretation of the results. For instance, the stack emission limit of $115\,\mathrm{mg\,Nm^{-3}}$ is associated, on the best fit correlation between mass loading and obscuration, with one particular output value from the Erwin Sick transmissometer. However, in practice there is a range of uncertainty based on the scatter in the calibration data. At Redcar it has been decided to take, as the criterion for interpretation, the value for which it is 95 % certain that a given obscuration represents a given mass loading. Although this procedure may not seem as direct as the use of a gravimetric mass loading, it is the only way in which an analogue instrument such as a transmissometer can be incorporated into an emission limit based on particulate burden.

5. POLLUTION CONTROL AT SCUNTHORPE WORKS

BSC Scunthorpe Works was formed in 1967 on the amalgamation of three private works belonging to Lysaght, Richard, Thomas & Baldwin and the United Steel Company. The layout of the works and their relationship to Scunthorpe town is shown in Fig. 8. The historical development of the Works has resulted in a less coherent geographical structure than Redcar, although this is overcome to some degree by rail, conveyor belt and pipeline links to facilitate the transfer of raw materials and fuels.

The total steel output from the works is 3–4 Mt annum^{-1}, of which about 25 % is produced at Normanby Park.

The steelmaking and associated plant at Scunthorpe includes three sinter plants (April 1980).

1. *Seraphim 'E' Plant* (1962) has two strands, with an area of $250\,\mathrm{m^2}$ and a capacity of $35\,000\,\mathrm{t\,week^{-1}}$. The main strand gases are cleaned by two new three-zone electrostatic precipitators, having a flow rate of $17\,000\,\mathrm{Nm^3\,min^{-1}}$. The precipitators are designed to clean down to $27\,\mathrm{mg\,Nm^{-3}}$ operating on three zones, and still to be within $115\,\mathrm{mg\,Nm^{-3}}$ when one zone is out. Discharge end gases are again cleaned by precipitators.

2. *Redbourn Sinter Plant* (1962) has a capacity of $45\,000\,\mathrm{t\,week^{-1}}$ from two strands having a total area of $310\,\mathrm{m^2}$. Main and dedust gas streams are cleaned by precipitators.

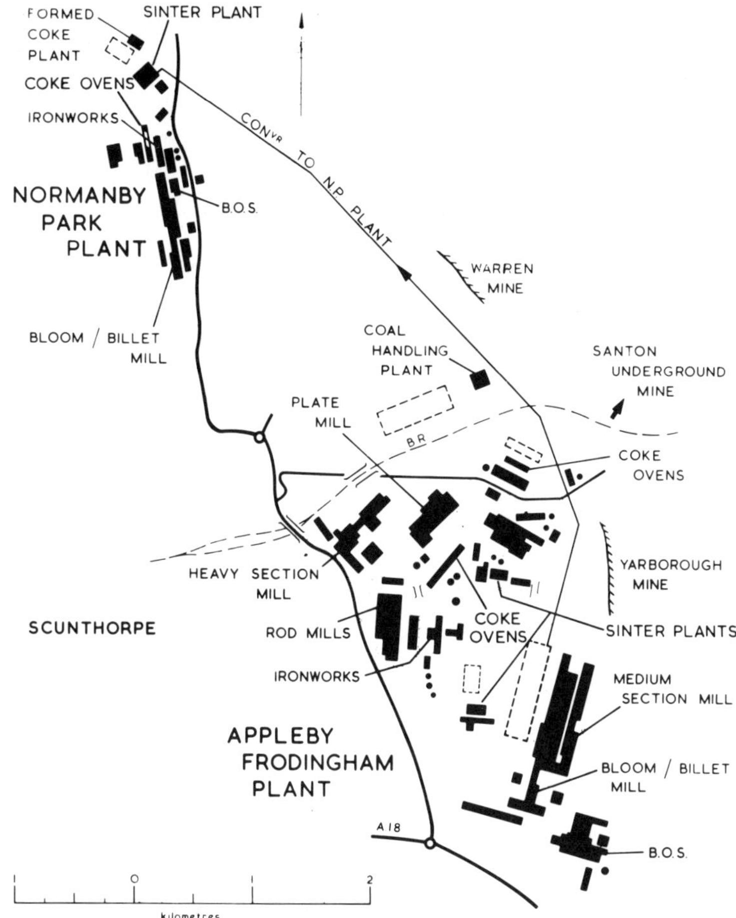

FIG. 8.   The location of the main production units at the Scunthorpe Works of BSC.

3.   *Normanby Park Sinter Plant* (1959/64) has a capacity of 35 000 t week^{-1} from three strands with a total area of 280 m². Although the main strand gases have no specific gas cleaning, the particulate emission has remained within the limit of 460 mg Nm^{-3} which prevailed at the time of construction. Dedust precipitators are fitted to this plant, and one of the pair is monitored by an Erwin Sick transmissometer to ensure the emission is less than 115 mg Nm^{-3}.

There are ten batteries of coke ovens at Scunthorpe, of which seven were built before 1960 and three were commissioned in 1979. The three most recent batteries are designed for wet charging or preheated pipeline charging, and have Gneisnau-type mobile gas cleaning units for controlling pushing emissions.

Steel is manufactured at two plants. The LD† plant at Normanby Park is a small, first generation oxygen lancing unit having two vessels of 85 t capacity. In contrast, the BOS (Basic Oxygen Steel) plant at Appleby Frodingham, with three vessels of 300 t, was commissioned in 1973 as part of the Anchor development involving the Immingham ore terminal and new rolling capacity. Both the LD plant and the BOS plant have high efficiency venturi scrubbers on the primary emissions. These scrubbers are chosen for their high reliability, so that primary emissions are seldom a problem. Both plants also have partial secondary ventilation schemes, although these collect less than half of the fume emitted into the building.

In addition to these main plants, there are subsidiary processes which can give rise to atmospheric emissions. For example, the desire for low sulphur steels has led to the desulphurisation of iron by lancing with calcium carbide, thereby forming a high sulphur slag which can then be separated. The process results in the emission of copious fume of very fine particle size, which must be extracted and cleaned. Secondly, billets of hot steel are descaled by application of an intense scarfing flame, which burns off the unwanted 3–4 mm outer layer. Again this produces dense fine fume and at Scunthorpe this is cleaned by an irrigated electrostatic precipitator.

6. MONITORING AT SCUNTHORPE

The fundamental reasons for the measurement of emissions and ambient concentrations of recognised pollutants have already been identified in Section 4.1., namely, the commitment by BSC to positive and socially responsible pollution control policies and protection of the local environment. Clearly the same reasoning applies to Scunthorpe as to Redcar, and indeed the monitoring activities are carried out to the same ends. However, Scunthorpe having been established as a works before the growth of awareness about environmental matters led to the continuation of labour intensive, low technology monitoring for both the emission and ambient cases in contrast to the capital intensive, high technology route

† Linz-Donawitz, the Austrian inventors of the oxygen lanced converter.

which was appropriate to Redcar. In the following two sections we will look at the impact of this difference on the effectiveness of the monitoring effort.

6.1. Emission Monitoring

Emission monitoring falls into two distinct categories—commissioning of new plant and the on-going programme to measure present emission performance.

Sophisticated emission measuring devices require initial gravimetric calibration, so their use is clearly not appropriate for testing the specification of new gas cleaning equipment. Such a test involves a relatively short programme—typically one month—of intensive measurement of gas flow rates, temperatures, velocities and mass loadings, in conjunction with other plant operating parameters, with the objective of tuning the gas cleaning system and ensuring that the emission is as specified. The only way to measure a mass loading to the required accuracy under these conditions is with a standard isokinetic gravimetric sampling train, using BCURA† or similar equipment. The exact technique may need to be adapted to meet specific sampling conditions, for example the presence of high water contents in the gas flow.

It may appear that there would be an overwhelming case for continuous monitors for the long-term routine measurement of emissions. In practice, however, the arguments are more finely balanced. Firstly, even an almost ideal emission such as the continuous, steady dry sinter plant waste gas does change its properties from time to time, and factors, such as size distribution, which are catered for automatically by gravimetric sampling may corrupt the calibration of a transmissometer. Secondly, there are many emissions on the works—particularly those following wet washers—where continuous monitors are not applicable. Thirdly, the works must maintain the capability and expertise for accurate commissioning measurements as described in the previous paragraph.

Since such measurements are not required continuously, the testing team is free to do routine stack tests during the intervening periods. In fact, Scunthorpe Works operates two such test teams, which can work independently to cover the range of measurements required.

Although Scunthorpe relies almost entirely on this manual sampling approach, it is anticipated that suitable continuous monitors will eventually be located on the sinter plant stacks. Several monitors have been evaluated

† Sampling equipment designed by the British Coal Utilisation Research Association and now manufactured under licence by Airflow Developments Limited.

in recent years; an Erwin Sick transmissometer is fitted to a dedust stack at Normanby Park; interesting results are being obtained at the time of writing with the Ikor 2710, which measures charge transfer when particles impact on a conducting probe and infers mass loading from the current generated.

The discussion so far has related to measurements on emissions that are confined to ducts or stacks. There are many emissions, however, which are released in clouds from poorly defined areas, yet which still require assessment. Examples are the secondary fume which eludes the steelmaking extraction system and subsequently escapes through ventilation slots in the roof, and black smoke emissions when charging coke ovens. In the latter situation, a charging car carrying four hoppers of crushed coal is aligned over four corresponding holes in the oven top. The hoppers are then emptied sequentially through telescopic chutes which are lowered to mate with the holes.

Contact of the finely divided coal with the hot oven generates a burst of gas and smoke, and emission of this is prevented by steam aspiration which creates a negative pressure environment in the oven. Nevertheless, smoke is often emitted at any or all of the four charging holes, the hoppers themselves, and sundry other openings. It is not possible to make any gravimetric measurements in such a complex situation. Nevertheless, it is possible to make a consistent semi-quantitative estimate of the emission, and thus to compare relative performance when operational or mechanical

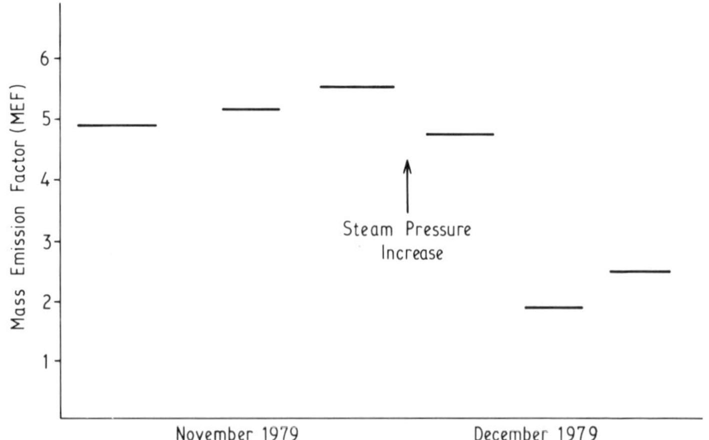

FIG. 9. Measurements of mass emission factor made over a six-week period at Dawes Lane Coke Ovens, Scunthorpe.

changes are made. The measurement made is called a mass emission factor (MEF)[6] and is derived simply by timing the periods of smoke emission by stop watch, assigning a weighting based on the visual appearance and summing the components to arrive at a factor. Application of this technique to a battery at Scunthorpe at which the aspiration steam pressure was being increased and the control improved shows clearly (Fig. 9) the fall in average MEF during the course of the improvements.

6.2. Ambient Monitoring

Ambient pollution monitoring began at the then United Steel Company in 1955, with one Warren Springs (Fuel Research Station) smoke and SO_2 apparatus and three deposit gauges. The aims of these measurements were stated to be:

(1) to provide basic information about the pollution on the works, its dependence on wind, rain, etc., and

(2) to accumulate records of atmospheric pollution with which it would be possible to estimate the effect of future plant modifications and future installation of dust collecting equipment.

In 1971–73, with increased environmental awareness and the imminent commissioning of the Anchor development, a full monitoring network was established in and around Scunthorpe Works. By 1973 the network, with 20 sites involving 20 deposit gauges and 16 smoke/SO_2 apparatus, was complete. It has remained essentially the same since then, with a small turnover as sites become unsuitable or unavailable. Figure 10 shows the locations of the sites in relation to the main works production units.

The Warren Springs apparatus measures SO_2 (as net acid gas) from the pH change in a hydrogen peroxide bubbler, and smoke from the change in reflectance of a filter paper. The instrument cost per site is around £400 as against perhaps £14 000 (1980 prices) for continuous equivalents, although this is balanced to some extent by the greater routine maintenance and analytical costs of the Warren Springs apparatus. The greatest disadvantage in practice is that a 24 h average is produced, making it very difficult to distinguish concentration changes brought about by changing wind directions or other short-term events.

The National Survey of smoke and SO_2, which involves over 1300 measurement sites, has provided a yardstick against which the Scunthorpe results can be judged. The Scunthorpe sites are averaged into three groups: works (all sites actually within works boundaries), perimeter (a ring of sites round the outside of the works) and town (three sites in Scunthorpe). For

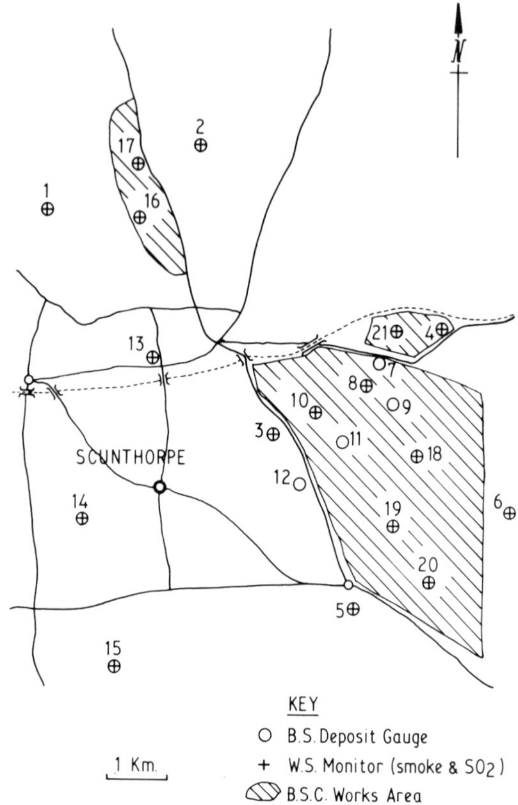

FIG. 10.   Location of the Warren Spring (smoke/SO$_2$) monitors and deposit gauges in and around BSC Scunthorpe Works.

each of these groups, a baseline figure is compiled from the results from sites in corresponding categories of the National Survey (e.g. industrial, urban centre) and this national average is used to assess trends in the Scunthorpe figures. Over the past decade the relevant National Survey averages have fallen quite steadily: the average smoke results by about $3\cdot5\,\mu\mathrm{g\,m}^{-3}$ annually, SO$_2$ by about $4\,\mu\mathrm{g\,m}^{-3}$ annually, and deposits by about $5\,\mathrm{mg\,m}^{-2}\,\mathrm{day}^{-1}$.[7] Such a national improvement must clearly influence any judgement of the local Scunthorpe results.

The corresponding Scunthorpe results for the works, perimeter and town annual averages are shown in Figs. 11(a), (b) and (c) for smoke, SO$_2$ and deposits, respectively. The works average smoke concentration has

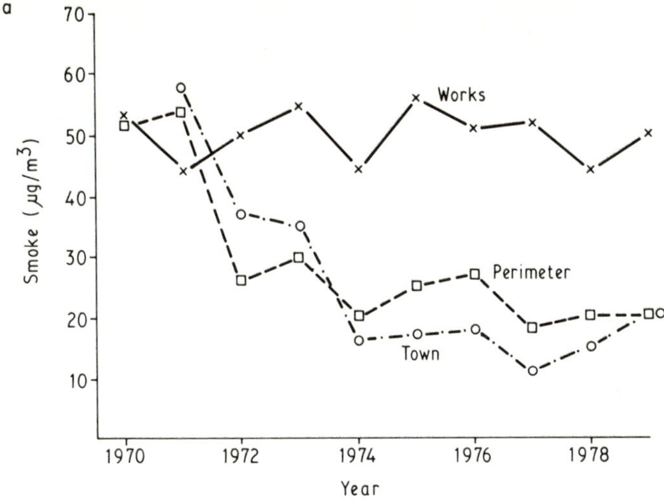

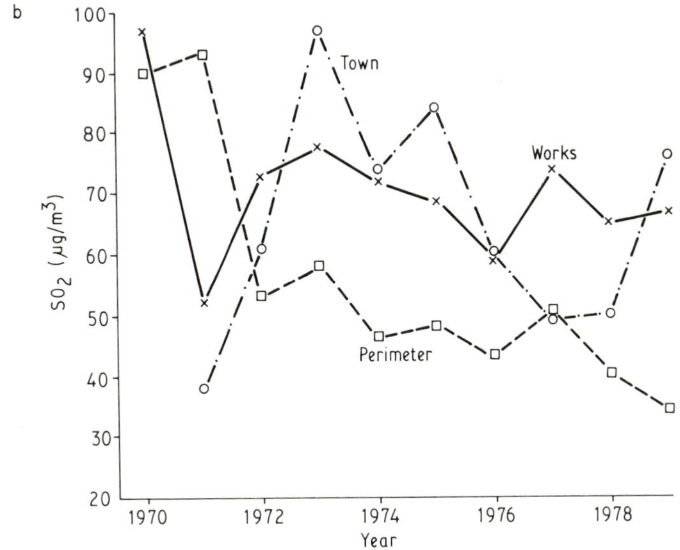

FIG. 11. Annual average levels of (a) smoke, (b) SO_2 and (c) deposits at Scunthorpe over the period 1970–79.

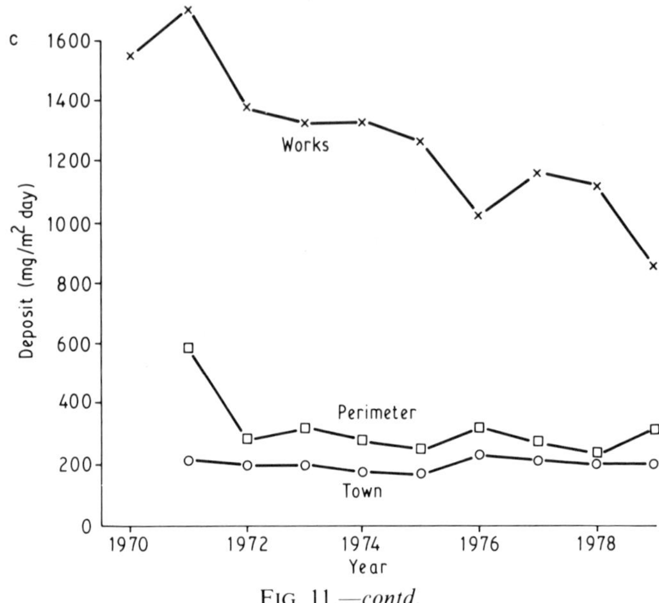

Fig. 11.—*contd.*

remained constant at about $50\,\mu\mathrm{g\,m^{-3}}$. Town and perimeter smoke concentrations dropped steadily to 1974, reflecting the successful application of a 12-stage domestic smoke control programme which now covers the majority of Scunthorpe. The SO_2 situation is more confused, with wide fluctuations in the town average which is now higher than works or perimeter. Works deposits have decreased steadily to their present level of about $900\,\mathrm{mg\,m^{-2}\,day^{-1}}$, and the relative level of works deposits confirms the impression that most of the coarse grit and dust created by the works drops out within the works boundaries.

The major changes in Scunthorpe which may be reflected in pollution trends have been the Anchor development of 1973 which brought foreign ore practice and replaced open hearth steelmaking with BOS, the Local Authority smoke control programme and improvements in pollution control practices. It is extremely difficult to make a quantitative estimate of the smoke or particulates tonnage emitted from year to year. Sulphur dioxide emissions, however, are calculable directly from records of sulphur contents, gas flow rates and oil usage. Figure 12 shows the estimated annual total sulphur dioxide emissions since 1970. There was a sharp reduction in 1973 with the introduction of foreign ore, followed by a gradual decline associated with a reduced consumption of coke oven gas.

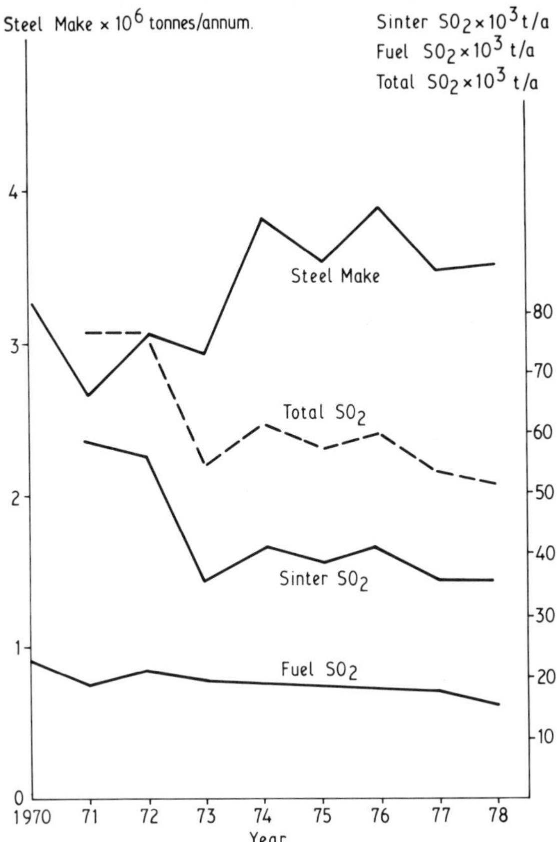

FIG. 12.   Annual average emissions of SO_2 from sintering and the combustion of oil or coke oven gas. The annual steel production is given for reference.

A detailed comparison has been made between Scunthorpe ambient concentrations and standards recently proposed by the Commission for the European Communities.[8] These CEC standards are given as follows.

a. Daily mean smoke not to exceed $150 \, \mu g \, m^{-3}$ with SO_2 not to exceed $250 \, \mu g \, m^{-3}$ for more than 7 days year^{-1}, unless the daily mean smoke is less than $150 \, \mu g \, m^{-3}$, when SO_2 is not to exceed $350 \, \mu g \, m^{-3}$. If SO_2 is below $250 \, \mu g \, m^{-3}$, smoke can reach $250 \, \mu g \, m^{-3}$.

b. Winter medians of daily smoke and SO_2 not to exceed $130 \, \mu g \, m^{-3}$ unless the median smoke is less than $60 \, \mu g \, m^{-3}$, when median SO_2 is not to exceed $180 \, \mu g \, m^{-3}$.

c.   Annual medians of daily smoke and SO_2 not to exceed $80\,\mu\mathrm{g\,m}^{-3}$ unless the median smoke is less than $40\,\mu\mathrm{g\,m}^{-3}$, when the median SO_2 is not to exceed $120\,\mu\mathrm{g\,m}^{-3}$.

The complex format of these limits is brought about by interaction between smoke and SO_2, whereby a given concentration of SO_2 is more harmful in the presence of a high smoke concentration, and vice versa. The analysis (Table 1) shows that no health hazard exists in the works in general, and that perimeter and town sites are substantially cleaner than even these stringent limits.

TABLE 1

NUMBER OF SMOKE/SO_2 MEASUREMENT SITES EXCEEDING CEC STANDARDS a, b AND c DURING THE FOUR YEARS 1976–79

Standard	Year			
	1976/77	1977/78	1978/79	1979/80[a]
Standard a Works	4	3	2	1
Perimeter	0	0	0	0
Town	0	0	0	0
Standard b Works	0	0	0	1
Perimeter	0	0	0	0
Town	0	0	0	0
Standard c Works	0	1	0	1
Perimeter	0	0	0	0
Town	0	0	0	0

[a] Estimated from 9 months data.

Despite the limitations on time resolution mentioned above, it is possible by means of multiple linear regressions to show the directional dependence of pollution measurements. In Fig. 13, for example, it can be seen that the main sources of smoke at Site 10 are coke ovens to the east, while the SO_2 contribution also comes from rod mills to the south.

It is clear from the analyses given in this section that a low-technology approach to pollution monitoring does provide the capability to answer the basic questions. What is the pollution level now? Are the concentrations increasing or decreasing? Are they a health risk? Which sources dominate ground level concentrations? The initial remit has been satisfied, and there is consequently no immediate need to enhance the system despite the availability of more advanced equipment.

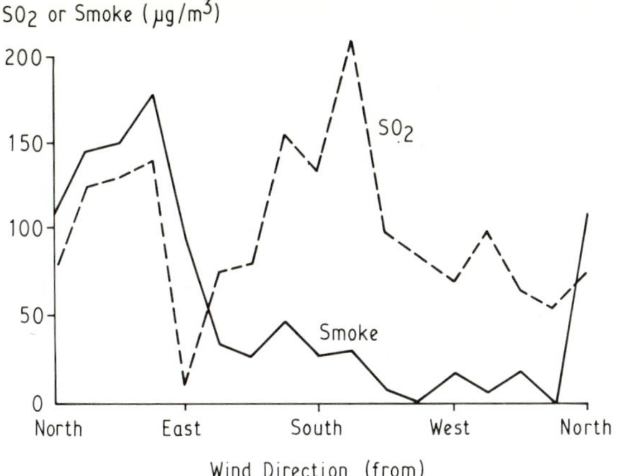

FIG. 13.   Dependence of smoke and SO_2 concentrations measured at Site 10 (from Fig. 10) on wind direction.

7.   CONCLUSION

At this critical stage in the development of the Redcar Works, with several plants only recently commissioned, it is premature to give any judgement on the overall effectiveness of the air pollution control and monitoring arrangements. They are certainly the most comprehensive and sophisticated that BSC has yet installed. The emphasis on continuous monitors results in a deluge of information, and it has been important to set up proper machinery for logging, analysing, summarising and interpreting this information. Quality assurance involving instrument maintenance, calibration and numerical techniques is being closely supervised.

Personnel are available to consider output values or changes of value obtained. Had BSC not made such provisions at Redcar, the final destination of the data would have been the filing cabinet rather than the action list.

Scunthorpe Works have continued their reliance on older methods of measurement. In the case of emission measurements, these methods are essential in the commissioning phase and adequate in the long term, except that they do not provide rapid warning of control equipment efficiency reduction or failure. In the case of ambient measurements, the methods provide all the information which is necessary for environmental decision making, at a low cost and high data availability. As with Redcar, it is important that the correct machinery exists to follow up results.

ACKNOWLEDGEMENT

I am grateful to the Management of BSC Scunthorpe Division for permission to publish this contribution.

REFERENCES

1. Redcar Stage II Review of Environmental Control Measures, British Steel Corporation, Planning and Capital Developments Division (Redcar Development), 1977.
2. Alkali & c. Works Regulation Act, HMSO, London, 1906.
3. Control of Pollution Act, HMSO, London, 1974.
4. Dark Smoke (Permitted Periods) Regulations, HMSO, London, 1958.
5. COLLS, J. J. *Environ. Technol. Letts*, 1980, **1**, 209–24.
6. British Carbonisation Research Assn. Special publication No. 5, 3rd edn, 1974.
7. The Investigation of Air Pollution: (a) National Survey of Smoke and Sulphur Dioxide; (b) Deposit Gauge, Warren Spring Laboratory (annual publications).
8. ANON. Proposal for a Council directive concerning health protection standards for sulphur dioxide and suspended particulate matter, *Official J. of the European Communities*, Mar. 1976.

INDEX